# Medical Inpatients: Nutritional Therapy and Care

# Medical Inpatients: Nutritional Therapy and Care

Editor: Natasha Parsons

AMERICAN
MEDICAL PUBLISHERS
www.americanmedicalpublishers.com

AMERICAN
MEDICAL PUBLISHERS
www.americanmedicalpublishers.com

**Cataloging-in-Publication Data**

Medical inpatients : nutritional therapy and care / edited by Natasha Parsons.
p. cm.
Includes bibliographical references and index.
ISBN 978-1-63927-718-6
1. Diet therapy. 2. Nutrition. 3. Diet in disease. 4. Diseases--Nutritional aspects.
5. Therapeutics, Physiological. 6. Dietetics. 7. Medical care. I. Parsons, Natasha.
RM216 .M43 2023
615.854--dc23



American Medical Publishers,
41 Flatbush Avenue,
1st Floor, New York,
NY 11217, USA

ISBN 978-1-63927-718-6 (Hardback)

# Contents

# Preface

Medical inpatient is the term used to refer to someone who is admitted to a hospital for a brief or extended stay. Along with proper medication and treatment, it is critical that the inpatients are provided with the right type of nutrition and care since food is the primary source of nutrition. Nutritional therapy refers to the treatment based on nutrition, which involves checking a patient's nutritional status, and prescribing and providing the right foods or nutrients to treat different medical conditions. The human body breaks down the food to receive the molecules, such as carbohydrates, minerals, proteins, vitamins and fats. A patient's body must be able to metabolize and utilize the nutrients for supporting all body functions. If the body does not receive these nutrients, it becomes difficult for it to work properly. This book explores all the important aspects of nutritional therapy in the modern day. It covers in detail some strategies for the management of medical inpatients. Those in search of information to further their knowledge will be greatly assisted by this book.

Various studies have approached the subject by analyzing it with a single perspective, but the present book provides diverse methodologies and techniques to address this field. This book contains theories and applications needed for understanding the subject from different perspectives. The aim is to keep the readers informed about the progresses in the field; therefore, the contributions were carefully examined to compile novel researches by specialists from across the globe.

Indeed, the job of the editor is the most crucial and challenging in compiling all chapters into a single book. In the end, I would extend my sincere thanks to the chapter authors for their profound work. I am also thankful for the support provided by my family and colleagues during the compilation of this book.

**Editor**

# Changes in Nutritional Status in Pulmonary Tuberculosis: Longitudinal Changes in BMI According to Acid-Fast Bacilli Smear Positivity

**Yousang Ko [1,2,*,†], Changwhan Kim [3,†], Yong Bum Park [1,2], Eun-Kyung Mo [1,2] and Jin-Wook Moon [1,2]**

1 Department of Internal Medicine, Division of Pulmonary, Allergy and Critical Care Medicine, Kangdong Sacred Heart Hospital, Hallym University College of Medicine, Seoul 05355, Korea; bfspark2@gmail.com (Y.B.P.); ekmopark@gmail.com (E.-K.M.); cozybar@hanmail.net (J.-W.M.)
2 College of Medicine, Lung Research Institute of Hallym University, Chuncheon 24253, Korea
3 Department of Internal Medicine, School of Medicine, Jeju National University Hospital, Jeju National University, Jeju 63241, Korea; masque70@naver.com
* Correspondence: koyus@naver.com
† Yousang Ko and Changwhan Kim contribute equally to this work.

**Abstract:** Malnutrition is closely associated with pulmonary tuberculosis (PTB). However, changes before and after treatment remain unclear. We aimed to investigate the longitudinal changes in nutritional status from treatment to follow-up of TB in 215 PTB cases in South Korea. First, we evaluated the trend in body mass index (BMI) from the time of diagnosis to a 2-year follow-up. Second, we compared the BMIs of our cases with 5694 controls who participated in a Korean national survey after treatment. During the treatment period, the BMI of the smear-positive group ($n = 72$) significantly increased compared with that of the smear-negative group ($n = 143$) (+1.9 kg/m$^2$ vs. +0.4 kg/m$^2$, $p = 0.001$). Almost all the changes occurred in the early phase, with unremarkable differences in the rest of the treatment period and up to the 2-year follow-up period. When compared with controls, the smear-positive PTB group also had a lower BMI than the smear-negative PTB group, which, however, was lower than that of the general population, though all the participants regained their BMIs during treatment. These results clarify the nutritional aspects of PTB and enable better strategies to support patients with PTB.

**Keywords:** pulmonary tuberculosis; body mass index; smear positivity; malnutrition

---

## 1. Introduction

Tuberculosis (TB), caused by *Mycobacterium tuberculosis* (MTB), is the most lethal infectious disease in the world and has afflicted humans for centuries. Pulmonary TB (PTB) is the most common TB infection in humans [1]. The association between the development of active TB and malnutrition has been described on the basis of geographical correlation, animal models, and observational studies in humans [2–5].

The mechanism by which malnutrition leads to PTB occurrence is not yet clear. Malnutrition may reduce the proliferation of T lymphocytes and impair cell-mediated immunity, which in turn may lead to increased susceptibility to infection [2]. In contrast, obesity is considered a protective factor against active PTB [6,7]. Moreover, malnutrition is an important factor in the development of PTB and is also considered to be associated with the relapse risk and treatment response rate of PTB [8,9].

Efforts have been made to terminate TB infections under the banner of the WHO End TB strategy under the Stop TB plan. The WHO predicted that malnutrition is responsible for 18% of the global TB burden, attributable for 1.9 million cases. Moreover, it is the most powerful risk factor as compared to human immunodeficiency virus (HIV) infection, smoking, diabetes, and alcohol consumption [1]. Thus, a better understanding of malnutrition-related TB infections will help us reach the goal we desire.

Malnutrition status can be measured using diverse methods. Among these, body mass index (BMI) and mid-upper arm circumference are commonly used to assess nutritional status [2]. In adults, BMI has been extensively used in clinical practice despite its limitations, as it has the advantage of easy accessibility. Previous studies have shown correlations between BMI and TB infections [2,10,11].

Previous research has focused on body weight and its changes in patients with PTB [8,12–14]. Body weight loss is often observed in patients with tuberculosis at the time of diagnosis and, for centuries, has been considered to be an important risk factor for tuberculosis. On the contrary, body weight gain is a useful biomarker of treatment outcome and relapse [8]. However, there are problems of inter-personal variability and inter-racial differences. Previous studies have investigated the effect of anti-TB treatment on body weight gain, but they were mostly based on patients with smear-positive PTB. However, smear-negative PTB is more common in developed countries, including South Korea.

In the present study, we hypothesized that the changes in malnutrition status differ according to disease severity, because of "nothing to lose nothing to gain". We aimed to evaluate longitudinal changes in BMI in patients with PTB with positive and negative sputum acid-fast bacilli (AFB) smears at the time of diagnosis, on treatment completion, and up to 2 years after treatment completion. Moreover, we compared changes in serologic markers with changes in BMI.

## 2. Experimental Section

### 2.1. Study Population and Design

This study was a retrospective analysis of protocol-based collective data form the TB clinic of Hallym University Kangdong Sacred Heart Hospital (Seoul, Korea) from January 2015 to December 2016. The hospital is situated in an area with intermediate TB burden, with a reported estimated prevalence of 101/100,000 persons in 2015. We enrolled all consecutive patients aged >20 years who had been diagnosed with culture-positive PTB. All the patients with PTB received anti-TB medication daily. Patients were excluded if they were transferred to another hospital, if they died or were lost to follow-up during anti-TB treatment, if they showed poor adherence to anti-TB treatment, or if they had incomplete medical records. We also excluded cases with multi-drug or rifampicin-resistant PTB because of the long duration of anti-TB treatment.

Another group was recruited for comparison. We aimed to determine whether the nutritional status of patients with PTB could be completely recovered to match that of the general population. Thus, we compared the nutritional status of the enrolled patients at the time of TB treatment completion with that of the subjects who participated in the Korea National Health and Nutrition Examination Surveys (KNHANES) in 2013. KNHANES is a nationwide survey of the health and nutritional status of the Korean population (https://knhanes.cdc.go.kr/knhanes). We evaluated BMI after treatment completion to compare it with normal subjects in the general population. Finally, 5694 subjects who participated in the survey were selected after excluding those with previous ($n$ = 223) and current ($n$ = 4) TB infections.

The protocol for this study was approved by the Institutional Review Board of Hallym University Kangdong Sacred Heart Hospital (IRB 2020-04-008). Informed consent was waived because of the retrospective nature of the study.

### 2.2. Data Collection

We reviewed the medical records of the patients at our TB clinics. Finally, 215 adult patients with PTB were included in this study (Figure 1).

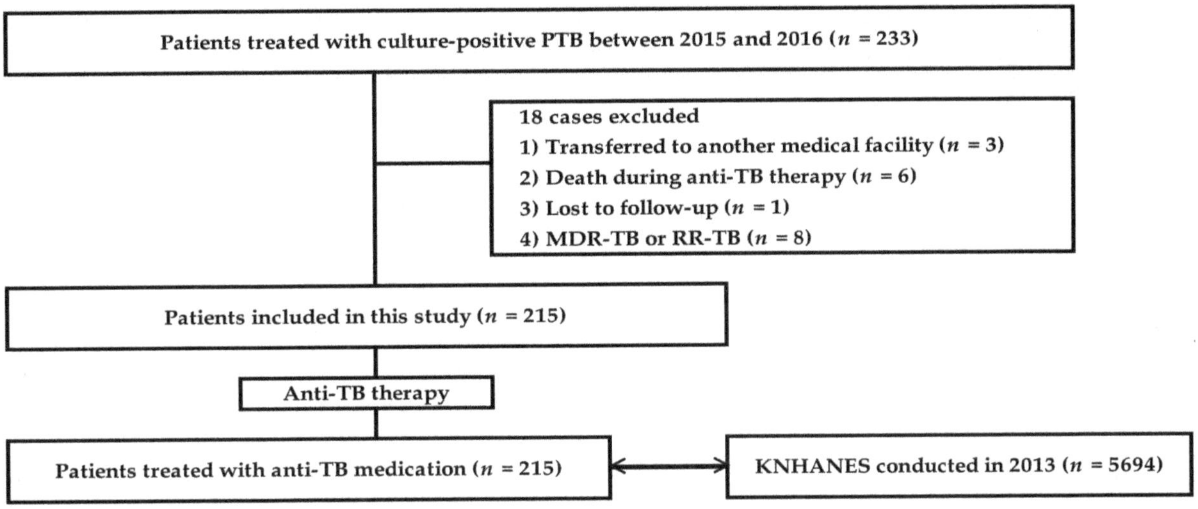


**Figure 1.** Flow chart of the study. PTB, pulmonary tuberculosis; MDR, multi-drug resistant; TB, tuberculosis; RR, rifampicin resistance; KNHANES, Korea National Health and Nutrition Examination Survey.

### 2.3. *Radiographic Data*

Chest radiographs and computerized tomographic scans of the patients were reviewed for the presence of cavities and to determine the extent of the disease. The extent of each lesion was categorized based on lobar involvement. Uni-lobar and multi-lobar involvement of PTB were defined by the involvement of ≤1 and ≥2 lobes, respectively.

### 2.4. *Microbiological Data*

The AFB smears were examined after auramine-rhodamine fluorescent staining and were graded on a scale from 0 to 4+ [15]. MTB culturing was simultaneously performed with solid media, 3% Ogawa media (Eiken Chemical, Tokyo, Japan) and liquid media in the mycobacteria growth indicator tube 960 system (BD Biosciences, Franklin Lakes, NJ, USA).

### 2.5. *Assessment of BMI*

BMI was used to assess nutritional status, calculated as the weight in kilograms divided by the height in meters squared. Individuals were categorized into five BMI groups: severely underweight (<16), underweight (16–18.4), normal weight (18.5–24.9), overweight (25–29.9), and obese (≥30) [2]. Malnutrition is defined as BMI less than 18.5 kg/m$^2$ [16].

### 2.6. *Treatment Outcomes of PTB*

Treatment outcomes were categorized based on WHO definitions as follows: (1) cured PTB patients who had bacteriologically confirmed TB at the beginning of treatment and who were smear- or culture-negative in the last month of treatment and on at least one previous occasion; (2) patients with TB who completed the treatment (without evidence of failure, but with no record of being cured); (3) patients whose treatments failed (patients with TB whose sputum smears or cultures were positive at month 5 or later during the treatment); (4) patients who died (patients with TB who died due to any reason before or during the course of treatment) [17].

### 2.7. *Statistical Analysis*

Data are presented as means and standard deviations (SD) for continuous variables and numbers (percentage) for categorical variables. Data were compared using Student's t-test for continuous variables and Pearson's chi-square test or Fisher's exact test for categorical variables. Longitudinal changes in BMI were analyzed by mixed-effect linear regressions. All the tests were two-sided and $p$-values < 0.05 were considered to be statistically significant. Data were analyzed using IBM SPSS Statistics, version 26 (IBM, Armonk, NY, USA) and Graph Pad Prism 8.0 (GraphPad, San Diego, CA, USA).

## 3. Results

### 3.1. Patient Characteristics

During the 2-year-long study period, 227 patients were treated for PTB, and subsequently 12 were excluded in accordance with the exclusion criteria (Figure 1). A total of 215 patients with PTB, consisting of 72 (33.5%) AFB smear-positive cases and 143 (66.5%) AFB smear-negative cases were included for analysis. The demographic and clinical characteristics of the enrolled cases are summarized in Table 1. The mean age of the population was 50.9 ± 18.9 years, of which 136 (63.3%) were men. The mean body weight and BMI were 58.3 ± 11.4 kg and 21.2 ± 3.2 kg/m$^2$, respectively. The patients with PTB were concomitantly affected by TB pleuritis in 34 cases (15.8%), TB lymphadenitis, 4 cases (1.9%); and, TB epididymitis, 1 case (0.4%).

**Table 1.** Demographic and clinical characteristics of the enrolled 215 patients with PTB.

| | **All Patients** | **AFB-S (+) PTB** | **AFB-S (−) PTB** | ***p*-Value** |
|---|---|---|---|---|
| | $n$ = 215 | $n$ = 72 | $n$ = 143 | |
| Age, years | 50.9 ± 18.9 | 54.2 ± 17.1 | 49.3 ± 19.6 | 0.075 |
| Male gender, % | 136 (63.3) | 52 (72.2) | 84 (58.7) | 0.036 |
| Height, cm | 165.3 ± 9.5 | 166.2 ± 8.8 | 164.9 ± 9.8 | 0.347 |
| Body Weight, kg | 58.0 ± 11.4 | 57.9 ± 11.3 | 58.7 ± 11.4 | 0.643 |
| BMI, kg/m$^2$ | 21.2 ± 3.2 | 20.6 ± 3.3 | 21.5 ± 3.1 | 0.033 |
| severely underweight (<16) | 6 (2.8) | 3 (4.2) | 3 (2.1) | |
| underweight (16–18.4) | 38 (17.7) | 22 (30.6) | 16 (11.2) | |
| normal weight (18.5–24.9) | 144 (67.0) | 41 (56.9) | 103 (72.0) | 0.006 |
| overweight (25–29.9) | 25 (11.6) | 6 (8.3) | 19 (13.3) | |
| obese (>30) | 2 (0.9) | 0 | 2 (1.4) | |
| Comorbidity | | | | |
| COPD or asthma | 9 (3.8) | 1 (1.4) | 8 (5.6) | 0.278 |
| Thyroid disease | 2 (0.9) | 0 | 2 (1.4) | 0.552 |
| Cardiovascular disease | 32 (13.7) | 12 (16.7) | 20 (14.0) | 0.685 |
| Malignancy | 11 (4.7) | 5 (6.9) | 6 (4.2) | 0.513 |
| Hematologic disease | 2 (0.9) | 2 (2.8) | 0 | 0.111 |
| Chronic liver disease | 19 (8.1) | 8 (11.1) | 11 (7.7) | 0.449 |
| Rheumatic disease | 6 (2.6) | 1 (1.4) | 5 (3.5) | 0.666 |
| CKD | 2 (0.9) | 1 (1.4) | 1 (0.7) | 0.559 |
| Diabetes | 44 (14.8) | 22 (30.6) | 22 (15.4) | 0.012 |
| Neurologic disease | 6 (2.6) | 0 | 6 (4.2) | 0.182 |
| Cerebrovascular disease | 2 (0.9) | 1 (1.4) | 1 (0.7) | 1.000 |
| Immunologic disease | 1 (0.4) | 0 | 1 (0.7) | 1.000 |
| Silicosis | 1 (0.4) | 0 | 1 (0.7) | 1.000 |
| KTP | 2 (0.9) | 1 (1.4) | 1 (0.7) | 1.000 |
| Smoking status | | | | 0.223 |
| Never smoker | 92 (39.3) | 26 (36.1) | 66 (46.2) | |
| Former smoker | 47 (20.1) | 15 (20.8) | 32 (22.4) | |
| Current smoker | 76 (32.5) | 31 (43.1) | 45 (31.5) | |
| Alcohol use | | | | <0.001 |
| Heavy drinker | | 9 (12.5) | 11 (7.7) | |

AFB-S, acid-fast bacilli smear; PTB, pulmonary tuberculosis; BMI, body mass index; CKD, chronic kidney disease; KTP, kidney transplantation, COPD, chronic obstructive lung disease.

### *3.2. Clinical, Radiological, and Microbiological Differences between the AFB Smear-Positive and AFB Smear-Negative Groups*

There were unremarkable differences in age, height, body weight, comorbidities, and smoking status according to AFB smear status before anti-TB treatment at baseline. However, the proportions of male patients (72.2% vs. 58.7, $p = 0.036$) and heavy alcohol drinkers (12.5 vs. 7.7%, $p < 0.001$) were higher in the AFB smear-positive group (Table 1).

Although all the enrolled patients predominantly had localized PTB, the AFB smear-positive group had more extensive PTB than the smear-negative group (63.9 vs. 39.0%, $p < 0.001$) (Table 2). The frequency of cavitation was also considerably higher in the smear-positive group (61.2 vs. 18.1%, $p < 0.001$). In the patients with drug-resistant PTB, there were unremarkable differences between the two groups except for the proportion of patients resistant to pyrazinamide.

**Table 2.** Clinical, radiological and microbiological characteristics of the enrolled 215 cases of PTB.

| | **All Patients** | **AFB-S (+) PTB** | **AFB-S (−) PTB** | ***p*-Value** |
|---|---|---|---|---|
| | $n = 215$ | $n = 72$ | $n = 143$ | |
| New cases | 187 (87) | 61 (84.7) | 126 (88.1) | 0.523 |
| Previously treated cases | 28 (13.0) | 11 (15.3) | 17 (11.9) | |
| Radiographic feature | | | | |
| Cavity | 64 (29.8) | 41 (61.2) | 23 (18.1) | <0.001 |
| Extent of lung lesion | | | | |
| Uni-lobar involvement | 116 (54.0) | 26 (36.1) | 91 (70.0) | <0.001 |
| Multi-lobar involvement | 85 (39.5) | 46 (63.9) | 39 (30.0) | |
| AFB smear status | | | | |
| Positive | 72 (33.5) | | | |
| 4+ | 16 (7.4) | 16 (22.2) | | |
| 3+ | 19 (8.8) | 19 (26.4) | | |
| 2+ | 18 (8.4) | 18 (25.0) | | |
| 1+ | 19 (8.8) | 19 (26.4) | | |
| Negative | 143 (66.5) | | | |
| DST profiles | | | | |
| Resistant to isoniazid | 20 (9.3) | 10 (13.9) | 10 (7.0) | 0.134 |
| Resistant to pyrazinamide | 7 (3.3) | 5 (6.9) | 2 (1.4) | 0.043 |
| Resistant to ethambutol | 2 (0.9) | 2 (2.8) | 0 | 0.111 |
| Resistant to streptomycin | 5 (2.3) | 1 (1.4) | 4 (2.8) | 0.666 |
| Resistant to fluoroquinolone | 2 (0.9) | 1 (1.4) | 1 (0.7) | 1.000 |
| Resistant to protionamide | 3 (1.4) | 1 (1.4) | 2 (1.4) | 1.000 |
| Resistant to PAS | 4 (1.9) | 3 (4.2) | 1 (0.7) | 0.110 |

AFB-S, acid-fast bacilli smear; PTB, pulmonary tuberculosis; DST, drug sensitivity test; PAS, para-amino salicylic acid.

In terms of nutrition status, the AFB smear-positive group had a lower BMI ($20.6 \pm 3.3$ kg/m$^2$ vs. $21.5 \pm 3.1$ kg/m$^2$, $p = 0.033$) than the AFB smear-negative group. Moreover, in the severely underweight, underweight, normal weight, overweight, and obese categories of BMI, the AFB smear-positive group had more undernourished patients ($p = 0.006$) (Table 1). Biochemically, the AFB smear-positive group had a lower albumin level than the smear-negative group ($3.7 \pm 0.6$ g/dL vs. $4.0 \pm 0.6$ g/dL, $p < 0.001$) at the time of diagnosis (Table 3).

**Table 3.** Sequential changes of the nutritional status in enrolled 215 cases after anti-TB treatment.

| | All Patients | AFB-S (+) PTB | AFB-S (−) PTB | *p*-Value |
|---|---|---|---|---|
| | *n* = 215 | *n* = 72 | *n* = 143 | |
| Treatment duration, months | 8.3 ± 3.4 | 9.2 ± 3.8 | 7.2 ± 1.2 | 0.003 |
| BMI, baseline | 21.2 ± 3.2 | 20.6 ± 3.3 | 21.5 ± 3.1 | 0.033 |
| Severely underweight (<16) | 6 (2.8) | 3 (4.2) | 3 (2.1) | |
| Underweight (16–18.4) | 38 (17.7) | 22 (30.6) | 16 (11.2) | |
| Normal weight (18.5–24.9) | 144 (67.0) | 41 (56.9) | 103 (72.0) | 0.006 |
| Overweight (25–29.9) | 25 (11.6) | 6 (8.3) | 19 (13.3) | |
| Obese (>30) | 2 (0.9) | 0 | 2 (1.4) | |
| BMI, 1st trimester | 21.6 ± 3.1 | 21.6 ± 3.4 | 21.6 ± 2.9 | 0.737 |
| BMI, 2nd trimester | 21.9 ± 3.1 | 22.1 ± 3.4 | 21.9 ± 2.9 | 0.722 |
| BMI, completion | 22.1 ± 3.1 | 22.5 ± 3.4 | 21.9 ± 2.9 | 0.254 |
| Severely underweight (<16) | 3 (1.4) | 1 (1.4) | 2 (1.4) | |
| Underweight (16–18.4) | 16 (7.4) | 6 (8.3) | 10 (7.0) | |
| Normal weight (18.5–24.9) | 155 (75.5) | 47 (65.3) | 108 (75.7) | 0.316 |
| Overweight (25–29.9) | 37 (17.2) | 15 (20.8) | 22 (15.4) | |
| Obese (>30) | 4 (1.9) | 3 (4.2) | 1 (0.7) | |
| Protein, baseline | 6.9 ± 0.8 | 6.8 ± 0.8 | 7.0 ± 0.7 | 0.108 |
| Protein, 1st trimester | 7.1 ± 0.6 | 7.2 ± 0.6 | 7.0 ± 0.5 | 0.137 |
| Protein, 2nd trimester | 7.0 ± 0.5 | 7.0 ± 0.5 | 6.9 ± 0.5 | 0.47 |
| Protein, completion | 7.0 ± 0.5 | 7.1 ± 0.4 | 7.0 ± 0.6 | 0.086 |
| Albumin, baseline | 3.9 ± 0.6 | 3.7 ± 0.6 | 4.0 ± 0.6 | <0.001 |
| Albumin, 1st trimester | 4.2 ± 0.4 | 4.1 ± 0.3 | 4.1 ± 0.4 | 0.323 |
| Albumin, 2nd trimester | 4.2 ± 0.5 | 4.2 ± 0.3 | 4.2 ± 0.5 | 0.995 |
| Albumin, completion | 4.3 ± 0.4 | 4.3 ± 0.3 | 4.3 ± 0.4 | 0.648 |

AFB-S, acid-fast bacilli smear; BMI, body mass index.

### *3.3. Sequential Changes in Body Weight, BMI, Serum Protein Levels, and Albumin Levels during Anti-TB Therapy*

The mean changes in body weight, body weight percentages compared with baseline, BMIs, serum protein levels, and serum albumin levels from initiation to completion of anti-TB therapy are presented in Figure 2 and Table 3. The curves of observed changes from baseline in the BMI, and in serum albumin levels in the two groups, separated early but did not continue to diverge after the first trimester. In other words, the AFB smear-positive group had more malnutrition in the baseline compared with the negative group, but these differences were not observed after the first trimester. After first trimester, mean values of body weight and BMI in the AFB smear-positive group were higher, but not statistically different. This indicates that catch-up recovery of undernutrition in AFB smear-positive PTB occurred in the early period of anti-TB therapy. During the treatment period, the patients with AFB smear-positive PTB had significantly higher regains of BMI than the patients with AFB smear-negative PTB (+1.9 kg/m$^2$ vs. +0.4 kg/m$^2$, $p = 0.001$).

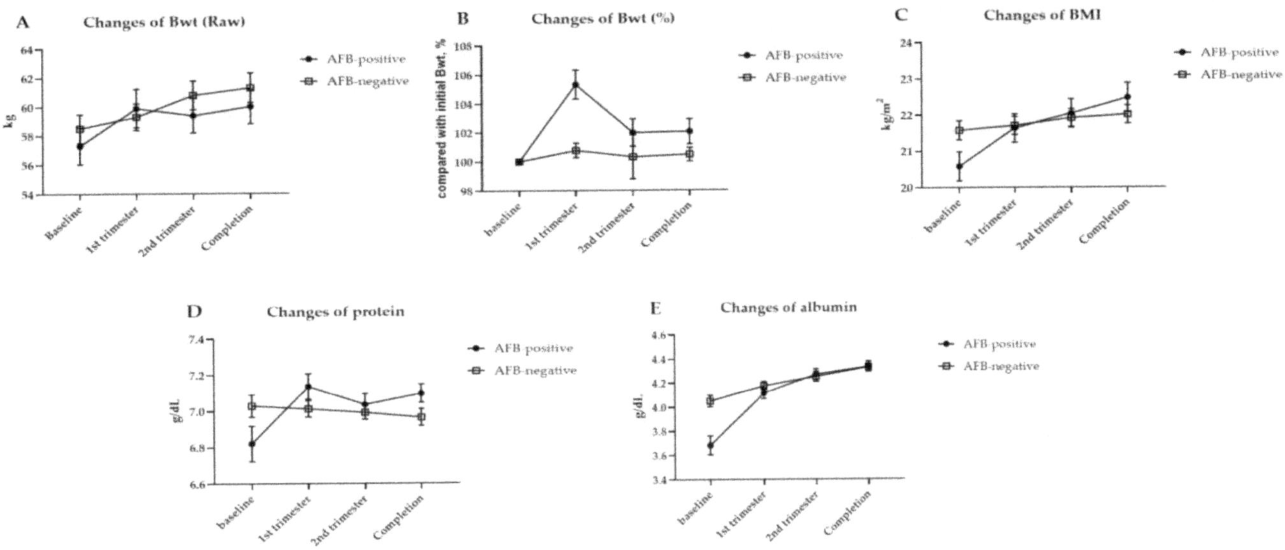


**Figure 2.** Changes from baseline in body weight (**A**), % changes in body weight compared with baseline (**B**), body mass index (**C**), serum protein levels (**D**), and serum albumin levels (**E**) during anti-TB treatment; the observed mean changes from baseline over the period of anti-TB therapy in the AFB smear-positive and negative groups. Bwt, body weight; BMI, body mass index; AFB, acid-fast bacilli.

### *3.4. Sequential Changes in Body Weight and BMI after Anti-TB Therapy*

The changes in body weight, percentages of body weight change compared with the baseline, and BMIs from enrolment to 2 years after anti-TB therapy are presented in Figure 3. The trend observed after treatment completion did not differ between the two groups. Furthermore, there were unremarkable changes in body weight and BMI.

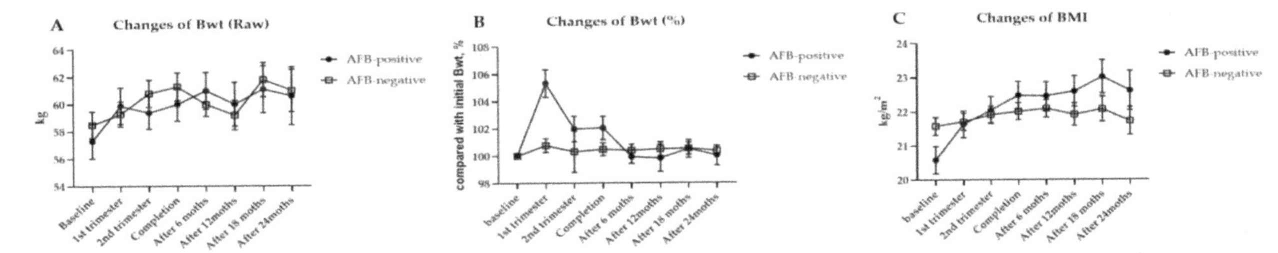


| | baseline | 1st trimester | 2nd trimester | completion | After 6 moths | After 12 months | After 18 months | After 24 months |
|---|---|---|---|---|---|---|---|---|
| AFB-positive | 72 | 72 | 72 | 72 | 72 | 50 | 37 | 24 |
| AFB-negative | 143 | 143 | 143 | 143 | 143 | 90 | 59 | 40 |

**Figure 3.** Changes from baseline in body weight (**A**), % change of body weight compared with baseline (**B**) body mass index (**C**) from the time of diagnosis to 2 years follow-up after treatment completion; the observed mean change from baseline over the period of anti-TB therapy in the AFB smear-positive and negative groups. Bwt, body weight; BMI, body mass index; AFB, acid-fast bacilli.

Additionally, we compared the BMIs and nutritional statuses, according to the BMI categories, of patients at treatment completion and at the restoration point from TB infection with subjects who participated in the KNHANES in 2013 ($n$ = 5694) (Table 4). Despite the successful completion of treatment for TB, the PTB group had a lower BMI and the patients were more undernourished than the general population.

**Table 4.** Comparison of demographics between enrolled 215 cases on completion of anti-TB treatment and 5694 cases of KHANES data in 2013.

| | In This Study | KNHANES 2013 | $p$-Value |
|---|---|---|---|
| | $n$ = 215 | $n$ = 5694 | |
| Age, years | 51.5 ± 18.9 | 50.3 ± 16.3 | 0.345 |
| Male gender, % | 136 (63.3) | 2240 (42.9) | <0.001 |
| Height, cm | 165.3 ± 9.5 | 162.3 ± 9.4 | <0.001 |
| Body Weight, kg | 60.9 ± 11.5 | 62.8 ± 11.9 | 0.015 |
| BMI, completion, kg/m2 | 22.1 ± 3.1 | 23.7 ± 3.5 | <0.001 |
| severely underweight (<16) | 3 (1.4) | 10 (0.2) | |
| underweight (16–18.4) | 16 (7.4) | 232 (4.1) | |
| normal weight (18.5–24.9) | 155 (75.5) | 3295 (57.9) | <0.001 |
| overweight (25–29.9) | 37 (17.2) | 1853 (32.5) | |
| obese (>30) | 4 (1.9) | 304 (5.3) | |

KNHANES, Korea National Health and Nutrition Examination Surveys; BMI, body mass index.

## 4. Discussion

We investigated the longitudinal changes in BMI as a marker of malnutrition in patients with PTB. The factors that may affect malnutrition were analyzed by clinical, radiological, and laboratory examination according to the microbiological burden. Our study showed that undernutrition was more prevalent in patients with positive AFB smears and in those who had more advanced disease, and that patients almost recovered from TB infection-related undernutrition in the early phase after initiation of anti-TB treatment. This is remarkable in patients with AFB smear-positive, and not in AFB smear-negative patients. However, nutritional status did not reach that of the general population despite the completion of anti-TB treatment. Moreover, this phenomenon was maintained for a follow-up period of 2 years.

TB and malnutrition have been traditionally considered to be strongly associated [11]. However, it is unclear whether malnutrition leads to TB infection or whether it results from TB infection. Moreover, one previous study showed that this phenomenon is only observed in PTB and not in extra-PTB [18]. This could be affected by the characteristics of extra-PTB such as its occurrence in relatively young and pauci-bacillary infections. This means that the correlation between TB infections and malnutrition may be more complex than we think and expect [2,11]. Therefore, long-term observations in the general population need to be performed to thoroughly investigate changes in nutritional statuses before and after TB infection. However, this poses a challenge in real-world settings.

In our study, the nutritional status of TB patients, as measured by BMI, improved in the early phase but did not change in at least two years in the AFB smear-positive group. This indirectly suggests that malnutrition may predispose patients to PTB infection. However, there were unremarkable changes in the AFB smear-negative group. They had no remarkable BMI recovery during or after anti-TB treatment. This means that there was no remarkable malnutrition in the AFB smear-negative group. It also raises the assumption that PTB infection can cause malnutrition due to it being a consumptive disease. Furthermore, the BMI after 2 years of treatment completion was relatively lower in the AFB smear-negative group than that in the general population. The present finding that malnutrition was not fully repleted during anti-TB treatment is consistent with the results of a previous study in a small group of 30 subjects in the United Kingdom [19]. In addition, in our study, recovery was not satisfactory after treatment. Therefore, it indicates that there is insufficient understanding about the relationship between TB infections and nutrition. Thus, a well-designed prospective study is needed for better understanding.

TB infection remains a major health problem worldwide, including in South Korea. Fortunately, in South Korea, it has steadily declined to 46.4 per 100,000 population, which was the estimated incidence in 2019 [20]. South Korea is constantly moving toward being a low-TB burden country.

However, the TB burden is still not as low as that in other OECD (Organization for Economic Co-operation and Development) countries. TB-related mortality is also continuously decreasing in South Korea [20]; however, PTB survivors face other malnutrition-related medical problems in the future even after the end of treatment [21]. Thus, it is necessary to better understand not only anti-TB treatment but also host-related responses, including nutritional changes. A comprehensive understanding of TB and TB-related phenomena could lead us one step forward towards the real end of TB in the world.

There were several limitations to this study. First, given its retrospective nature, selection bias may have influenced our findings. For example, we included and analyzed cases from TB outpatient clinics because they could measure BMI and they conducted follow-ups regularly. This means that severe cases with prolonged hospitalization due to advanced PTB or other combined diseases such as malignancies, bedridden states, or deaths during treatment were not included because the trend of malnutrition could not be identified in them. Therefore, this could underestimate our results. However, advanced cases of PTB that may lead to fatality, or complex cases with other medical problems, are also important to overcome TB infection, but these are not a major proportion. Second, this study was conducted in a high-income country with a very low HIV infection rate. Thus, this limitation could also underestimate our results. Third, our results were based on a relatively small sample size. For these reasons, our results may not be generalized to other clinical situations, and further studies are needed to determine whether these results can be applied.

The current study provides new data on the association between PTB and nutrition changes. Malnutrition-related TB is usually found in advanced disease, and is recovered in the early stages of treatment. However, the recovery of nutritional state is not sufficiently comparable to the general population after the end of treatment ended and after 2 years of follow-up. Therefore, the completion of anti-TB treatment might be the beginning, but not the end, from a social health perspective.

**Author Contributions:** Study conception and design: Y.K. and C.K.; Acquisition of data, Y.K., C.K., Y.B.P., E.-K.M. and J-W.M.; Data analysis and interpretation, Y.K., C.K., Y.B.P., E.-K.M. and J.-W.M.; Writing-Original draft preparation, Y.K. and C.K.; Writing-Review and Editing, Y.K., C.K., Y.B.P., E.-K.M. and J.-W.M. All authors have read and agreed to the published version of the manuscript.

**Acknowledgments:** The authors thank Youn Jung Lee and Shin ye ju for their help in the data collection.

## References

1. World Health Organization. *Global Tuberculosis Report*; World Health Organization: Geneva, Switzerland, 2017.
2. Sinha, P.; Davis, J.; Saag, L.; Wanke, C.; Salgame, P.; Mesick, J.; Horsburgh, C.R.; Hochberg, N.S. Undernutrition and tuberculosis: Public health implications. *J. Infect. Dis.* **2019**, *219*, 1356–1363. [CrossRef] [PubMed]
3. Cegielski, J.P.; McMurray, D.N. The relationship between malnutrition and tuberculosis: Evidence from studies in humans and experimental animals. *Int. J. Tuberc. Lung Dis.* **2004**, *8*, 286–298. [PubMed]
4. Mahuad, C.; Bozza, V.; Pezzotto, S.M.; Bay, M.L.; Besedovsky, H.; Del Rey, A.; Bottasso, O. Impaired immune responses in tuberculosis patients are related to weight loss that coexists with an immunoendocrine imbalance. *Neuroimmunomodulation* **2007**, *14*, 193–199. [CrossRef] [PubMed]
5. Padmapriyadarsini, C.; Shobana, M.; Lakshmi, M.; Beena, T.; Swaminathan, S. Undernutrition & tuberculosis in India: Situation analysis & the way forward. *Indian J. Med. Res.* **2016**, *144*, 11–20. [CrossRef] [PubMed]
6. Yen, Y.F.; Hu, H.Y.; Lee, Y.L.; Ku, P.W.; Lin, I.F.; Chu, D.; Lai, Y.J. Obesity/overweight reduces the risk of active tuberculosis: A nationwide population-based cohort study in Taiwan. *Int. J. Obes.* **2017**, *41*, 971–975. [CrossRef] [PubMed]

7. Leung, C.C.; Lam, T.H.; Chan, W.M.; Yew, W.W.; Ho, K.S.; Leung, G.; Law, W.S.; Tam, C.M.; Chan, C.K.; Chang, K.C.; et al. Lower risk of tuberculosis in obesity. *Arch. Intern. Med.* **2007**, *167*, 1297–1304. [CrossRef] [PubMed]
8. Khan, A.; Sterling, T.R.; Reves, R.; Vernon, A.; Horsburgh, C.R. Lack of weight gain and relapse risk in a large tuberculosis treatment trial. *Am. J. Respir. Crit. Care Med.* **2006**, *174*, 344–348. [CrossRef] [PubMed]
9. Ter Beek, L.; Alffenaar, J.C.; Bolhuis, M.S.; Van der Werf, T.S.; Akkerman, O.W. Tuberculosis-related malnutrition: Public health implications. *J. Infect. Dis.* **2019**, *220*, 340–341. [CrossRef] [PubMed]
10. Mupere, E.; Malone, L.; Zalwango, S.; Okwera, A.; Nsereko, M.; Tisch, D.J.; Parraga, I.M.; Stein, C.M.; Mugerwa, R.; Boom, W.H.; et al. Wasting among Uganda men with pulmonary tuberculosis is associated with linear regain in lean tissue mass during and after treatment in contrast to women with wasting who regain fat tissue mass: Prospective cohort study. *BMC Infect. Dis.* **2014**, *14*, 24. [CrossRef] [PubMed]
11. Casha, A.R.; Scarci, M. The link between tuberculosis and body mass index. *J. Thorac. Dis.* **2017**, *9*, E301–E303. [CrossRef] [PubMed]
12. Krapp, F.; Veliz, J.C.; Cornejo, E.; Gotuzzo, E.; Seas, C. Bodyweight gain to predict treatment outcome in patients with pulmonary tuberculosis in Peru. *Int. J. Tuberc. Lung Dis.* **2008**, *12*, 1153–1159. [PubMed]
13. Bernabe-Ortiz, A.; Carcamo, C.P.; Sanchez, J.F.; Rios, J. Weight variation over time and its association with tuberculosis treatment outcome: A longitudinal analysis. *PLoS ONE* **2011**, *6*, 18474. [CrossRef] [PubMed]
14. Hoa, N.B.; Lauritsen, J.M.; Rieder, H.L. Changes in body weight and tuberculosis treatment outcome in Viet Nam. *Int. J. Tuberc. Lung Dis.* **2013**, *17*, 61–66. [CrossRef] [PubMed]
15. Council of the Infectious Disease Society of America. Diagnostic standards and classification of Tuberculosis in adults and children. This official statement of the American thoracic society and the centers for disease control and prevention was adopted by the ATS board of directors, July 1999. This statement was endorsed by the, September 1999. *Am. J. Respir. Crit. Care Med.* **2000**, *161*, 1376–1395. [CrossRef]
16. Cederholm, T.; Barazzoni, R.; Austin, P.; Ballmer, P.; Biolo, G.; Bischoff, S.C.; Compher, C.; Correia, I.; Higashiguchi, T.; Holst, M.; et al. ESPEN guidelines on definitions and terminology of clinical nutrition. *Clin. Nutr.* **2017**, *36*, 49–64. [CrossRef] [PubMed]
17. World Health Organization. *Definitions and Reporting Framework for Tuberculosis-2013 Revision*; World Health Organization: Geneva, Switzerland, 2013.
18. Tverdal, A. Body mass index and incidence of tuberculosis. *Eur. J. Respir. Dis.* **1986**, *69*, 355–362. [PubMed]
19. Onwubalili, J.K. Malnutrition among tuberculosis patients in Harrow, England. *Eur. J. Clin. Nutr.* **1988**, *42*, 363–366. [PubMed]
20. Korea Centers for Disease Control and Prevention. *Annual Report on the Notified Tuberculosis in Korea 2019*; Korea Centers for Disease Control and Prevention: Cheongju, Korea, 2020.
21. Choi, C.J.; Choi, W.S.; Kim, C.M.; Lee, S.Y.; Kim, K.S. Risk of sarcopenia and osteoporosis in male tuberculosis survivors: Korea national health and nutrition examination survey. *Sci. Rep.* **2017**, *7*, 13127. [CrossRef] [PubMed]

2

# Key Aspects in Nutritional Management of COVID-19 Patients

**Alfredo Fernández-Quintela [1,2,3,†], Iñaki Milton-Laskibar [1,2,3,†], Jenifer Trepiana [1,2,3,*], Saioa Gómez-Zorita [1,2,3,*], Naroa Kajarabille [1,2,3], Asier Léniz [1,3,4], Marcela González [5] and María P. Portillo [1,2,3]**

1 Nutrition and Obesity Group, Department of Pharmacy and Food Science, University of the Basque Country (UPV/EHU) and Lucio Lascaray Research Institute, 01006 Vitoria, Spain; alfredo.fernandez@ehu.eus (A.F.-Q.); inaki.milton@ehu.eus (I.M.-L.); naroa.kajarabille@ehu.eus (N.K.); asier.leniz@gmail.com (A.L.); mariapuy.portillo@ehu.eus (M.P.P.)
2 CIBEROBN Physiopathology of Obesity and Nutrition, Institute of Health Carlos III, 01006 Vitoria, Spain
3 Bioaraba Health Research Institute, 01009 Vitoria, Spain
4 Basque Health Service (Osakidetza), Integrated Health Care Organization Araba, 01009 Álava, Spain
5 Nutrition and Food Science Department, Faculty of Biochemistry and Biological Sciences, National University of Litoral and National Scientific and Technical Research Council (CONICET), Santa Fe 3000, Argentina; maidagon@fbcb.unl.edu.ar
* Correspondence: jenifer.trepiana@ehu.eus (J.T.); saioa.gomez@ehu.eus (S.G.-Z.)

† These authors contributed equally to this work.

**Abstract:** This review deals with the relationship among nutrition, the immune system, and coronavirus disease 2019 (COVID-19). The influence of nutrients and bioactive molecules present in foodstuffs on immune system activity, the influence of COVID-19 on the nutritional status of the patients, and the dietary recommendations for hospitalized patients are addressed. Deficient nutritional status is probably due to anorexia, nausea, vomiting, diarrhea, hypoalbuminemia, hypermetabolism, and excessive nitrogen loss. There is limited knowledge regarding the nutritional support during hospital stay of COVID-19 patients. However, nutritional therapy appears as first-line treatment and should be implemented into standard practice. Optimal intake of all nutrients, mainly those playing crucial roles in immune system, should be assured through a diverse and well-balanced diet. Nevertheless, in order to reduce the risk and consequences of infections, the intakes for some micronutrients may exceed the recommended dietary allowances since infections and other stressors can reduce micronutrient status. In the case of critically ill patients, recently published guidelines are available for their nutritional management. Further, several natural bioactive compounds interact with the angiotensin-converting enzyme 2 (ACE2) receptor, the gateway for severe acute respiratory syndrome (SARS) and severe acute respiratory syndrome coronavirus 2 (SARS-CoV-2). Natural bioactive compounds can also reduce the inflammatory response induced by SARS-CoV-2. These compounds are potential beneficial tools in the nutritional management of COVID-19 patients.

**Keywords:** COVID-19; SARS-CoV-2; nutrition; malnutrition; nutritional support; bioactive compounds

---

## 1. Introduction

In December 2019, there was an outbreak of pneumonia of unknown cause in Wuhan, Hubei Province, China, which affected more than 60 people on the twentieth of that month. On 31 December, the Wuhan Municipal Health Committee informed the World Health Organization (WHO) that 27 people had been diagnosed with pneumonia of unknown cause, being 7 of them critically ill [1].

By January, the first cases of coronavirus disease 2019 (COVID-19) had been reported outside China: two in Thailand and one in Japan. Then, the rapid spread of the disease prompted the WHO to declare it as a health emergency of international concern, based on the impact the virus could have on underdeveloped countries with fewer health infrastructure. By that date, the disease had been detected in all provinces of mainland China, and cases were also diagnosed in 15 other countries. In March, the disease was already in more than 100 territories worldwide, and recognized as a pandemic by the WHO. At present, the number of confirmed cases continues to grow.

The virus that produced COVID-19 is the severe acute respiratory syndrome coronavirus 2 (SARS-CoV-2), an enveloped positive-sense RNA virus that mainly affects the respiratory system, being the spread of droplets generated by an infected subject the main route of transmission. When SARS-CoV-2 binds angiotensin-converting enzyme 2 (ACE2) receptors in the alveolar epithelial cells, the immune system responds through inflammation-related manifestation as well as antigen-presenting cell recruitment (Figure 1). The disease can be asymptomatic or present mild affection of the upper respiratory tract, while in the most severe cases is characterized by acute respiratory distress syndrome, heart failure, and septic shock [2]. Moreover, as the disease advances, multi-organ failure has also been reported as the result of uncontrolled acute inflammation. Indeed, the immune response against the virus triggered by this uncontrolled inflammation results in pulmonary tissue damage, which in turn reduces lung capacity. The tissue damage produced by SARS-CoV-2 at the alveolar level is characterized by pathological changes of the tissue, infiltration, and hyperplasia. Besides respiratory failure, other features have also been described as common in critically ill patients of COVID-19, among them infiltration of immune cells into lung injuries, high levels of inflammatory response, thrombosis, and multi-organ failure [3].

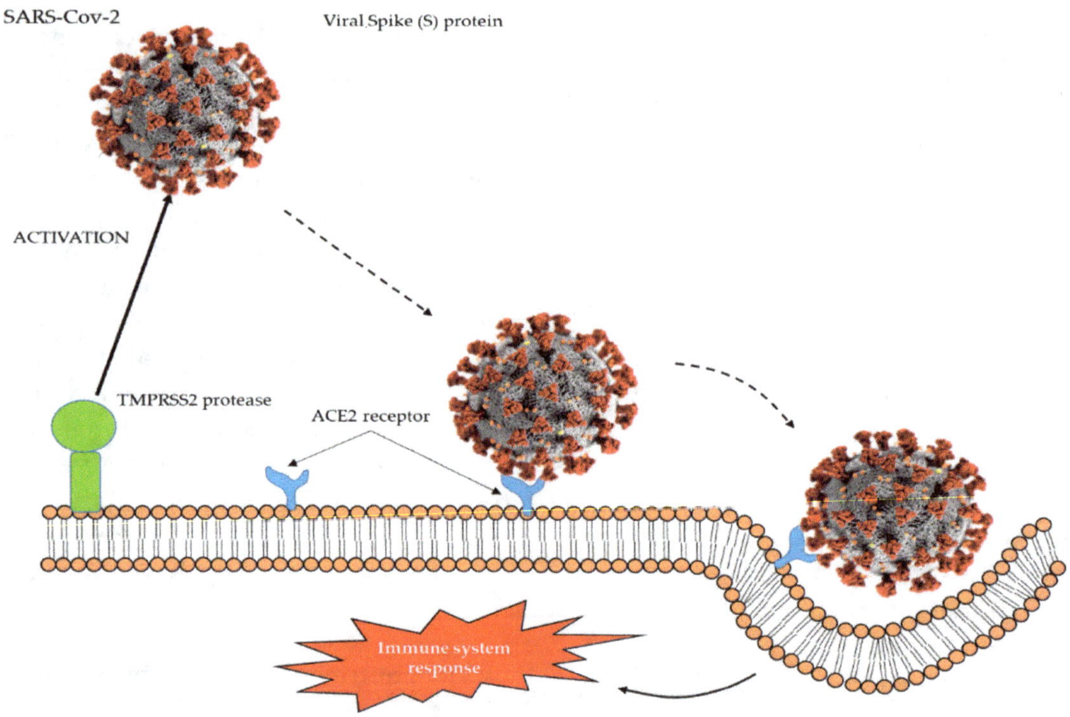


**Figure 1.** Severe acute respiratory syndrome coronavirus 2 (SARS-CoV-2) virus uses the angiotensin-converting enzyme 2 (ACE2) receptor to enter the host cell and the transmembrane protease serine 2 (TMPRSS2) for Spike (S) protein priming.

Additionally, the presence of other chronic diseases in the patient may exacerbate the inflammatory response derived from COVID-19, increasing the risk for adverse effects and mortality. In this regard, the systemic inflammation present in subjects with non-communicable diseases (NCDs), such as diabetes, tend to make the respiratory symptoms of the infection more severe [4]. On the other hand, it has been reported that excessive body mass index (BMI) and/or adiposity are considered risk factors for complications derived from COVID-19 infection, especially in patients with compromised heart and lung function [5]. Similarly, the damage in blood vessels that commonly exist in patients with diabetes and/or high-blood pressure increases the risk of these subjects to suffer COVID-19 derived thrombotic complications.

Due to the novelty of this pandemic, scientific community is currently looking for effective vaccines, as well as drugs to treat the pathology. One of the biggest challenges is focused on reducing inflammation, without compromising the correct immune response of the patient. In this scenario, science should focus not only in effective drugs but also in nutrition. The importance of an adequate nutritional status and dietary habits has been extensively highlighted in the COVID-19 pandemic, not only as a matter of avoiding the presence of NCDs that can result in more severe infections, but also as a way to modulate the inflammatory status of the patients. Indeed, the underestimation of the importance of nutrition in COVID-19 patients can dramatically affect the outcome of these patients [3,6].

The aim of the present review is to analyze the current knowledge on the relationship among nutrition, the immune system, and COVID-19 in order to formulate clinical advice and to highlight the directions for future research. Thus, the influence of nutrients and bioactive molecules present in foodstuffs on immune system activity, the influence of COVID-19 on nutritional status of patients and the dietary recommendations for COVID-19 hospitalized patients are addressed in this manuscript.

## 2. The Role of Specific Dietary Nutrients on Immune System Function and COVID-19 Disease

The influence of nutrition in the immune system has been widely reported. In addition, recent studies have also highlighted the influence of both, an adequate nutritional status and the appropriate intake of specific nutrients in COVID-19. Nevertheless, due to the novelty of the disease, information regarding the effects of some nutrients is scarce, and in some cases, this information comes from ecological studies. Therefore, it seems plausible that part of the information included in this section may be updated in the upcoming months as the result of the research that is currently ongoing. Protein deficiency is linked to impaired immune system function, mainly due to its negative effects on both, the amount of functional immunoglobulins and gut-associated lymphoid tissue (GALT). Besides quantity, the quality of proteins is also an important factor with regard to the relationship of this macronutrient with immune system. In this line, it has been highlighted that including proteins of high biological value (those present in eggs, lean meat, fish, and dairy) containing all the essential amino acids may exert an anti-inflammatory effect. In addition, some amino acids, such as arginine and glutamine are well known for their ability to modulate the immune system [7].

Among lipids, the omega-3 fatty acids eicosapentaenoic acid (EPA) and docosahexaenoic acid (DHA) can inactivate enveloped viruses by modulating the optimal host lipid conditions for viral replication. On the other hand, EPA and DHA inhibit cyclooxygenase enzymes (COX) and, thus, may help suppressing prostaglandin (pro-inflammatory) production [3]. Moreover, they are enzymatically converted to pro-resolving mediators (SPMs), such as protectins, resolvins, and maresins, alleviating inflammation [8]. According to these effects, the supplementation with DHA and EPA may be useful to reduce the severity and/or improve the recovery of patients with COVID-19. On the other hand, polar lipids, such as phospholipids, glycolipids or sphingolipids (also present in food sources of omega 3 fatty acids, such as fish and fish oils) have the ability to block platelet-activating factor (PAF) as well as its receptor, exerting anti-inflammatory effects that may be beneficial in COVID-19. Moreover, it has also been described that these lipid species can also down-regulate the enzymes involved in PAF biosynthesis, as well as up-regulate those involved on its degradation [9]. The blockage of platelet activation may also be useful to prevent the thrombotic complications associated to COVID-19 [3].

Carbohydrates and dietary fiber have also been reported to be related to immune system function. As far as carbohydrates is concerned, the consumption of those with higher glycemic indexes (highly processed carbohydrates) can result in mitochondrial overload and subsequent free radical synthesis.

Indeed, increased circulating levels of inflammatory cytokines such as C reactive protein (CRP), tumor necrosis factor alpha (TNF-α), and interleukin-6 (IL-6) have been reported with the consumption of these kind of carbohydrates [10]. Due to the aforementioned inflammatory status that usually occurs in respiratory infections such as COVID-19, limiting the consumption of foods rich in these carbohydrates may be advisable.

With regard to fiber, its importance for a correct metabolic functioning has been widely reported. Several studies have revealed that an adequate fiber intake (25–35 g/day) may help reducing both, systemic and gut inflammation. Indeed, the consumption of foods that are source of fiber has been related to lower levels of inflammatory cytokines (CRP, TNF-α, and IL-6), as well as enhanced levels of short chain fatty acids (SCFAs) [7]. In this regard, it has been described that different SCFAs (acetate, propionate, and butyrate) have a direct anti-inflammatory effect by inhibiting the release of pro-inflammatory molecules and by decreasing the expression of nuclear factor kB (NF-kB). Moreover, SCFAs also play an important role in the maintenance of an adequate gut microbiota by increasing the diversity, as well as enhancing the presence of specific health-associated bacteria [11]. Besides gut microbiota, nasopharyngeal microbiota may also be involved in respiratory infections. Indeed, it has been reported that this kind of infections may result in altered gut microbiota and innate immune system response [12]. Taking into account that COVID-19 has been related to respiratory and gastrointestinal symptoms, it seems plausible that gut microbiota impairment may occur, which in turn can result in an enhanced inflammatory status.

Vitamins A, C, D, E, B6, B12, and folate, iron, magnesium and trace elements including zinc, selenium and copper [13,14] play a pivotal role in disease susceptibility and the maintenance of immune function (Table 1) [15]. Deficiencies and/or inadequate status in these nutrients may negatively affect immune system, resulting in decreased resistance against infections.

**Table 1.** Recommended intakes of certain nutrients with key roles in disease susceptibility and the maintenance of an adequate immune function.

| Nutrient | Immune Function | Recommendation | | References |
|---|---|---|---|---|
| | | Healthy Individuals | Diseased/Infected Patients | |
| Vitamin C | Maintenance of functional and structural integrity of mucosal cells in innate barriers<br>Normal functioning of T cells<br>Antimicrobial, anti-inflammatory and antioxidant effects<br>Antibody production<br>Reduction of respiratory tract and lung infection risk | 200 mg/day | 1–2 g/day | [16,17] |
| Vitamin D | Maintenance of functional and structural integrity of mucosal cells in innate barriers<br>Normal functioning of T cells<br>Antimicrobial, anti-inflammatory and antioxidant effects<br>Antibody production and antigen responses<br>Reduction of respiratory tract and lung infection risk<br>Alleviation of the inflammatory response | 2000 IU/day (50 μg/day) | 10,000 IU during few weeks, followed by 5000 IU (until 25–hydroxyvitamin D concentrations rise above 40–60 ng/mL (equivalent to 100–150 nmol/L)) | [16,18,19] |

**Table 1.** *Cont.*

| Nutrient | Immune Function | Recommendation | | References |
|---|---|---|---|---|
| | | Healthy Individuals | Diseased/Infected Patients | |
| Vitamin E | Maintenance of functional and structural integrity of mucosal cells in innate barriers<br>Differentiation, and functioning of innate immune cells<br>Anti-inflammatory and antioxidant effects<br>Antibody production and antigen responses<br>Reduction of respiratory tract and lung infection risk<br>Support of T cell-mediated immunity | 15 mg/day (RDA) | 200 IU/day | [16] |
| Selenium | Differentiation, and functioning, of innate immune cells<br>Normal functioning of T cells<br>Antibody production<br>Antimicrobial, anti-inflammatory and antioxidant effects | 50 μg/day | Up to 200 μg/day | [17,20] |
| Zinc | Maintenance of functional and structural integrity of mucosal cells in innate barriers.<br>Differentiation, and functioning, of innate immune cells.<br>Antimicrobial, anti-inflammatory and antioxidant effects.<br>Antibody production and antigen response.<br>Support of lymphocyte and cytokine functions, and innate immunity overall.<br>Inhibits the activity and replication of coronavirus (SARS-CoV which caused an outbreak in 2002) | Men: 8 mg/day<br>Women: 11 mg/day<br>(RDA) | Zinc lozenges: over 75 mg/day administered within 24 h (divided into 6–8 doses, each separated by 2–3 h when awake)<br>Zinc gluconate: 13.3 mg/day within 3 days (at least) | [16–18,21–23] |
| Iron | Maintenance of functional and structural integrity of mucosal cells in innate barriers<br>Differentiation, and functioning, of innate immune cells<br>Normal functioning of T cells.<br>Antimicrobial, anti-inflammatory and antioxidant effects | Men: 8 mg/day<br>Women age 19–50: 18 mg/day<br>Women age > 51: 8 mg/day<br>(RDA) | Ferrous iron salts (ferrous sulfate and ferrous gluconate): 60 mg Fe/day (taken with food to avoid gastric discomfort) | [17,24] |
| Omega-3 fatty acids (EPA + DHA) | Conversion to specialized pro-resolving mediators (SPMs) such as, protectins, resolvins and maresins to relieve the inflammation and enhance lung injury | 250–300 mg/day of EPA + DHA | 1500–3000 mg/day EPA + DHA | [16,25] |
| Multivitamin supplements including vitamins (A, B6, B12, C, D, E and folate) and trace elements (Zn, Fe, Se, Mg and Cu) | Support of the cells and tissues of the immune system overall<br>Maintenance and development of in innate barriers<br>Growth and differentiation of innate cells<br>Antibody production and generation of memory cells<br>Production and activity of antimicrobial proteins<br>Phagocytic activities of neutrophils and macrophages | Supplying nutrient requirements according to the 100% RDA for age and gender<br>This is in addition to a well-balanced diet | | [16,25,26] |

DHA: docosahexaenoic acid, EPA: eicosapentaenoic acid, RDA: Recommended Dietary Allowances.

The mentioned vitamins and minerals are essential for adaptive immunity as they are involved in cytokine production, lymphocyte differentiation and proliferation, antibody production, and generation of memory cells. Regarding to innate immunity, they also contribute to the maintenance and development of physical barriers and differentiation of innate cells, production, and activity of antimicrobial proteins, phagocytic activities of neutrophils and macrophages, and regulation of the overall inflammatory response.

Significant research has been conducted over decades regarding the usage of vitamin C as a remedy for colds [3]. In the case of COVID-19, there is no evidence so far to recommend its supplementation. In this regard, a clinical trial devoted to analyzing the effect of vitamin C (24 g/day for 7 days) in 140 patients with severe COVID-19 is being carried out in Wuhan (China) (Identifier: NCT04264533) [27].

The relationship between vitamin A and infections has been extensively described. In the case of respiratory infections, vitamin A plays a pivotal role due to its involvement in healthy mucus layer formation, as well as enhancing antigen non-specific immune response [28]. Indeed, histopathological alterations have been described in pulmonary epithelium and parenchyma in subjects with vitamin A deficiency, resulting in impaired respiratory function [29]. Consequently, adequate intakes of this vitamin should be guaranteed in order to avoid further complications in the case of COVID-19.

The association of vitamin D deficiency with respiratory tract infections and lung injury has been widely reported. Indeed, the usage of vitamin D agonists has shown effectiveness ameliorating the aforementioned conditions [30]. Furthermore, previous investigations have demonstrated that high-dose supplementation of vitamin D (250,000–500,000 IU/day) is safe and effective in improving the health status of mechanically ventilated critically ill patients (enhancing the capacity of blood for oxygen transport and increasing hemoglobin levels), which resulted in shorter hospital stays [31,32]. With regard to COVID-19, Ilie et al. have studied the role of vitamin D levels on the prevention of this infection and the mortality induced by this disease [33]. The authors have determined the mean levels of 25(OH)D in subjects from 20 European countries, as well as the number of positive cases and deaths caused by COVID-19. They have found a negative association between the mean levels of vitamin D and the number of COVID-19 cases, as well as with the mortality. They also observed that vitamin D levels are severely low in the aging population, which is the most vulnerable population group for COVID-19.

In the same line, a retrospective study carried out in Switzerland has shown that patients positive for SARS-CoV-2 have lower levels of 25(OH)D than non-infected subjects [34]. However, when patients were stratified by age, the mentioned difference was only significant among patients older than 70 years, who are the subjects in higher risk to suffer clinical complications in COVID-19. Based on the results obtained, the authors proposed to reach a plasma concentration of 30 ng/mL 25(OH)D in this population, in order to reduce the risk in case of serious disease.

Nevertheless, not all the results go in the same direction. Thus, taking into account that black and minority ethnic individuals seem to be more affected by COVID-19, vitamin D deficiency is being studied to explain this fact. In a study conducted by the UK Biobank, 1474 participants were submitted to COVID-19 test, being positive 449 of them. Among the 1474 subjects, 95% were white people (12% of them were vitamin D deficient), 1% were black people (36% of them were vitamin D deficient), 2% were South Asian subjects (57% of them were vitamin D deficient) and the remaining 2% belonged to other ethnic groups (29% of them were vitamin D deficient). Among all the participants, 25(OH)D concentration was lower in those patients who subsequently had confirmed COVID-19 infection. Moreover, 25(OH)D predicted COVID-19 infection when displayed an univariate analysis, but not after it was adjusted for potential confounders. Univariate analysis showed that black and South Asian ethnicities were associated with confirmed COVID-19 infection compared with whites, although adjustment for 25(OH)D serum concentrations showed no significant associations between vitamin D nutritional status, ethnicity, and an increased susceptibility to COVID-19 infection. Authors concluded that the potential role of 25-hydroxyvitamin D concentration to explain susceptibility to COVID-19 infection could not be supported overall or in blacks and minority ethnic populations [35]. Nevertheless, it should be highlighted that after the publication of these results, two letters to the editor showing some weak points of this study have been published [36,37].

As shown in the previous lines, the studies carried out to date have reported controversial results regarding vitamin D levels and the risk to develop COVID-19. Consequently, there is no enough evidence to recommend supplementation of this vitamin in those subjects who do not exhibit deficits. In this regard, meeting the recommended dietary allowances for this vitamin would be the best advice.

By contrast, higher doses of vitamin D are advisable for vulnerable subjects in order to avoid deficits, especially in situations of lockdown [3].

Vitamin E has been related to the correct function of the humoral and innate immune functions. Indeed, the ability of vitamin E to scavenge reactive oxygen species (ROS) plays an important role in oxidative stress reduction, exerting anti-inflammatory effects. In addition, vitamin E also protects polyunsaturated fatty acids (PUFAs) and immune cells from oxidation. To date, there is little evidence regarding the use and/or dosage of vitamin E as a prophylactic or therapeutic agent against COVID-19.

Iron is a nutrient with diverse implications in COVID-19. On the one hand, it is well known the importance of iron for the correct functioning of the immune system. However, it is also well established that iron-containing enzymes are essential for the completion of virus replication process, particularly coronaviruses [21]. Thus, it has been pointed out that iron chelation could be an alternative adjuvant strategy to treat COVID-19 patients, via manipulation of key iron regulators (still needs further research) or via venous injection or oral administration of iron chelators. In this sense, previous treatments with iron chelator deferiprone (DFP, Ferriprox®) prolonged the survival of patients with acquired immunodeficiency syndrome (AIDS) after human immunodeficiency virus (HIV) infection [38,39]. Evidence also suggests that iron chelators can exhibit antiviral effect on HIV through the elevation of intracellular iron efflux and increasing iron exporter ferroportin expression [40]. Despite to date little is known about iron regulation in COVID-19 patients, it could be deduced from other viral infections that iron chelation might be an alternative beneficial adjuvant in treating COVID-19. However, it is important to point out that there is no empirical research to date, so further investigation is needed.

Selenium plays an essential role in the immune system due to its anti-inflammatory effect. Zhang et al. (2020) have identified a positive association between higher recovery rate from COVID-19 infection and adequate selenium status in 17 cities outside the region of Hubei (China) [20]. This effect is in line with the significant benefits of selenium supplementation demonstrated against other viral infections, including HIV [41,42], hepatitis B linked liver cancer linked [43] or epidemic hemorrhagic fever [44].

Interestingly, the amount of trace elements present in food varies according to the geographical differences of the soil. In this regard, soils in different regions of China have been reported to have the highest and lowest selenium levels in the world. Zhang et al. (2020) have found that infected patients from the areas with high selenium levels were more prone to recover from COVID-19 [20]. Indeed, the cure rate (percentage of COVID-19 patients declared as recovered) was almost threefold higher on the city of Enshi in Hubei Province, which has the highest selenium intake in China, compared to the other cities in Hubei. By contrast, in Heilongjiang Province, where selenium intake is among the lowest in the world, the death rate from COVID-19 was almost fivefold higher than the average of all the other provinces outside of Hubei. These observations suggest that selenium intake seem to be related to the clinical outcome in COVID-19 patients. However, further research is still needed in order to provide more specific advice regarding the adequate intake of this mineral.

With regard to zinc, te Velthuis et al. (2010) demonstrated that increasing $Zn^{2+}$ concentration inhibits the replication of SARS-coronavirus (SARS-CoV) [45]. On the other hand, zinc deficiency is linked with defective cell-mediated immune response, as well as with increased susceptibility for various infections. Indeed, it has been suggested that increased zinc intake may exert beneficial effects on COVID-19 infections by reducing gastrointestinal and lower respiratory symptoms. In addition, it has been suggested that zinc intakes of 30–50 mg/d may exert beneficial effects on RNA viruses [46].

Copper is essential to maintain DNA integrity by preventing oxidative DNA damage. Studies conducted in rodent models with chronic TNF-$\alpha$-induced lung inflammation proposed that copper supplementation may ameliorate such inflammation [47]. However, no substantial evidence is available in order to recommend copper supplementation against COVID-19.

Figure 2 shows the effects of several nutrients on immune system function and other important aspects on COVID-19 infection, such as oxidative stress, inflammation, and thrombosis.

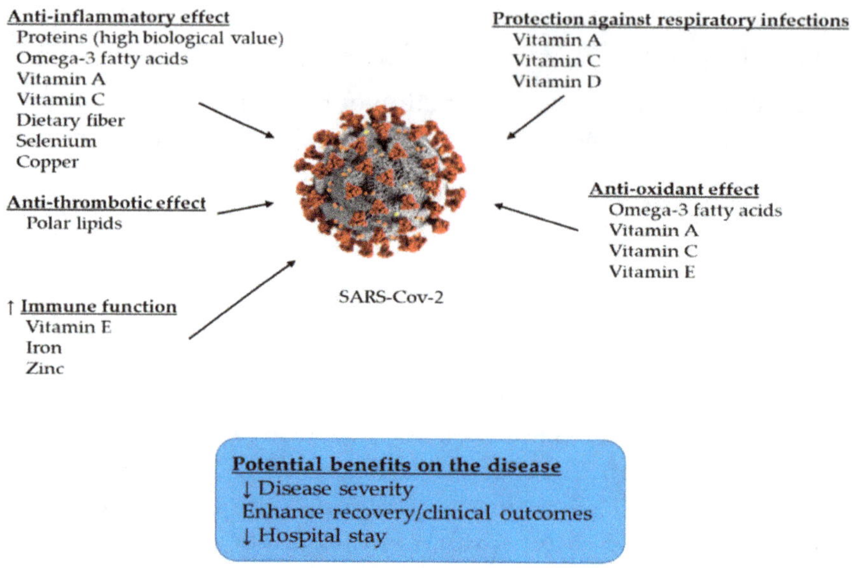


**Figure 2.** Effects of several nutrients on aspects of COVID-19 infection. ↑: increase, ↓: decrease.

## 3. The Role of Specific Bioactive Compounds Present in the Diet on Immune System Function and COVID-19 Disease

Nowadays, there is an urgent need to identify molecules effective to prevent COVID-19 disease and/or to reduce its severity. In this regard, it has been found that several natural bioactive compounds interact with ACE2 receptor, which is the gateway for SARS and SARS-CoV-2, and thus regulates the viral infection. Natural bioactive compounds can also reduce the inflammatory response induced by SARS-CoV-2 infection. Taking into account that a great number of the patients with COVID-19 present "pro-inflammatory cytokine storm", which drive to a worse prognosis, these molecules could represent a promising target for immunomodulatory therapies. In the following lines, the potential benefits of resveratrol (3,5,4′-trihydroxy-*trans*-stilbene), celastrol, oleoylethanolamide, and natural peroxisome proliferator-activated receptor $\gamma$ (PPAR-$\gamma$) agonists (Figure 3) are described. Nevertheless, it should be pointed out that the vast majority of these results have been obtained in animal models; thus, further studies are still needed to check them in humans.

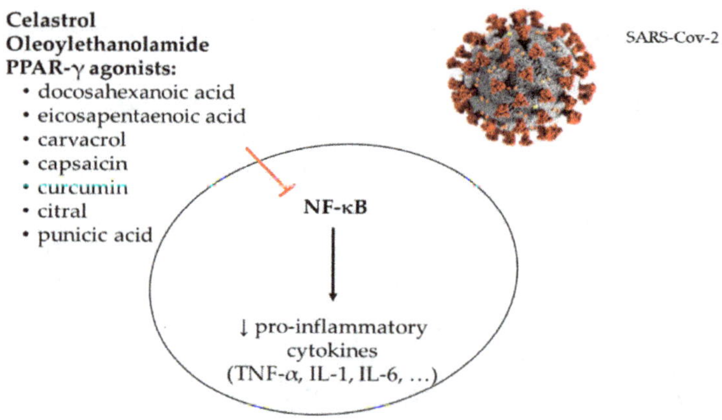


**Figure 3.** Anti-inflammatory effect of bioactive compounds present in foodstuffs. PPAR: peroxisome proliferator-activated receptor, TNF: tumor necrosis factor, IL: interleukin, ↓: decrease.

### 3.1. *Resveratrol*

Resveratrol is a polyphenol belonging to the group of stilbenes, naturally found in red wine, berries, grapes, nuts, and other foodstuffs. Horne et al. (2020) reviewed the biological interaction between resveratrol and the ACE2 receptor described in four studies that have been published to date [48]. As explained in the Introduction section, SARS-CoV-2 uses the ACE2 receptor to enter the mammalian cells, as well as the transmembrane protease serine 2 (TMPRSS2), involved in the viral spike-(S) protein cleavage, which in turn mediates the fusion of virus and cellular membranes necessary for viral entry (Figure 1). Therefore, due to the role of ACE2 in SARS-CoV-2 infection, it could be thought that nutrients or molecules (such as some bioactive compounds and antihypertensive drugs) that may enhance the expression/synthesis of this enzyme should be avoided in order to reduce the risk of infection. However, it must be noted that ACE2 activation also exerts beneficial effects on the lung injury produced by SARS-CoV-2 infection [3]. Thus, due to the dual role that ACE2 may play in COVID-19, further research is needed in order to better understand whether its activation represents a beneficial or a detrimental effect in the development of the disease.

Tiao et al. (2018) observed, in a study carried out in rats, that resveratrol increases ACE2 protein levels in the liver, at a dose of 50 mg/kg/day [49]. Oliveira Andrade et al. (2014) reported that mice fed a high-fat diet supplemented with resveratrol revealed increased ACE2 gene expression in adipose tissue compared with mice fed the high-fat diet alone [50]. Kim et al. (2018) studied the effect of this natural compound in thoracic aortas of 24-month-old mice, observing an increased expression of ACE2 protein and an enhanced protection against arterial aging [51]. There is also an in vitro study carried out in human aortic smooth muscle cells, in which resveratrol incubation for 24 h up-regulated ACE2 protein [52].

### 3.2. *Celastrol*

Habtemariam et al. (2020) reviewed the effect of celastrol, a pentacyclic triterpenoid, which has shown anti-inflammatory benefits on lung diseases, in animal models, by suppressing NF-kB signaling [53] (Figure 4). In the study reported by Shi et al. (2018), this compound improved chronic obstructive pulmonary disease by decreasing interleukin-8 (IL-8), TNF-$\alpha$, and monocyte chemoattractant protein-1 (MCP1) levels, as well as by increasing enzymatic antioxidant defenses in mice [54]. These results are in good accordance with those previously reported by Wei and Wang (2017), who observed that celastrol reduced these pro-inflammatory cytokines and NF-kB activation in rats, showing lipopolysaccharide (LPS)-induced acute respiratory distress syndrome [55]. More recently, Iwata-Yoshikawa et al. (2019) showed that NF-kB pathway was regulated by TMPRSS2 protein in the airway of a TMPRSS2 knockout murine model, after coronavirus infection [56]. In this sense, the authors suggested that celastrol could be a promising candidate for COVID-19 treatment due to its capacity to inhibit TMPRSS2 protein and, thus, reduce the cleavage of S protein and the subsequent viral entry.

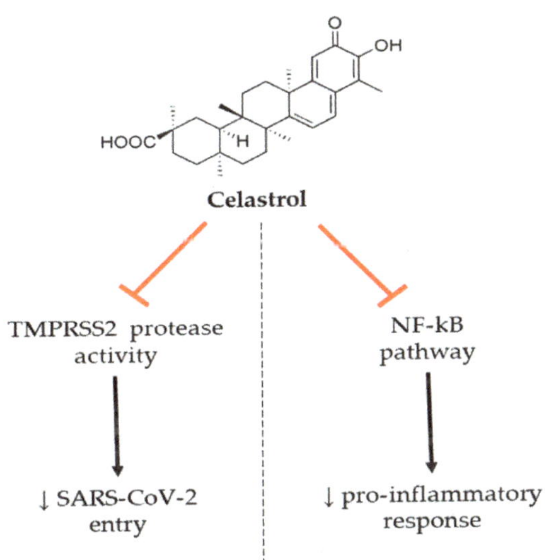


**Figure 4.** Anti-inflammatory activity of celastrol. NF-κB: nuclear factor *kappa* B, TMPRSS2: transmembrane protease serine 2, ↓: decrease.

### 3.3. *Oleoylethanolamide*

It is well known that the activation of immune system receptors called toll like receptors (TLRs) reduces the expression levels of PPARs, thus activating the NF-kB pathway and leading to the release of cytokines IL-6 and interleukin-1β (IL-1β) [57,58]. Ghaffari et al. (2020) suggested that oleoylethanolamide (OEA), derived from oleic acid (omega-9 monounsaturated fatty acid) and synthesized in the gastro-intestinal tract, may activate PPAR-α receptors and thus prevent gene expression of inflammatory cytokines [59]. This is supported by the results observed in a recent clinical trial where OEA decreased serum levels of IL-6 and TNF-α in obese patients [60]. These facts have encouraged the authors to conduct a clinical trial to evaluate this hypothesis on patients infected with COVID-19 in Iran.

### 3.4. *Natural PPAR-γ Agonists*

In viral infections, pro-inflammatory cytokines (e.g., TNF-α and IL-1) are released by lung-epithelial cells, endothelial cells and immune cells. PPAR-γ, a transcription factor member belonging to the PPAR family, is known as a regulator of inflammatory response. It suppresses the expression of the pro-inflammatory M1 macrophages and activates the proliferation of anti-inflammatory M2 macrophages. Moreover, it acts on the transcription of inflammatory cytokine genes and inhibits the production of cyclooxygenase-2 (COX-2), an enzyme that induces inflammatory response [61].

In this context, natural PPAR-γ agonists present in foodstuffs could also act as anti-inflammatory molecules by inhibiting the expression of pro-inflammatory cytokines. Ciavarella et al. (2020) have published a review where the anti-inflammatory effect of several natural compounds are summarized [62]: (a) EPA and DHA, provided by sea food and fish oil [63], (b) carvacrol, a monoterpenic phenol present in thyme and oregano, two plants of the Mediterranean area [64], (c) capsaicin, contained in hot pepper, one of the most used spices around the world [65], (d) carnosic acid and carnosol, two dipertenoids present in rosemary and sage [66,67], (e) punicic acid, contained in pomegranate seed oil [68], (f) citral, present in lemongrass oil [69], and (g) curcumin [70,71].

The effects of curcumin on SARS-CoV-2 infection have been addressed by several research groups. As early as 2007, Wen et al. determined the quantity of spike proteins in cultures of Vero E6 cells infected with SARS-CoV, and observed that this compound was able to significantly decrease the virus replication [72]. Later on, Ting et al. (2018), using porcine epidemic diarrhea virus (PEDV) as a coronavirus model, showed that curcumin could suppress viral replication by inhibiting the synthesis of negative-strand RNA virus [73]. Recently, Zahedipour et al. (2020) have shown that curcumin may target critical steps of the viral infection by reducing the penetration of the virus and attacking the components necessary for the viral replication cycle [74].

It is important to point out that some patients infected with COVID-19 develop pulmonary fibrosis, which is mediated by the transforming growth factor β (TGF-β) pathway. With regard to this signaling pathway, it has been reported that curcumin induces a reduction in a mouse model of viral-induced acute respiratory distress syndrome [75]. Moreover, curcumin can reduce type I collagen protein and TGF-β mRNA levels in rodent models with fibrosis [76]. Although the anti-fibrotic effects of curcumin have not been tested in a model of COVID-19, similar effects in this case may be hypothesized.

### 3.5. *Probiotics*

The gut microbiota is in continuous bidirectional interaction with the host, regulating both adaptive and innate immune systems. It is well known that alterations in intestinal microbiota composition and its metabolites influence organs involved in metabolism, such as adipose tissue or liver, producing metabolic inflammation [77]. Nowadays, great attention is paid to the presence of microorganisms in the lung, an organ rich in bacterial colonies. Indeed, a crosstalk between both organs known as "gut-lung axis" has been proposed [78]. Consequently, exogenous factors, such as antibiotics, diet, or exposition to toxics, that alter gut microbiota, could cause lung inflammation through the mentioned axis, thus increasing morbidity of fibrosis or pneumonia, which are clinical outcomes of COVID-19. Taking this into account, it has been recently postulated that probiotics can exert protection against viral infections at three different levels: (a) providing a stronger innate immune response in the gut, (b) decreasing the gut permeability, and (c) regulating the acquired immune response [79].

In a pilot study, fecal samples of patients diagnosed with SARS-CoV-2 infection (confirmed via polymerase chain reaction (PCR) tests) were collected during hospitalization and compared with samples of healthy individuals [80]. COVID-19 patients presented more opportunistic pathogens and a depletion of commensals in the gut, while healthy subjects maintained a higher prevalence of *Eubacterium, Roseburia, Lachnospiraceae Eubacterium, Faecalibacterium prausnitzii, Roseburia*, and *Lachnospiraceae*. Right now, there are three registered clinical trials devoted to studying the effect of probiotics on COVID-19 patients [79]. One of them is a preventive study that evaluates the beneficial effects of *Lactobacillus coryniformis* on the incidence of COVID-19 illness in healthcare workers exposed to SARS-Cov-2 (NCT04366180). Other clinical trial is evaluating the effect of bacteriotherapy in the treatment of patients with acute diarrhea, and in the prevention of intensive cares in COVID-19 patients (NCT04368351). In the third one, the adjuvant use of oxygen-ozone therapy, along with probiotic supplementation, is investigated in patients with COVID-19 (NCT04366089).

Based on these ideas, probiotics could be proposed as potential tools to be included in the nutritional treatment of COVID-19 patients. Thus, Renzo et al. (2020) have suggested the potential therapeutic use of probiotics such as *Lactobacillus rhamnosus* and *Bifidobacterium lactis*, which exhibit anti-inflammatory effects, and prebiotics for restoring the innate and adaptive immunity [81].

## 4. Protein-Energy Malnutrition

When addressing COVID-19 disease, the study of nutritional status is very relevant since it plays an important role on the functionality of immune system, necessary to face the virus infection. Indeed, malnutrition is associated with immune dysfunction and thus it is likely to assume that this condition could make individuals more vulnerable to the viral infection [82,83].

On the other hand, nutritional status can be negatively affected by the SARS-CoV-2 itself, as well as by the applied treatments. Hospitalized patients with COVID-19 tend to present malnutrition at the time of hospitalization. Chronic diseases that are commonly present in patients with COVID-19 (mainly diabetes, chronic obstructive pulmonary disease, renal insufficiency, cardiovascular diseases or dementia), as well as other risk factors such as socio-economic status or frailty, have negative effects on the nutritional status of these patients. In addition, during hospital stay, the prolonged immobilization, mainly in long stays in intensive care units (ICU), leads to muscle mass losses, making the recovery of these subjects harder. Furthermore, the need for assisted breathing during prolonged periods also contributes to the development of sarcopenia and malnutrition [84–88]. This deteriorated nutritional status seems to be involved in the virulence of the virus, and probably in the clinical outcome. In this regard, studies conducted in Italy have demonstrated the importance of maintaining/recovering an adequate nutritional status in the clinical outcomes of the patients [89,90].

Due to fluid administration and rapid wasting of lean tissues, weight and BMI changes do not accurately reflect malnutrition in COVID-19 patients. Thus, the loss of lean body mass is of more concern than that of the BMI. Indeed, loss of muscle and sarcopenia have to be detected, since the larger the muscle mass decrease is, the more severe the malnutrition will be [91].

Malnutrition is probably due to anorexia, nausea, vomiting, and diarrhea (which impair food intake and absorption), hypoalbuminemia, hypermetabolism, and excessive nitrogen loss [92,93]. These effects are clearly associated with the increase in pro-inflammatory cytokines observed in these patients. Moreover, anorexia can also be related to dysgeusia. Lechien et al. conducted a study devoted to analyzing the effect of COVID-19 infection on gustatory disorders [94]. For this purpose, 417 mild-to-moderate COVID-19 patients (164 males and 263 females) with a mean age of 37 years old were recruited from 12 European hospitals. More than 88% of the patients reported gustatory dysfunction, which was characterized by impairment of salty, sweet, bitter, and sour tastes.

The gustatory disturbance consisted of reduced/discontinued or inaccurate capability to taste flavors in 79% and 21% of patients, respectively. In these subjects, olfactory and gustatory dysfunctions were positively correlated. In summary, this study identified gustatory dysfunction as symptom of the European COVID-19 infection. In addition, Zayet et al. (2020) carried out a retrospective study in 217 adults in France, where patients were divided in 2 groups: patients infected by COVID-19 confirmed by a positive PCR on nasopharyngeal sample (95 patients) and patients with a negative PCR result on nasopharyngeal sample (122 patients) [95]. In patients positive in COVID-19, 65% had dysgeusia, whereas in patients negative in COVID-19, only 16% had this symptom. This difference in the frequency was statistically significant. The authors concluded that dysgeusia is frequently reported in patients consulting from COVID-19. Other authors also showed similar results [96–99]. It is still unknown the mechanism by which gustatory dysfunction takes place, but according to Printza et al. (2020), SARS-CoV-2 may enter into tongue taste cells via the ACE-2 receptor, which not only is present in pulmonary tissue but also in taste organs (at least in mice) [100]. Accordingly, the usual function of the sensory cells can be disturbed.

Several studies have shown the results of nutritional status assessment in various cohorts of COVID-19 patients. Li et al. (2020) carried out the first study aimed to evaluate the nutritional status in elderly patients suffering COVID-19 [101]. For that purpose, a cross-sectional study was designed including 182 patients (65 male and 117 female) from a hospital in Wuhan (China), with a mean age of 69 years and positive in COVID-19. The nutritional assessment of the participants was performed by using the Mini Nutritional Assessment (MNA), a tool for institutionalized geriatric patients. MNA takes into account food intake, weight loss, BMI, morbidity, major or acute psychological diseases, and cognitive status. In these patients, MNA mean score was 22.9, which means a risk of malnutrition; in fact, among the patients, 53% were malnourished, 28% at risk of malnutrition and 20% non-malnourished. There were no differences in age, gender, triceps skin-fold thickness, mid-arm circumference, hypertension, or cerebrovascular, cardiovascular, and chronic lung diseases among the three groups. However, there were statistical differences in the incidence of diabetes mellitus, BMI, calf circumference, albumin, hemoglobin, and lymphocyte counts among the three groups, being the highest values in the group without malnutrition and the lowest in malnourished group. Finally, the multivariate regression analysis showed that diabetes, low calf circumference, and low albumin levels were independent risk factors for malnutrition in these subjects. In view of these results, the authors concluded that in Wuhan (China) there was a high prevalence of malnutrition in elderly patients with COVID-19.

Liu et al. (2020) aimed to evaluate the nutritional risk, as well as their associated clinical outcomes, in older patients with COVID-19. To do so, a retrospective study was carried out in 141 patients (68 males and 73 females), older than 65 years (average age 72 years), 77 of them with hypertension or/and diabetes, showing different status of COVID-19 (46 common COVID-19, 73 severe COVID-19 and 22 extremely severe COVID-19), treated in a hospital from Wuhan (China) [102]. Participants were classified as normal group (no nutritional risk) or as nutritional risk group, according to the criteria of each nutritional risk tool used. The nutritional screening risk methods used by researchers were Nutrition Risk Screening 2002 (NRS 2002), Malnutrition Universal Screening Tool (MUST), MNA short form (MNA-sf), and Nutrition Risk Index (NRI). NRS 2002 predicts patients who would benefit from nutritional treatment in hospital settings and takes into account the BMI, body weight loss, food intake and the severity of the disease. MUST is useful for identifying the necessity of nutritional treatment and for assessing the risk of malnutrition based on different factors like BMI, unintentional weight loss and the presence of acute disease factors to detect disease related malnutrition. NRI is a screening tool that predicts patient's malnutrition status, based on serum albumin, as well as, on current and usual body weight.

Depending on the used nutritional screening risk method, the assignation to each tool to normal or nutritional risk groups was as follows: 85% of the patients with NRS 2002, 41% with MUST, 77% with MNA-sf and 60% with NRI were assigned to the risk group. These results show that, independently of the used nutritional assessment method, a high percentage of the older patients suffering COVID-19 showed malnutrition.

As far as anthropometric measurements and clinical outcomes are concerned, statistical analysis did not show differences between the normal group and the nutritional risk group. By contrast, with MUST tool BMI was lower in nutritional risk group than in normal group. When using NRS 2002, the fever duration was measured, which resulted to be longer in the nutritional risk group when compared to the control group. Serum albumin and total protein levels were also higher in the control group than in the nutritional risk group, by using all the nutritional risk tools, with the exception of MUST.

When data were adjusted for age, sex, presence of co-morbidities and BMI, NRS 2002, MNA-sf, and NRI methods demonstrated that patients from the nutritional risk group showed longer hospital stay, lower appetite, worse severity of the disease, and greater weight loss than the patients in the normal group. By using NRS 2002 and NRI methods, patients with nutritional risk also showed higher hospital expenses than normal patients.

## 5. Recommendations for Nutritional Treatment

Although nowadays, the knowledge regarding the nutritional support during hospital stay of COVID-19 patients is still limited, nutritional therapy appears as first-line treatment and should be implemented into standard practice [7,103,104]. In spite of that, due to the priority assigned to urgent pathologies like respiratory issues, the nutritional status of patients has been relegated to a second place. In fact, almost half of the hospitalized polymorbid and 23–60% of patients in acute care are not correctly nourished [105,106]. Other facts that have also exacerbated this situation are that medical teams cannot invest enough time to grant an optimal nourishment due to work overload, staff shortages (healthcare personnel have suffered a high infection rate) or insufficient availability of personal protective equipment. Additionally, a restriction to family visits has been applied in most affected countries, removing a support in nourishment. Moreover, in most hospitals clinical teams and structures have been reorganized resulting in provisional limitations of dietetic support.

The general recommendation for COVID-19 patients is to follow healthy diets to maintain a correct immune function [3]. Optimal intake of all nutrients, mainly those that play crucial roles in immune system, should be assured through a diverse and well-balanced diet. However, current data suggest that there is a prevalent micronutrient and omega-3 fatty acid deficiency in several population groups [107–109]. On the other hand, in the review reported by Calder et al. (2020) [16], based on several meta-analysis [110–118], the authors state that in order to promote the optimum functioning of the immune system and to reduce the risk and consequences of infections, the intakes for some micronutrients may exceed the recommended dietary allowances since infections and other stressors can reduce micronutrient status. Thus, supplements may help restoring their normal blood levels [16,119–121]. With regard to supplementation, it is important to advise the general public to always consult a medical doctor prior consuming such products, as they can interact with other nutrients, drugs, and medical treatments; indeed, they can turn into toxic elements causing several disorders and aggravating certain conditions.

### 5.1. *Nutritional Therapy in Non-Critically Ill Hospitalized COVID-19 Patients*

Cintoni et al. (2020) described the nutritional management strategy adopted in Fondazione Policlinico A. Gemelli-IRCCS (Rome, Italy), which is considered a reference center for COVID-19 in the region [122]. Due to the mean age of their patients (65 years), their nutritional status is usually not optimal. Moreover, the low palatability of hospital meals makes the energy and protein intake low, which can exacerbate the bad nutritional status of the patients. In this scenario, the orally feedable patients of COVID-19 receive a personalized meal provision, which is completed with oral nutritional supplements in order to meet the energy and protein requirements. In the case of patients who are unable to eat, enteral/parenteral nutritional formulas, rich in protein and poor in glucose, are provided. In this regard, previous studies conducted in China have demonstrated that the inclusion of nutritional support in the treatment of symptomatic COVID-19 patients is of major importance. The conclusion of these studies is that the design of specific nutritional strategies are needed in hospitals [123].

Caccialanza et al., (2020) have also proposed an empirical protocol to promptly and pragmatically implement nutritional care in hospitalized non-ICU COVID-19 patients [89]. The authors recognized that their protocol might be debatable, since it may not be in total agreement with the current guidelines on clinical nutrition [124]. However, they do believe that nutritional care in hospitalized non-ICU COVID-19 patients might be overlooked despite being potentially effective in preventing the consequences of malnutrition and beneficial to clinical outcomes in this patient population [89]. The authors have based their protocol on the observation of the symptoms shown by the patients at hospital admission (severe inflammation, anorexia leading to a major reduction of food intake, and respiratory failure). Since a significant number of patients reported severe eating difficulties, they decided to start with an oral supplementation with whey proteins (20 g/d) and intravenous multivitamin, multi-mineral, and trace element solutions, in order to match the recommended dietary allowances upon admission. Whey proteins were selected based on their high digestibility, anabolic and antioxidant properties [125], immunomodulatory [126], and potential antiviral activities [127]. Further, since specific vitamin and micronutrient deficits have been reported to be harmful during viral infections, including COVID-19 patients [7], the authors justify the micronutrient intravenous administration to meet recommended dietary allowances. The most debatable aspect of their protocol might be the election of parenteral nutrition over enteral nutrition. This election is due to the respiratory difficulties of COVID-19 patients. Certainly, enteral nutrition requires the presence of a nasogastric tube, which may compromise the effectiveness of non-invasive ventilation or continuous positive airway pressure [89]. Further, enteral feeding implies an increased risk of aspiration of the nutritional solution [128]. Indeed, this protocol shows debatable limitations, but taking into account that underfeeding occurs in patients hospitalized for COVID-19, a rapid intervention in non-critically ill patients can improve their prognosis, therefore reducing the pressure on the limitation in ICU availability detected in hospitals worldwide [129].

Once the acute phase of the pneumonia is over, COVID-19 patients need specific rehabilitation, not only to recover the respiratory capacity but also to improve disability and quality of life. Brugliera et al. (2020) describe their experience working in the COVID-19 rehabilitation unit in the Hospital of San Raffaele Scientific Unit (Milan, Italy) with 50 COVID-19 patients [6]. According to the authors, the majority (90%) of the patients showed some degree of dysphagia, mainly due to previous orotracheal intubation, making necessary the use of diets with modified consistency or nasogastric feeding, and highlighting the importance of nutritional support, as well as of swallowing training to improve the recovery of these patients. Due to the direct relationship between nutritional status and the risk of suffering from different illnesses (among them the COVID-19), this parameter was studied by means of the MUST, and the results showed that 45% of the studied population were in high risk of malnutrition, while 26% had moderate risk.

Based on the knowledge acquired by the authors while working with patients who were recovering from COVID-19, a 3-step nutritional protocol has been designed. The first step of this protocol would be focused on the nutritional assessment and malnutrition screening of the patient. For this purpose, different anthropometric parameters, as well as the body composition of the patients are studied. Further, the weight loss is monitored and a hematochemical analysis of blood parameters (including, among others, blood count, total protein, ferritin, blood sugar and markers of liver function) carried out. Finally, the swallowing capacity of the patients (in order to determine whether a specific diet is needed) is evaluated and their intake assessment monitored. Once this first step is completed, a second step devoted to setting the nutritional treatment of the patient takes place. In this regard, the energy and macronutrient requirements of the patient are assessed, using the meal management computerized system of the hospital. In this scenario, energy requirements are calculated using predictive equations, which are adapted to the nutritional status of the patients (clinical status, physical activity, or stress). As far as macronutrients are concerned, a protein intake of >1 g/kg/day (up to

1.5 g/kg/day) is guaranteed, as well as carbohydrate and lipid requirements stablished based on the non-protein energy (30:70 in patients with no respiratory insufficiency and 50:50 in patients with respiratory insufficiency). In addition, maintaining an adequate hydration of the patient is another aspect of the intervention that must be taken into account. In this regard, the clinical history of the patient (heart or renal failure, vomiting or diarrhea) must be analyzed. Moreover, additional supportive therapy (adequate vitamin and oligoelement intake, essential and branched amino acids and probiotics) is also provided. Similarly, nutritional advice that can be useful for the patient (while in the hospital as well as once they are discharged) is provided. As far as the third step is concerned, this is based in continuous monitoring of the patient by a multidisciplinary team over time, which allows modifying the treatment according to the status of the patient.

Using this protocol, the MUST improved in 5 of the 32 patients (out of the 50 patients that were included in the rehabilitation unit) that stayed at least for 10 days in the COVID-19 rehabilitation unit. Moreover, 14 of these patients improved their BMI while in 15 patients this parameter remained stable. Based on these observations, the authors conclude that nutritional status plays a pivotal role in the clinical outcomes of patients recovering from COVID-19, and that nutritional support along with rehabilitation may improve the chances of recovery in patients of COVID-19.

*5.2. Nutritional Therapy in Critically Ill Hospitalized COVID-19 Patients*

Some COVID-19 patients experience severe respiratory symptoms and/or multi-organ failure, being very ill at hospital admission and thus needing specialized support [99,123]. Indeed, acute respiratory complications, requiring prolonged ICU stays, are a major cause of morbidity and mortality in COVID-19 patients. Most of these patients rapidly progress from cough to dyspnea, and then to respiratory failure requiring mechanical ventilation. Consequently, the timing of nutritional intervention appears to be critical [130]. Therefore, nutritionists should choose the most appropriate way to recover the subject's health.

As with any other critically ill patients, nutritional management is an integral component of good supportive care. The European Society for Clinical Nutrition and Metabolism (ESPEN) has recently published some guidelines for the nutritional management of patients with SARS-CoV-2 infection. In these guidelines specific recommendations are included for patients hospitalized in ICUs, among them early enteral nutrition (when possible), use of agents that promote gastric emptying, initiation of peripheral nutrition in situations in which enteral nutrition is not possible/tolerated and use of enteral nutrition after extubation when oral feeding is not tolerated. According to these ESPEN guidelines, enteral nutrition is preferred for patients in the ICU who receive mechanical ventilation [91]. However, the specific needs of patients with COVID-19 may require the adoption of prone ventilation or neuromuscular blockade, and consequently enteral nutrition implementation in daily practice could be difficult [128]. Further, a delay of enteral nutrition can be mandatory when life-threatening hypoxemia occurs [91].

On the other hand, the changes induced by the disease itself in the gastrointestinal tract of the patients, along with the elevated sedation required for these patients, makes difficult to provide adequate nutritional support. Bearing this in mind, Arkin et al. (2020) provided information regarding several of the considerations that have to be taken into account when nutrition is provided to critically ill patients of COVID-19 [131]. One such consideration is related to the gastrointestinal hypomotility that is commonly found in these patients, which in turn results in enteral feeding intolerance. Indeed, this situation seems not to be derived from the high-doses of sedatives and opioids that are needed to facilitate mechanical ventilation, since other patients under similar conditions do not present feeding intolerance. Thus, the authors suggest that the enteral feeding intolerance is related to the infection produced by the SARS-CoV-2. Moreover, despite several pharmacological agents devoted to promoting gastrointestinal motility are provided to COVID-19 patients at the time of ICU admission, their intestinal motility remains impaired. Additionally, even in the cases in which gastrointestinal motility is maintained/recovered (by studying gastric residuals and stool output), impaired nutrient absorption has been described. In the case of the patients in which gastric residuals are >500 mL, the use of a post-pyloric feeding tube is recommended by the ESPEN guidelines. However, this approach involves technical challenges in the placement as well as increased exposure of the staff to viral infection and obvious difficulties when proning of the patient is required. Besides the gastrointestinal features of critically ill COVID-19 patients, severe lung injury is also common in these subjects. This condition makes necessary strategies devoted to avoiding aspirations. In this regard, the authors suggest holding tube feeding 1-h prior proning as an effective approach to avoid aspirations. Indeed, the authors state that due to the challenges related to aspiration in prone patients, continuous tube feeding is maintained (instead of using bolus tube feeding).

As far as diet is concerned, the ESPEN guidelines recommend hypocaloric nutrition in the first week of ICU stay. However, since the patients normally spend days/weeks sick at their homes before being admitted in a hospital, the risk of developing malnutrition increases. Moreover, the life-threatening features that are common on these patients at the time of ICU admission produces further delay in enteral nutrition, increasing even more the risk of malnutrition. Due to these facts, critically ill COVID-19 patients may have poor nutritional status, which in turn may increase the severity of the infection. In this regard, the authors point towards the necessity of a more aggressive early total parenteral nutritional support in these patients.

Taking all that into account, and considering that COVID-19 patients need more energy than normal, the nutritional management of the critically ill patient in the long-term should avoid underfeeding or overfeeding. It is recommended to supply around 20 or 30 kcal/kg body weight/day for polymorbid patients aged >65 years or for severely underweight polymorbid patients respectively [124,132]. These values should be adjusted with regard to nutritional status, disease status, and tolerance [133]. It is important to take into account that in severely underweight patients, the target of 30 kcal/kg body weight/day should be slowly achieved (in the case of artificial nutrition, target speed must be reached in 3–4 days) due to the high risk of refeeding syndrome of this population [104,132].

Protein needs are higher in the critically ill patient due to the protein catabolism driven by inflammatory mediators [132]. It is estimated as 1 g protein/kg body weight/day in older people [133], or 1.3 g protein/kg body weight/day with increased supply of branched chain amino acids (up to 50% in polymorbid medical inpatients), in order to prevent muscle loss and to strength respiratory muscles [132]. Other authors increased these recommendations to 1.5 g protein/kg body weight/day [89]). These amounts should be individually adjusted with regard to nutritional status, disease status, and tolerance [124].

The needs of fat and carbohydrate have to be adapted to the energy requirements, considering an energy ratio from fat and carbohydrates between 30:70% for individuals with no respiratory deficiency and to 50:50% for ventilated patients [104]. Fat requirement in the critically ill patient is around 1.5 g/kg body weight/day, giving priority to the usage of medium and long chain fatty acids. As far as carbohydrates requirement is concerned, a supply of 2 g/kg body weight/day, not exceeding 150 g/day, must be considered. This is due to their high CO2 production rate that should be limited in case of respiratory failure [132].

With regard to micronutrients in ICU patients, mineral and vitamin supply with routine supplements must be considered depending on the nutritional therapy used. Administration of doses higher than recommendations of vitamin D can be used because of their positive effects [132]. Certainly, it has been reported that high doses of Vitamin D in infected patients may improve immunologic recovery during antiretroviral treatment, reduce levels of inflammation and immune activation, and increase immunity against pathogens [89]. In turn, vitamin C supplementation significantly reduces mortality in critically ill patients [134].

In the case of enteral nutrition, attention must be paid to the needs of specific nutrients to be included in the formula. Thus, enteral diets containing EPA, gamma-linolenic acid, and antioxidant agents may offer a clinical benefit in oxygenation and days of ventilation in patients with acute respiratory distress syndrome [91]. Further, specific lipid emulsions could offer additional benefits over corticosteroid and anti-IL-6 drugs in the modulation of the inflammatory response. However, COVID-19 patients' response to specific enteral diets remains to be determined [130].

## 6. Future Research

In the present review, we provide data about key aspects in nutritional management of COVID-19 patients, based on the current knowledge. Nevertheless, due to the novelty of the disease, information regarding the effects of some nutrients is still scarce.

Regarding the role of specific nutrients in COVID-19 disease, very often the nutritional advice is based on their effects in infections caused by other viruses with symptoms similar to those caused by SARS-CoV-2. On the other hand, in some cases the studies reported are ecological studies, which are the first step in the investigation of a possible relationship between a disease and a determined exposure. Their great advance is that they are carried out very quickly, practically without cost and with information that is usually available. However, their main limitations are that they cannot determine if there is an association between an exposure and disease at the individual level, and their inability to control for potentially confounding variables. Consequently, further research based on analytical instead of descriptive studies, such as randomized controlled clinical trials, are warranted.

Regarding the effects of bioactive compounds present in foodstuffs on COVID19, the vast majority of the results have been obtained in preclinical studies. One advantage of these studies is that animals can be directly exposed to the virus under treatments with various bioactive compounds, as a first step to know if some of these substances could reduce or even prevent infection with the SARS-CoV-2 virus. Moreover, they allow the researchers to determine the mechanism involved. In this field of research, studies addressed in humans are needed to confirm the beneficial effects observed in animals.

Another important aspect is to focus the research on specific age groups, paying special attention to the elderly, since it is known that the evolution of the disease depends largely on age. In the same way, it would be important to carry out separate studies in men and women since it appears that men are more negatively affected by this disease. All this will contribute to making a personalized nutritional approach, and therefore more successful.

**Author Contributions:** Conceptualization, M.P.P.; project administration and funding acquisition, M.P.P.; writing—original draft preparation, A.F.-Q., S.G.-Z., I.M.-L., N.K., J.T., A.L., M.G., and M.P.P.; writing—reviewing and editing, A.F.-Q., S.G.-Z., I.M.-L., N.K., J.T., A.L., M.G., and M.P.P. All authors have read and agreed to the published version of the manuscript.

## References

1. International Society for Infectious Diseases. ProMed «PRO/AH/EDR> COVID-19 update (59): Global, cruise ship, more countries, WHO. *Int. Soc. Infect. Dis.* **2020**. Available online: https://promedmail.org (accessed on 9 August 2020).
2. Zhou, F.; Yu, T.; Du, R.; Fan, G.; Liu, Y.; Liu, Z.; Xiang, J.; Wang, Y.; Song, B.; Gu, X.; et al. Clinical course and risk factors for mortality of adult inpatients with COVID-19 in Wuhan, China: A retrospective cohort study. *Lancet* **2020**, *395*, 1054–1062. [CrossRef]
3. Zabetakis, I.; Lordan, R.; Norton, C.; Tsoupras, A. COVID-19: The inflammation link and the role of nutrition in potential mitigation. *Nutrients* **2020**, *12*, 1466. [CrossRef] [PubMed]
4. Gupta, R.; Hussain, A.; Misra, A. Diabetes and COVID-19: Evidence, current status and unanswered research questions. *Eur. J. Clin. Nutr.* **2020**, *74*, 864–870. [CrossRef] [PubMed]
5. Wu, Z. Characteristics of and important lessons from the coronavirus disease 2019 (COVID-19) outbreak in China: Summary of a report of 72314 cases from the chinese center for disease control and prevention. *JAMA* **2020**, *323*, 1239–1242. [CrossRef] [PubMed]

6. Brugliera, L.; Spina, A.; Castellazzi, P.; Cimino, P.; Arcuri, P.; Negro, A.; Houdayer, E.; Alemanno, F.; Giordani, A.; Mortini, P.; et al. Nutritional management of COVID-19 patients in a rehabilitation unit. *Eur. J. Clin. Nutr.* **2020**, *74*, 860–863. [CrossRef] [PubMed]
7. Iddir, M.; Brito, A.; Dingeo, G.; Fernandez Del Campo, S.S.; Samouda, H.; La Frano, M.R.; Bohn, T. Strengthening the immune system and reducing inflammation and oxidative stress through diet and nutrition: Considerations during the COVID-19 crisis. *Nutrients* **2020**, *12*, 1562. [CrossRef] [PubMed]
8. Duvall, M.G.; Levy, B.D. DHA-and EPA-derived resolvins, protectins, and maresins in airway inflammation. *Eur. J. Pharmacol.* **2016**, *785*, 144–155. [CrossRef]
9. Lordan, R.; Tsoupras, A.; Zabetakis, I. Platelet activation and prothrombotic mediators at the nexus of inflammation and atherosclerosis: Potential role of antiplatelet agents. *Blood Rev.* **2020**, 100694. [CrossRef]
10. Monnier, L.; Mas, E.; Ginet, C.; Michel, F.; Villon, L.; Cristol, J.P.; Colette, C. Activation of oxidative stress by acute glucose fluctuations compared with sustained chronic hyperglycemia in patients with type 2 diabetes. *JAMA* **2006**, *295*, 1681–1687. [CrossRef]
11. Carlson, J.L.; Erickson, J.M.; Lloyd, B.B.; Slavin, J.L. Health effects and sources of prebiotic dietary fiber. *Curr. Dev. Nutr.* **2018**, *2*, nzy005. [CrossRef] [PubMed]
12. Marsland, B.J.; Trompette, A.; Gollwitzer, E.S. The gut-lung axis in respiratory disease. *Ann. Am. Thorac. Soc.* **2015**, *12* (Suppl. 2), S150–S156. [PubMed]
13. Maggini, S.; Beveridge, S.; Sorbara, P.J.P.; Senatore, G. Feeding the immune system: The role of micronutrients in restoring resistance to infections. *CAB Rev.* **2008**, *3*, 1–21. [CrossRef]
14. Maggini, S.; Pierre, A.; Calder, P.C. Immune function and micronutrient requirements change over the life course. *Nutrients* **2018**, *10*, 1531. [CrossRef]
15. Calder, P.C. Omega-3 polyunsaturated fatty acids and inflammatory processes: Nutrition or pharmacology? *Br. J. Clin. Pharmacol.* **2013**, *75*, 645–662. [CrossRef]
16. Calder, P.C.; Carr, A.C.; Gombart, A.F.; Eggersdorfer, M. Optimal nutritional status for a well-functioning immune system is an important factor to protect against viral infections. *Nutrients* **2020**, *12*, 1181. [CrossRef]
17. Gombart, A.F.; Pierre, A.; Maggini, S. A review of micronutrients and the immune system-working in harmony to reduce the risk of infection. *Nutrients* **2020**, *12*, 236. [CrossRef]
18. Muscogiuri, G.; Barrea, L.; Savastano, S.; Colao, A. Nutritional recommendations for CoVID-19 quarantine. *Eur. J. Clin. Nutr.* **2020**, *74*, 850–851. [CrossRef]
19. Grant, W.B.; Lahore, H.; McDonnell, S.L.; Baggerly, C.A.; French, C.B.; Aliano, J.L.; Bhattoa, H.P. Evidence that vitamin D supplementation could reduce risk of Influenza and COVID-19 infections and deaths. *Nutrients* **2020**, *12*, 988. [CrossRef]
20. Zhang, J.; Taylor, E.W.; Bennett, K.; Saad, R.; Rayman, M.P. Association between regional selenium status and reported outcome of COVID-19 cases in China. *Am. J. Clin. Nutr.* **2020**, *111*, 1297–1299. [CrossRef]
21. Liu, W.; Zhang, S.; Nekhai, S.; Liu, S. Depriving iron supply to the virus represents a promising adjuvant therapeutic against viral survival. *Curr. Clin. Microbiol. Rep.* **2020**, *7*, 13–19. [CrossRef] [PubMed]
22. Singh, M.; Das, R.R. Zinc for the common cold. *Cochrane Database Syst. Rev.* **2013**, *6*. [CrossRef]
23. Mossad, S.B.; Macknin, M.L.; Medendorp, S.V.; Mason, P. Zinc gluconate lozenges for treating the common cold. A randomized, double-blind, placebo-controlled study. *Ann. Intern. Med.* **1996**, *125*, 81–88. [CrossRef] [PubMed]
24. Abbaspour, N.; Hurrell, R.; Kelishadi, R. Review on iron and its importance for human health. *J. Res. Med. Sci.* **2014**, *19*, 164–174. [PubMed]
25. Fenton, J.I.; Hord, N.G.; Ghosh, S.; Gurzell, E.A. Immunomodulation by dietary long chain omega-3 fatty acids and the potential for adverse health outcomes. *Prostaglandins Leukot. Essent. Fat. Acids* **2013**, *89*, 379–390. [CrossRef] [PubMed]
26. Naja, F.; Hamadeh, R. Nutrition amid the COVID-19 pandemic: A multi-level framework for action. *Eur. J. Clin. Nutr.* **2020**, *20*, 1–5. [CrossRef]
27. Carr, A.C. A new clinical trial to test high-dose vitamin C in patients with COVID-19. *Crit. Care* **2020**, *24*, 1–2. [CrossRef]
28. McCullough, F.S.; Northrop-Clewes, C.A.; Thurnham, D.I. The effect of vitamin A on epithelial integrity. *Proc. Nutr. Soc.* **1999**, *58*, 289–293. [CrossRef]
29. Timoneda, J.; Rodriguez-Fernandez, L.; Zaragoza, R.; Marin, M.P.; Cabezuelo, M.T.; Torres, L.; Vina, J.R.; Barber, T. Vitamin A deficiency and the lung. *Nutrients* **2018**, *10*, 1132. [CrossRef]

30. Xu, J.; Yang, J.; Chen, J.; Luo, Q.; Zhang, Q.; Zhang, H. Vitamin D alleviates lipopolysaccharideinduced acute lung injury via regulation of the reninangiotensin system. *Mol. Med. Rep.* **2017**, *16*, 7432–7438. [CrossRef]
31. Han, J.E.; Jones, J.L.; Tangpricha, V.; Brown, M.A.; Brown, L.A.S.; Hao, L.; Hebbar, G.; Lee, M.J.; Liu, S.; Ziegler, T.R.; et al. High dose vitamin D administration in ventilated intensive care unit patients: A pilot double blind randomized controlled trial. *J. Clin. Transl. Endocrinol.* **2016**, *4*, 59–65. [CrossRef] [PubMed]
32. Smith, E.M.; Jones, J.L.; Han, J.E.; Alvarez, J.A.; Sloan, J.H.; Konrad, R.J.; Zughaier, S.M.; Martin, G.S.; Ziegler, T.R.; Tangpricha, V. High-Dose vitamin D3 administration is associated with increases in hemoglobin concentrations in mechanically ventilated critically ill adults: A pilot double-blind, randomized, placebo-controlled trial. *JPEN J. Parenter. Enter. Nutr.* **2018**, *42*, 87–94. [CrossRef] [PubMed]
33. Ilie, P.C.; Stefanescu, S.; Smith, L. The role of vitamin D in the prevention of coronavirus disease 2019 infection and mortality. *Aging Clin. Exp. Res.* **2020**, *32*, 1195–1198. [CrossRef] [PubMed]
34. D'Avolio, A.; Avataneo, V.; Manca, A.; Cusato, J.; De Nicolo, A.; Lucchini, R.; Keller, F.; Cantu, M. 25-hydroxyvitamin D concentrations are lower in patients with positive PCR for SARS-CoV-2. *Nutrients* **2020**, *12*, 1359. [CrossRef] [PubMed]
35. Hastie, C.E.; Mackay, D.F.; Ho, F.; Celis-Morales, C.A.; Katikireddi, S.V.; Niedzwiedz, C.L.; Jani, B.D.; Welsh, P.; Mair, F.S.; Gray, S.R.; et al. Vitamin D concentrations and COVID-19 infection in UK Biobank. *Diabetes Metab. Syndr.* **2020**, *14*, 561–565. [CrossRef]
36. Grant, W.B.; McDonnell, S.L. Letter in response to the article: Vitamin D concentrations and COVID-19 infection in UK biobank (Hastie et al.). *Diabetes Metab. Syndr.* **2020**, *14*, 893–894. [CrossRef]
37. Roy, A.S.; Herlekar, R. Response to 'Vitamin D concentrations and COVID-19 infection in UK Biobank'. *Diabetes Metab. Syndr.* **2020**, *14*, 777. [CrossRef]
38. Costagliola, D.G.; de Montalembert, M.; Lefrere, J.J.; Briand, C.; Rebulla, P.; Baruchel, S.; Dessi, C.; Fondu, P.; Karagiorga, M.; Perrimond, H. Dose of desferrioxamine and evolution of HIV-1 infection in thalassaemic patients. *Br. J. Haematol.* **1994**, *87*, 849–852. [CrossRef]
39. Kaufmann, S.H.; McMichael, A.J. Annulling a dangerous liaison: Vaccination strategies against AIDS and tuberculosis. *Nat. Med.* **2005**, *11*, S33–S44. [CrossRef]
40. Green, D.A.; Antholine, W.E.; Wong, S.J.; Richardson, D.R.; Chitambar, C.R. Inhibition of malignant cell growth by 311, a novel iron chelator of the pyridoxal isonicotinoyl hydrazone class: Effect on the R2 subunit of ribonucleotide reductase. *Clin. Cancer Res.* **2001**, *7*, 3574–3579.
41. Baum, M.K.; Shor-Posner, G.; Lai, S.; Zhang, G.; Lai, H.; Fletcher, M.A.; Sauberlich, H.; Page, J.B. High risk of HIV-related mortality is associated with selenium deficiency. *J. Acquir. Immune Defic. Syndr. Hum. Retrovirol.* **1997**, *15*, 370–374. [CrossRef] [PubMed]
42. Taylor, E.W.; Ruzicka, J.A.; Premadasa, L.; Zhao, L. Cellular selenoprotein mRNA tethering via antisense Interactions with ebola and HIV-1 mRNAs may impact host selenium biochemistry. *Curr. Top. Med. Chem.* **2016**, *16*, 1530–1535. [CrossRef] [PubMed]
43. Steinbrenner, H.; Al-Quraishy, S.; Dkhil, M.A.; Wunderlich, F.; Sies, H. Dietary selenium in adjuvant therapy of viral and bacterial infections. *Adv. Nutr.* **2015**, *6*, 73–82. [CrossRef] [PubMed]
44. Hou, J.C. Inhibitory effect of selenite and other antioxidants on complement-mediated tissue injury in patients with epidemic hemorrhagic fever. *Biol. Trace Elem. Res.* **1997**, *56*, 125–130. [CrossRef] [PubMed]
45. Te Velthuis, A.J.; van den Worm, S.H.; Sims, A.C.; Baric, R.S.; Snijder, E.J.; van Hemert, M.J. Zn(2+) inhibits coronavirus and arterivirus RNA polymerase activity in vitro and zinc ionophores block the replication of these viruses in cell culture. *PLoS Pathog.* **2010**, *6*, e1001176. [CrossRef] [PubMed]
46. McCarty, M.F.; DiNicolantonio, J.J. Nutraceuticals have potential for boosting the type 1 interferon response to RNA viruses including influenza and coronavirus. *Prog. Cardiovasc. Dis.* **2020**, *63*, 383–385. [CrossRef]
47. Liu, L.; Geng, X.; McDermott, J.; Shen, J.; Corbin, C.; Xuan, S.; Kim, J.; Zuo, L.; Liu, Z. Copper deficiency in the lungs of TNF-alpha transgenic mice. *Front. Physiol.* **2016**, *7*, 234. [CrossRef]
48. Horne, J.R.; Vohl, M.C. Biological plausibility for interactions between dietary fat, resveratrol, ACE2, and SARS-CoV illness severity. *Am. J. Physiol. Endocrinol. Metab.* **2020**, *318*, E830–E833. [CrossRef]
49. Tiao, M.M.; Lin, Y.J.; Yu, H.R.; Sheen, J.M.; Lin, I.C.; Lai, Y.J.; Tain, Y.L.; Huang, L.T.; Tsai, C.C. Resveratrol ameliorates maternal and post-weaning high-fat diet-induced nonalcoholic fatty liver disease via renin-angiotensin system. *Lipids Health. Dis.* **2018**, *17*, 178. [CrossRef]

50. Andrade, J.M.O.; Paraiso, A.F.; Garcia, Z.M.; Ferreira, A.V.; Sinisterra, R.D.; Sousa, F.B.; Guimaraes, A.L.; de Paula, A.M.; Campagnole-Santos, M.J.; dos Santos, R.A.; et al. Cross talk between angiotensin-(1-7)/Mas axis and sirtuins in adipose tissue and metabolism of high-fat feed mice. *Peptides* **2014**, *55*, 158–165. [CrossRef]
51. Kim, E.N.; Kim, M.Y.; Lim, J.H.; Kim, Y.; Shin, S.J.; Park, C.W.; Kim, Y.S.; Chang, Y.S.; Yoon, H.E.; Choi, B.S. The protective effect of resveratrol on vascular aging by modulation of the renin-angiotensin system. *Atherosclerosis* **2018**, *270*, 123–131. [CrossRef] [PubMed]
52. Moran, C.S.; Biros, E.; Krishna, S.M.; Wang, Y.; Tikellis, C.; Morton, S.K.; Moxon, J.V.; Cooper, M.E.; Norman, P.E.; Burrell, L.M.; et al. Resveratrol inhibits growth of experimental abdominal aortic aneurysm associated with upregulation of angiotensin-converting enzyme 2. *Arterioscler. Thromb. Vasc. Biol.* **2017**, *37*, 2195–2203. [CrossRef] [PubMed]
53. Habtemariam, S.; Nabavi, S.F.; Berindan-Neagoe, I.; Cismaru, C.A.; Izadi, M.; Sureda, A.; Nabavi, S.M. Should we try the antiinflammatory natural product, celastrol, for COVID-19? *Phytother. Res.* **2020**, *34*, 1189–1190. [CrossRef] [PubMed]
54. Shi, K.; Chen, X.; Xie, B.; Yang, S.S.; Liu, D.; Dai, G.; Chen, Q. Celastrol alleviates chronic obstructive pulmonary disease by inhibiting cellular inflammation induced by cigarette smoke via the Ednrb/Kng1 signaling pathway. *Front. Pharmacol.* **2018**, *9*, 1276. [CrossRef] [PubMed]
55. Wei, Y.; Wang, Y. Celastrol attenuates impairments associated with lipopolysaccharide-induced acute respiratory distress syndrome (ARDS) in rats. *J. Immunotoxicol.* **2017**, *14*, 228–234. [CrossRef]
56. Iwata-Yoshikawa, N.; Okamura, T.; Shimizu, Y.; Hasegawa, H.; Takeda, M.; Nagata, N. TMPRSS2 contributes to virus spread and immunopathology in the airways of murine models after coronavirus infection. *J. Virol.* **2019**, *93*. [CrossRef] [PubMed]
57. Youssef, J.; Badr, M. Role of peroxisome proliferator-activated receptors in inflammation control. *J. Biomed. Biotechnol.* **2004**, *2004*, 156–166. [CrossRef]
58. Dana, N.; Vaseghi, G.; Haghjooy Javanmard, S. Crosstalk between peroxisome proliferator-activated receptors and toll-like receptors: A systematic review. *Adv. Pharm. Bull.* **2019**, *9*, 12–21. [CrossRef]
59. Ghaffari, S.; Roshanravan, N.; Tutunchi, H.; Ostadrahimi, A.; Pouraghaei, M.; Kafil, B. Oleoylethanolamide, a bioactive lipid amide, as a promising treatment strategy for coronavirus/COVID-19. *Arch. Med. Res.* **2020**, *51*, 464–467. [CrossRef]
60. Payahoo, L.; Khajebishak, Y.; Jafarabadi, M.A.; Ostadrahimi, A. Oleoylethanolamide supplementation reduces inflammation and oxidative stress in obese people: A clinical trial. *Adv. Pharm. Bull.* **2018**, *8*, 479–487. [CrossRef]
61. Han, S.; Inoue, H.; Flowers, L.C.; Sidell, N. Control of COX-2 gene expression through peroxisome proliferator-activated receptor gamma in human cervical cancer cells. *Clin. Cancer Res.* **2003**, *9*, 4627–4635. [PubMed]
62. Ciavarella, C.; Motta, I.; Valente, S.; Pasquinelli, G. Pharmacological (or synthetic) and nutritional agonists of ppar-gamma as candidates for cytokine storm modulation in COVID-19 disease. *Molecules* **2020**, *25*, 2076. [CrossRef] [PubMed]
63. Calder, P.C. N-3 fatty acids, inflammation and immunity: New mechanisms to explain old actions. *Proc. Nutr. Soc.* **2013**, *72*, 326–336. [CrossRef] [PubMed]
64. Hotta, M.; Nakata, R.; Katsukawa, M.; Hori, K.; Takahashi, S.; Inoue, H. Carvacrol, a component of thyme oil, activates PPARalpha and gamma and suppresses COX-2 expression. *J. Lipid Res.* **2010**, *51*, 132–139. [CrossRef]
65. Park, J.Y.; Kawada, T.; Han, I.S.; Kim, B.S.; Goto, T.; Takahashi, N.; Fushiki, T.; Kurata, T.; Yu, R. Capsaicin inhibits the production of tumor necrosis factor alpha by LPS-stimulated murine macrophages, RAW 264.7: A PPARgamma ligand-like action as a novel mechanism. *FEBS Lett.* **2004**, *572*, 266–270. [CrossRef]
66. Rau, O.; Wurglics, M.; Paulke, A.; Zitzkowski, J.; Meindl, N.; Bock, A.; Dingermann, T.; Abdel-Tawab, M.; Schubert-Zsilavecz, M. Carnosic acid and carnosol, phenolic diterpene compounds of the labiate herbs rosemary and sage, are activators of the human peroxisome proliferator-activated receptor gamma. *Planta Med.* **2006**, *72*, 881–887. [CrossRef]
67. Maione, F.; Cantone, V.; Pace, S.; Chini, M.G.; Bisio, A.; Romussi, G.; Pieretti, S.; Werz, O.; Koeberle, A.; Mascolo, N.; et al. Anti-inflammatory and analgesic activity of carnosol and carnosic acid in vivo and in vitro and in silico analysis of their target interactions. *Br. J. Pharmacol.* **2017**, *174*, 1497–1508. [CrossRef]

68. Bassaganya-Riera, J.; DiGuardo, M.; Climent, M.; Vives, C.; Carbo, A.; Jouni, Z.E.; Einerhand, A.W.; O'Shea, M.; Hontecillas, R. Activation of PPARgamma and delta by dietary punicic acid ameliorates intestinal inflammation in mice. *Br. J. Nutr.* **2011**, *106*, 878–886. [CrossRef]

69. Katsukawa, M.; Nakata, R.; Takizawa, Y.; Hori, K.; Takahashi, S.; Inoue, H. Citral, a component of lemongrass oil, activates PPARalpha and gamma and suppresses COX-2 expression. *Biochim. Biophys. Acta* **2010**, *1801*, 1214–1220. [CrossRef]

70. Aggarwal, B.B.; Harikumar, K.B. Potential therapeutic effects of curcumin, the anti-inflammatory agent, against neurodegenerative, cardiovascular, pulmonary, metabolic, autoimmune and neoplastic diseases. *Int. J. Biochem. Cell Biol.* **2009**, *41*, 40–59. [CrossRef]

71. Mazidi, M.; Karimi, E.; Meydani, M.; Ghayour-Mobarhan, M.; Ferns, G.A. Potential effects of curcumin on peroxisome proliferator-activated receptor-gamma in vitro and in vivo. *World J. Methodol.* **2016**, *6*, 112–117. [CrossRef] [PubMed]

72. Wen, C.C.; Kuo, Y.H.; Jan, J.T.; Liang, P.H.; Wang, S.Y.; Liu, H.G.; Lee, C.K.; Chang, S.T.; Kuo, C.J.; Lee, S.S.; et al. Specific plant terpenoids and lignoids possess potent antiviral activities against severe acute respiratory syndrome coronavirus. *J. Med. Chem.* **2007**, *50*, 4087–4095.

73. Ting, D.; Dong, N.; Fang, L.; Lu, J.; Bi, J.; Xiao, S.; Han, H. Correction to multisite inhibitors for enteric coronavirus: Antiviral cationic carbon dots based on curcumin. *ACS Appl. Nano Mater.* **2018**, *1*, 5451–5459. [CrossRef]

74. Zahedipour, F.; Hosseini, S.A.; Sathyapalan, T.; Majeed, M.; Jamialahmadi, T.; Al-Rasadi, K.; Banach, M.; Sahebkar, A. Potential effects of curcumin in the treatment of COVID-19 infection. *Phytother. Res.* **2020**. [CrossRef] [PubMed]

75. Avasarala, S.; Zhang, F.; Liu, G.; Wang, R.; London, S.D.; London, L. Curcumin modulates the inflammatory response and inhibits subsequent fibrosis in a mouse model of viral-induced acute respiratory distress syndrome. *PLoS ONE* **2013**, *8*, e57285. [CrossRef] [PubMed]

76. Chen, B.; Zhang, D.P.; Gao, W. Effect of curcumin on the expression of collagen type I protein and transforming growth factor-beta1 mRNA in pulmonary fibrosis rats. *Zhonghua Lao Dong Wei Sheng Zhi Ye Bing Za Zhi* **2008**, *26*, 257–261. [PubMed]

77. Tilg, H.; Zmora, N.; Adolph, T.E.; Elinav, E. The intestinal microbiota fuelling metabolic inflammation. *Nat. Rev. Immunol.* **2020**, *20*, 40–54. [CrossRef] [PubMed]

78. Enaud, R.; Prevel, R.; Ciarlo, E.; Beaufils, F.; Wieers, G.; Guery, B.; Delhaes, L. The gut-lung axis in health and respiratory diseases: A place for inter-organ and inter-kingdom crosstalks. *Front. Cell. Infect. Microbiol.* **2020**, *10*, 9. [CrossRef]

79. Infusino, F.; Marazzato, M.; Mancone, M.; Fedele, F.; Mastroianni, C.M.; Severino, P.; Ceccarelli, G.; Santinelli, L.; Cavarretta, E.; Marullo, A.G.M.; et al. Diet supplementation, probiotics, and nutraceuticals in SARS-CoV-2 infection: A scoping review. *Nutrients* **2020**, *12*, 1718. [CrossRef]

80. Zuo, T.; Zhang, F.; Lui, G.C.Y.; Yeoh, Y.K.; Li, A.Y.L.; Zhan, H.; Wan, Y.; Chung, A.; Cheung, C.P.; Chen, N.; et al. Alterations in gut microbiota of patients with COVID-19 during time of hospitalization. *Gastroenterology* **2020**, in press. [CrossRef]

81. Di Renzo, L.; Merra, G.; Esposito, E.; De Lorenzo, A. Are probiotics effective adjuvant therapeutic choice in patients with COVID-19? *Eur. Rev. Med. Pharmacol. Sci.* **2020**, *24*, 4062–4063. [PubMed]

82. Bourke, C.D.; Berkley, J.A.; Prendergast, A.J. Immune dysfunction as a cause and consequence of malnutrition. *Trends Immunol.* **2016**, *37*, 386–398. [CrossRef]

83. Ibrahim, M.K.; Zambruni, M.; Melby, C.L.; Melby, P.C. Impact of childhood malnutrition on host defense and infection. *Clin. Microbiol. Rev.* **2017**, *30*, 919–971. [CrossRef] [PubMed]

84. Wernerman, J. Intensive care unit nutrition—Nonsense or neglect? *Crit. Care* **2005**, *9*, 251–252. [CrossRef] [PubMed]

85. Kizilarslanoglu, M.C.; Kuyumcu, M.E.; Yesil, Y.; Halil, M. Sarcopenia in critically ill patients. *J. Anesth.* **2016**, *30*, 884–890. [CrossRef]

86. Singer, P. How could we make nutrition in the intensive care unit simple? *Rev. Bras. Ter. Intensiva* **2016**, *28*, 369–372. [CrossRef] [PubMed]

87. Diaz Ballve, L.P.; Dargains, N.; Urrutia Inchaustegui, J.G.; Bratos, A.; Milagros Percaz, M.; Bueno Ardariz, C.; Cagide, S.; Balestrieri, C.; Gamarra, C.; Paz, D.; et al. Weakness acquired in the intensive care unit. Incidence, risk factors and their association with inspiratory weakness. Observational cohort study. *Rev. Bras. Ter. Intensiva* **2017**, *29*, 466–475.
88. Brodsky, M.B.; Levy, M.J.; Jedlanek, E.; Pandian, V.; Blackford, B.; Price, C.; Cole, G.; Hillel, A.T.; Best, S.R.; Akst, L.M. Laryngeal injury and upper airway symptoms after oral endotracheal intubation with mechanical ventilation during critical care: A systematic review. *Crit. Care Med.* **2018**, *46*, 2010–2017. [CrossRef]
89. Caccialanza, R.; Laviano, A.; Lobascio, F.; Montagna, E.; Bruno, R.; Ludovisi, S.; Corsico, A.G.; Di Sabatino, A.; Belliato, M.; Calvi, M.; et al. Early nutritional supplementation in non-critically ill patients hospitalized for the 2019 novel coronavirus disease (COVID-19): Rationale and feasibility of a shared pragmatic protocol. *Nutrition* **2020**, *74*, 110835. [CrossRef]
90. Cena, H.; Chieppa, M. Coronavirus disease (COVID-19-SARS-CoV-2) and nutrition: Is infection in italy suggesting a connection? *Front. Immunol.* **2020**, *11*, 944. [CrossRef]
91. Singer, P. Preserving the quality of life: Nutrition in the ICU. *Crit. Care* **2019**, *23*, 139. [CrossRef] [PubMed]
92. Briguglio, M.; Pregliasco, F.E.; Lombardi, G.; Perazzo, P.; Banfi, G. The malnutritional status of the host as a virulence factor for new coronavirus SARS-CoV-2. *Front. Med.* **2020**, *7*, 146. [CrossRef] [PubMed]
93. Zhou, S.; Ye, B.; Fu, P.; Li, S.; Yuan, P.; Yang, L.; Zhan, X.; Chao, F.; Zhang, S.; Wang, M.Q.; et al. Double burden of malnutrition: Examining the growth profile and coexistence of undernutrition, overweight, and obesity among school-aged children and adolescents in urban and rural counties in Henan province, China. *J. Obes.* **2020**, *2020*, 2962138. [CrossRef] [PubMed]
94. Lechien, J.R.; Chiesa-Estomba, C.M.; De Siati, D.R.; Horoi, M.; Le Bon, S.D.; Rodriguez, A.; Dequanter, D.; Blecic, S.; El Afia, F.; Distinguin, L.; et al. Olfactory and gustatory dysfunctions as a clinical presentation of mild-to-moderate forms of the coronavirus disease (COVID-19): A multicenter European study. *Eur. Arch. Otorhinolaryngol.* **2020**, *277*, 2251–2261. [CrossRef] [PubMed]
95. Zayet, S.; Klopfenstein, T.; Mercier, J.; Kadiane-Oussou, N.J.; Wah, L.L.C.; Royer, P.Y.; Toko, L.; Gendrin, V. Contribution of anosmia and dysgeusia for diagnostic of COVID-19 in outpatients. *Infection* **2020**. [CrossRef] [PubMed]
96. Boscolo-Rizzo, P.; Borsetto, D.; Spinato, G.; Fabbris, C.; Menegaldo, A.; Gaudioso, P.; Nicolai, P.; Tirelli, G.; Da Mosto, M.C.; Rigoli, R.; et al. New onset of loss of smell or taste in household contacts of home-isolated SARS-CoV-2-positive subjects. *Eur. Arch. Otorhinolaryngol.* **2020**, *277*, 2637–2640. [CrossRef]
97. Carignan, A.; Valiquette, L.; Grenier, C.; Musonera, J.B.; Nkengurutse, D.; Marcil-Heguy, A.; Vettese, K.; Marcoux, D.; Valiquette, C.; Xiong, W.T.; et al. Anosmia and dysgeusia associated with SARS-CoV-2 infection: An age-matched case-control study. *CMAJ* **2020**, *192*, E702–E707. [CrossRef] [PubMed]
98. Lovato, A.; Galletti, C.; Galletti, B.; de Filippis, C. Clinical characteristics associated with persistent olfactory and taste alterations in COVID-19: A preliminary report on 121 patients. *Am. J. Otolaryngol.* **2020**, *41*, 102548. [CrossRef] [PubMed]
99. Sayin, I.; Yasar, K.K.; Yazici, Z.M. Taste and smell impairment in COVID-19: An aao-hns anosmia reporting tool-based comparative study. *Otolaryngol. Head Neck Surg.* **2020**, 194599820931820. [CrossRef] [PubMed]
100. Printza, A.; Constantinidis, J. The role of self-reported smell and taste disorders in suspected COVID19. *Eur. Arch. Otorhinolaryngol.* **2020**, *277*, 2625–2630. [CrossRef]
101. Li, T.; Zhang, Y.; Gong, C.; Wang, J.; Liu, B.; Shi, L.; Duan, J. Prevalence of malnutrition and analysis of related factors in elderly patients with COVID-19 in Wuhan, China. *Eur. J. Clin. Nutr.* **2020**, *74*, 871–875. [CrossRef] [PubMed]
102. Liu, G.; Zhang, S.; Mao, Z.; Wang, W.; Hu, H. Clinical significance of nutritional risk screening for older adult patients with COVID-19. *Eur. J. Clin. Nutr.* **2020**, *74*, 876–883. [CrossRef] [PubMed]
103. Alwarawrah, Y.; Kiernan, K.; MacIver, N.J. Changes in nutritional status impact immune cell metabolism and function. *Front. Immunol.* **2018**, *9*, 1055. [CrossRef] [PubMed]
104. Barazzoni, R.; Bischoff, S.C.; Breda, J.; Wickramasinghe, K.; Krznaric, Z.; Nitzan, D.; Pirlich, M.; Singer, P. Endorsed by the ESPEN Council ESPEN expert statements and practical guidance for nutritional management of individuals with SARS-CoV-2 infection. *Clin. Nutr.* **2020**, *39*, 1631–1638. [CrossRef] [PubMed]
105. Jie, B.; Jiang, Z.M.; Nolan, M.T.; Efron, D.T.; Zhu, S.N.; Yu, K.; Kondrup, J. Impact of nutritional support on clinical outcome in patients at nutritional risk: A multicenter, prospective cohort study in Baltimore and Beijing teaching hospitals. *Nutrition* **2010**, *26*, 1088–1093. [CrossRef]

106. Felder, S.; Lechtenboehmer, C.; Bally, M.; Fehr, R.; Deiss, M.; Faessler, L.; Kutz, A.; Steiner, D.; Rast, A.C.; Laukemann, S.; et al. Association of nutritional risk and adverse medical outcomes across different medical inpatient populations. *Nutrition* **2015**, *31*, 1385–1393. [CrossRef]
107. Bailey, R.L.; West, K.P., Jr.; Black, R.E. The epidemiology of global micronutrient deficiencies. *Ann. Nutr. Metab.* **2015**, *66* (Suppl. 2), 22–33. [CrossRef]
108. Bird, J.K.; Murphy, R.A.; Ciappio, E.D.; McBurney, M.I. Risk of deficiency in multiple concurrent micronutrients in children and adults in the United States. *Nutrients* **2017**, *9*, 655. [CrossRef]
109. Stark, K.D.; Van Elswyk, M.E.; Higgins, M.R.; Weatherford, C.A.; Salem, N., Jr. Global survey of the omega-3 fatty acids, docosahexaenoic acid and eicosapentaenoic acid in the blood stream of healthy adults. *Prog. Lipid Res.* **2016**, *63*, 132–152. [CrossRef]
110. Charan, J.; Goyal, J.P.; Saxena, D.; Yadav, P. Vitamin D for prevention of respiratory tract infections: A systematic review and meta-analysis. *J. Pharmacol. Pharmacother.* **2012**, *3*, 300–303. [CrossRef]
111. Bergman, P.; Lindh, A.U.; Bjorkhem-Bergman, L.; Lindh, J.D. Vitamin D and respiratory tract infections: A systematic review and meta-analysis of randomized controlled trials. *PLoS ONE* **2013**, *8*, e65835. [CrossRef] [PubMed]
112. Hemila, H.; Louhiala, P. Vitamin C for preventing and treating pneumonia. *Cochrane Database Syst. Rev.* **2013**, *8*, CD005532. [CrossRef] [PubMed]
113. Hemila, H.; Chalker, E. Vitamin C for preventing and treating the common cold. *Cochrane Database Syst. Rev.* **2013**, *1*, CD000980. [CrossRef] [PubMed]
114. Autier, P.; Mullie, P.; Macacu, A.; Dragomir, M.; Boniol, M.; Coppens, K.; Pizot, C.; Boniol, M. Effect of vitamin D supplementation on non-skeletal disorders: A systematic review of meta-analyses and randomised trials. *Lancet Diabetes Endocrinol.* **2017**, *5*, 986–1004. [CrossRef]
115. Martineau, A.R.; Jolliffe, D.A.; Greenberg, L.; Aloia, J.F.; Bergman, P.; Dubnov-Raz, G.; Esposito, S.; Ganmaa, D.; Ginde, A.A.; Goodall, E.C.; et al. Vitamin D supplementation to prevent acute respiratory infections: Individual participant data meta-analysis. *Health Technol. Assess.* **2019**, *23*, 1–44. [CrossRef] [PubMed]
116. Rejnmark, L.; Bislev, L.S.; Cashman, K.D.; Eiriksdottir, G.; Gaksch, M.; Grubler, M.; Grimnes, G.; Gudnason, V.; Lips, P.; Pilz, S.; et al. Non-skeletal health effects of vitamin D supplementation: A systematic review on findings from meta-analyses summarizing trial data. *PLoS ONE* **2017**, *12*, e0180512. [CrossRef] [PubMed]
117. Martineau, A.R.; Jolliffe, D.A.; Hooper, R.L.; Greenberg, L.; Aloia, J.F.; Bergman, P.; Dubnov-Raz, G.; Esposito, S.; Ganmaa, D.; Ginde, A.A.; et al. Vitamin D supplementation to prevent acute respiratory tract infections: Systematic review and meta-analysis of individual participant data. *BMJ* **2017**, *356*, i6583. [CrossRef]
118. Ran, L.; Zhao, W.; Wang, J.; Wang, H.; Zhao, Y.; Tseng, Y.; Bu, H. Extra dose of vitamin c based on a daily supplementation shortens the common cold: A meta-analysis of 9 randomized controlled trials. *BioMed Res. Int.* **2018**, *2018*, 183763. [CrossRef]
119. Mochalkin, N.I. Ascorbic acid in the complex therapy of acute pneumonia. *Voen Med. Zh.* **1970**, *9*, 17–21.
120. Hunt, C.; Chakravorty, N.K.; Annan, G.; Habibzadeh, N.; Schorah, C.J. The clinical effects of vitamin C supplementation in elderly hospitalised patients with acute respiratory infections. *Int. J. Vitam. Nutr. Res.* **1994**, *64*, 212–219.
121. Carr, A.C.; Maggini, S. Vitamin C and Immune Function. *Nutrients* **2017**, *9*, 1211. [CrossRef] [PubMed]
122. Cintoni, M.; Rinninella, E.; Annetta, M.G.; Mele, M.C. Nutritional management in hospital setting during SARS-CoV-2 pandemic: A real-life experience. *Eur. J. Clin. Nutr.* **2020**, *74*, 846–847. [CrossRef] [PubMed]
123. Li, X.Y.; Du, B.; Wang, Y.S.; Kang, H.Y.J.; Wang, F.; Sun, B.; Qiu, H.B.; Tong, Z.H. The keypoints in treatment of the critical coronavirus disease 2019 patient (2). *Zhonghua Jie He He Hu Xi Za Zhi* **2020**, *43*, 277–281. [PubMed]
124. Gomes, F.; Baumgartner, A.; Bounoure, L.; Bally, M.; Deutz, N.E.; Greenwald, J.L.; Stanga, Z.; Mueller, B.; Schuetz, P. Association of nutritional support with clinical outcomes among medical inpatients who are malnourished or at nutritional risk: An updated systematic review and meta-analysis. *JAMA Netw. Open* **2019**, *2*, e1915138. [CrossRef]
125. Rondanelli, M.; Faliva, M.A.; Gasparri, C.; Peroni, G.; Spadaccini, D.; Maugeri, R.; Nichetti, M.; Infantino, V.; Perna, S. Current opinion on dietary advice in order to preserve fat-free mass during a low-calorie diet. *Nutrition* **2020**, *72*, 110667. [CrossRef] [PubMed]

126. Gill, H.S.; Doull, F.; Rutherfurd, K.J.; Cross, M.L. Immunoregulatory peptides in bovine milk. *Br. J. Nutr.* **2000**, *84* (Suppl. 1), S111–S117. [CrossRef]
127. Ng, T.B.; Cheung, R.C.; Wong, J.H.; Wang, Y.; Ip, D.T.; Wan, D.C.; Xia, J. Antiviral activities of whey proteins. *Appl. Microbiol. Biotechnol.* **2015**, *99*, 6997–7008. [CrossRef]
128. Anderson, L. Providing nutritional support for the patient with COVID-19. *Br. J. Nurs.* **2020**, *29*, 458–459. [CrossRef]
129. Nardini, S.; Sanguinetti, C.M.; De Benedetto, F.; Baccarani, C.; Del Donno, M.; Polverino, M.; Annesi-Maesano, I. SARS-CoV-2 pandemic in Italy: Ethical and organizational considerations. *Multidiscip. Respir. Med.* **2020**, *15*, 672. [CrossRef]
130. Laviano, A.; Zanetti, M. Nutrition support in the time of SARS-CoV-2 (COVID-19). *Nutrition* **2020**, *74*, 110834. [CrossRef]
131. Arkin, N.; Krishnan, K.; Chang, M.G.; Bittner, E.A. Nutrition in critically ill patients with COVID-19: Challenges and special considerations. *Clin. Nutr.* **2020**, *39*, 2327–2328. [CrossRef] [PubMed]
132. Romano, L.; Bilotta, F.; Dauri, M.; Macheda, S.; Pujia, A.; De Santis, G.L.; Tarsitano, M.G.; Merra, G.; Di Renzo, L.; Esposito, E.; et al. Short Report-Medical nutrition therapy for critically ill patients with COVID-19. *Eur. Rev. Med. Pharmacol. Sci.* **2020**, *24*, 4035–4039. [PubMed]
133. Volkert, D.; Beck, A.M.; Cederholm, T.; Cruz-Jentoft, A.; Goisser, S.; Hooper, L.; Kiesswetter, E.; Maggio, M.; Raynaud-Simon, A.; Sieber, C.C.; et al. ESPEN guideline on clinical nutrition and hydration in geriatrics. *Clin. Nutr.* **2019**, *38*, 10–47. [CrossRef] [PubMed]
134. Wang, Y.; Lin, H.; Lin, B.W.; Lin, J.D. Effects of different ascorbic acid doses on the mortality of critically ill patients: A meta-analysis. *Ann. Intensive Care.* **2019**, *9*, 58. [CrossRef] [PubMed]

# 3

# Challenges and Perspectives in Nutritional Counselling and Nursing

**Maria F. Vasiloglou [1], Jane Fletcher [2] and Kalliopi-Anna Poulia [3,*]**

1 Diabetes Technology Research Group, ARTORG Center for Biomedical Engineering Research, University of Bern, Murtenstrasse 50, 3008 Bern, Switzerland; maria.vasiloglou@artorg.unibe.ch
2 Nutrition Nurses, Queen Elizabeth Hospital Birmingham, University Hospitals Birmingham NHS Foundation Trust, Mindelsohn Way, Edgbaston, Birmingham B15 2WG, UK; jane.fletcher@uhb.nhs.uk
3 Department of Nutrition and Dietetics, Laiko General Hospital of Athens, 11527 Athens, Greece
* Correspondence: lpoulia@gmail.com

**Abstract:** Nutritional counselling has been recognised as the first line approach in the management of numerous chronic diseases. Though usually carried out by dietitians, nutritional counselling may be used by nurses, or other healthcare professionals to improve nutritional status and meet healthcare goals. Healthcare professionals require training and education to facilitate a patient centred approach to effective counselling. Advances in digital technology have the potential to improve access to nutritional counselling for some patients such as those in primary care. However, caution is required to ensure that valuable interpersonal relationships are not lost, as these form the cornerstone of effective nutritional counselling. The aim of this narrative review is to explore aspects of effective nutritional counselling, including advances in e-counselling and areas where nursing input in nutritional counselling might enhance overall nutritional care.

**Keywords:** nutritional counselling; nursing; interventions; e-counselling

---

## 1. Introduction

Nutrition related chronic diseases—i.e., cancer, diabetes mellitus, chronic kidney disease, inflammatory bowel disease and so forth—and health problems that have significant implications on nutritional status, mainly by affecting digestion and absorption of food, place a significant burden on the overall health of a population and health care systems. As dietary modification can have a significant impact on biomarkers of non-communicable diseases and on symptoms of different clinical conditions, nutritional counselling has been recognised as the first line approach for their management [1]. Furthermore nutrition counselling is recommended as a key intervention in the management of malnutrition in older adults [2,3], and has been proven to be effective in chronic kidney disease, cancer and other clinical conditions [4–6].

Nutrition counselling is a two-way interaction through which a patient and the member of the medical team interpret the results of a nutritional assessment, identify patient's nutritional problems, needs and goals, discuss ways to meet these goals, and agree on future steps and the frequency of monitoring. It aims to help patients understand important information about the impact of nutrition on their health status and focuses on practical measures to cover nutritional needs. Moreover, it strengthens the importance of behavioural change [7–10]. However, nutrition counselling may present a time burden to patients, with high drop-out rates being a key challenge likely to affect outcomes [1], and face to face counselling having a significant impact on the use of resources in terms of clinic space and facilities. The development of new technology in e-counselling seeks to address these issues and expand access for patients.

Most of the time, nutrition counsellors are nutritionists or dietitians. However, other healthcare professionals such as nurses, community health workers or volunteers [3,7,11] play an essential role in nutritional counselling. The role of the nurse is recognised in nutrition screening but there is little evidence regarding the impact or effectiveness of the nurses' role in nutrition counselling. However, nurses form a core part of the team providing direct care to patients and as such are in a position to make positive behaviour changes [12], improving the effectiveness of nutritional interventions.

To meet the needs of an ever-changing healthcare environment, there is a need to explore the benefits of new technology in providing nutritional counselling to a wider audience. Although dietitians are key professionals in the nutritional counselling of patients, expanding the roles of other healthcare professionals may improve the impact and effectiveness of both counselling and interventions.

*Aims*

In this narrative review we aim to explore aspects of effective nutritional counselling including advances in technology and the role of the nurse in enhancing nutritional care.

## 2. Methodology

An electronic search was implemented in PubMed, Google Scholar Medline and Cinahl databases. Search terms included: 'Nutritional counselling', 'nurs* AND nutrition counselling' 'dietary counselling', 'patient education', 'nutrition education', 'nutrition AND nurse AND specialist' 'nursing', 'e-counselling', 'mHealth', 'eHealth', 'nutrition nurse specialist', 'patient-centred approach', 'nutritional care', 'remote nutrition counselling'. Publications were only included in the analysis if they were written in English and were related to humans. Articles were searched from January 2000 till May 2019. Non-peer reviewed literature, letters to the editor and studies performed on animals were excluded. From the articles retrieved in the first search round, additional references were identified by a manual search among the cited references. Moreover, additional references including characteristic and cornerstone references on nutrition counselling were added in introductory parts. As the review is narrative and not systematic, the references were selected according to the relevance to the subject of the manuscript.

## 3. Basic Characteristics of Effective Nutritional Counselling

As nutrition counselling can enhance health and nutrition outcomes, ideally it should be performed in a way that ensures patients' privacy and that the counsellor and the patient are feeling comfortable. This may be challenging in the hospital setting and measures should be taken towards this direction. Moreover, counsellors should be trained and use appropriate materials to enhance understanding and documentation, such as illustrations, food models, take-home brochures, data collection forms and referral forms.

Moreover, respecting the ethical aspects of nutritional counselling improves its outcomes. The main ethical values that should be followed are described in Table 1:

**Table 1.** Ethical values that underpin effective counselling [4].

| Ethical Values | Rationale |
|---|---|
| The provision of accurate information | Patients should develop a relation of trust with the counsellor, based on the fact that the words and actions are true and reliable. |
| Confidentiality | All information shared should be kept confidentially, except as needed for the nutritional treatment and recovery. |
| Respect of patients' autonomy | Patients, as long as they are mentally stable, keep the right to decide for themselves, without coercion. |
| Do no harm | Nutritional interventions in the hospital setting should always be based on evidence-based medicine. Any intervention that could harm or exploit patients emotionally, financially or medically should always be avoided. |
| Be fair | All patients should receive the same level of attention, according to their needs, without discrimination. Patient's rights dignity and differences should be respected. |

*Patient-Centered Approach in Nutrition Counselling*

The implementation of changes on nutrition behaviour is a complex procedure, as it combines elements of psychology, physiological needs, socioeconomic status and the level of the counsellor's ability to firstly identify the needs of the patients, and then to work co-operatively with them [3]. The patient-centred approach is generally accepted as efficient in managing nutritional counselling. It has been developed based on theoretical models developed in the late 40's by Rogers [13]. According to this theoretical model the patient has to identify the diet related problems and the nutritional counsellor will guide him towards the possible solutions.

The nutritionist/dietitian is the expert in the medical nutrition team, able to translate and combine the most current scientific information on food and health, food composition, psychological and physiological factors that could have an impact on dietary choices, and the relationship of those with health and diseases. He/she is the nutrition communicator, a skilled listener and a translator of emotions and abstract ideas on specific actions and steps towards dietary modification needed to enhance nutritional status, based on the individuals' life and biomedical requirements [14–16]. Gaining a better understanding of patients' preferences, attitudes and beliefs regarding their state of health and nutrition would allow interventions to be more focused, appropriate, sustainable and therefore, more effective [17]. The clinician–patient relationship has been associated with better patient attendance and adherence and greater patient satisfaction with care and treatment [18]. Moreover, patients' recall understanding, treatment adherence, and psychological wellbeing have been associated with effective doctor–patient communication. Therefore, an effective counselor refers not only to the expert nutrition knowledge but also to the privilege of having good communication skills. In this way, the development of a therapeutic relationship, characterized by mutual respect with the clients, will be easier to manage. However, this mode of practice requires organizational support and time, which are not always available to the dietitian in clinical practice. These dimensions may also be important in nutrition interventions, and future research should focus on the efficacy of nutritional counselling with these limitations in mind [19].

Under this spectrum, the main aim, and yet a great challenge, is to ensure that the patient has a full understanding of the relevant information of the nutritional problem and can work towards the development of specific skills to deal with the health challenges and their personal goals [20]. In order to have a successful outcome in patients receiving nutritional counselling, it is important to assess not only the patients' food choices and behavior, but also their access to health, environmental and social support systems. Therefore, the challenge is to be able to achieve essential and meaningful clinical outcomes, enhance the quality of life of the patient and, at the same time, encourage positive attitudes towards behavioral changes [21].

## 4. Challenges in Nutritional Counselling

Health professionals should always have in mind that patients are members of the community at large. At the community level, they receive multiple messages from different sources regarding nutritional behaviors that could enhance their wellbeing, their quality of life and improve health outcomes. Although health outcomes can be estimated by objective measurements, in terms of biochemical and physiological responses to interventions, the main issue is to identify what patients consider important as endpoints of quality of life and wellbeing [21]. Under the spectrum of the patient-centered approach, the bridging of biomedical imperatives and individual perspectives on health, quality of life and wellbeing is of paramount importance.

According to a recent systematic review by Mitchell et al. [1] of 26 randomized controlled studies (RCTs), representing 5500 adults, dietetic consultation in primary care appeared to be effective for the improvement of diet quality, the glycaemic control, and body weight control. One major limitation in analyzing RCTs that deals with nutrition consultations and dietary interventions though, is the fact that dietary assessment is subjected to errors and the available dietary assessment tools may not be too specific to identify qualitative improvements to the diet. Moreover, as nutrition is a factor influencing patients' life to a great extent, and at the same time is being influenced by personal, economic, psychological and emotional reasons, dietary interventions are usually characterized by high dropout rates and limited compliance. Therefore, measures to enhance adherence to dietetic interventions should always be considered [1].

Moving to more clinical settings, dietary interventions have been studied in environments that compromised health has a negative impact on nutritional status and raised the risk of malnutrition. In clinical cases health professionals providing nutrition consultations should always follow evidence-based medicine and established guidelines. As nutrition can be used as a complementary treatment that could be even harmful in some cases, i.e., in cancer patients, nutrition counselling should always be provided by specialized and qualified nutrition and dietetics professionals, to ensure the validity of the provided information. Lack of knowledge and misconceptions should be pointed out and scientific evidence should be provided. All non-justified and not scientific-based dietary theories should be addressed, under the spectrum of the individual perception of wellbeing [22,23].

In order to enhance compliance and adherence to nutritional interventions, other factors that could have an impact on the effectiveness of the intervention must be considered. The duration and the frequency of the consultations, the aims set on each consultation, the feedback that was given to the patients about their improvement or the achievement of the set goals can have an impact on the adherence to the nutritional intervention. More focused, clearly defined and measurable objectives increase effectiveness, whereas the use of vague objectives may limit the effectiveness of nutrition education due to the fact that it creates confusion and does not provide answers to the questions of the patients. Therefore, the design of the interventions should be clear and continued training for the trainers, with an emphasis on targeted interventions, should be available [24,25].

## 5. Nursing and Nutritional Care

Where studies have shown that patients benefit from receiving counselling and an individualised nutrition plan from a registered dietitian [26,27], the nurses' role is essential in reinforcing and facilitating nutritional plans and interventions in hospitalised patients. Observations suggest that nutritional outcomes may be enhanced with collaborative input from both dietitians and nurses [28]. As the daily providers of care, ward-based nurses are responsible for the direct delivery of nutritional interventions [29]. Additionally, nurses have a responsibility to pay special attention to promoting wellbeing, with nutrition being one of the fundamentals of care [30].

### *5.1. Ward-Based Nurses*

Perry et al. [31] report a systematic review identifying the range of nursing interventions implemented to improve nutritional outcomes in patients who have suffered a stroke. The review included 27 papers from 26 studies with five RCT's and five clinical trials. Due to the heterogeneity and poor quality of reported data, few interventions showed statistical significance. However, this review is important in highlighting the diversity of nursing activities in nutritional care. The Alliance to Advance Patient Nutrition [32] stresses the importance of multidisciplinary involvement in nutrition, with a focus on all stakeholders valuing nutritional care interventions. Important points for nursing intervention include nutrition screening, implementing early nutritional measures in those at risk and developing strategies to ensure patient compliance. Where dietitians carry out comprehensive assessment and patient education, the nurse's role is to reinforce this information and answer patient questions [32]. In this way, collaborative working between disciplines is essential.

Nevertheless, one of the key challenges in practice is the level of importance that nurses place on nutritional care. A study of the attitudes of 106 nurses found respondents felt strongly that it was the role of the nurse to carry out nutrition counselling [33]. Key nursing nutritional interventions were significantly positively associated with the overall nutrition knowledge score: Patient counselling ($r = 0.23$, $p = 0.02$) and nutrition screening/assessment ($r = 0.23$, $p = 0.02$). This finding indicated that the higher the overall nutrition knowledge score among nurses, the higher these tasks were ranked [4].

However, the same study found that nurses ranked tasks associated with nutrition lower than other nursing tasks, such as giving medication and carrying out wound dressings. A small ($n = 22$) focus group study of staff working in an acute medical ward found that nurses struggled to put nutritional priorities in to practice, with competing activities being a particular issue at mealtimes [34]. A nursing survey carried out in Canadian hospitals ($n = 346$) reported nurses' perceptions as one of the reasons for insufficient nutrition [35]. The study found that 17% of the respondents thought that a lack of assistance at mealtimes was a major contributor, and 14% thought that assisting with nutrition was time consuming [35].

Though nursing interventions such as screening and assistance with eating and drinking are crucial, there appears to be little recorded evidence of nurses carrying out nutritional counselling at the ward level in internal medicine. Studies suggest successful nurse involvement in nutritional counselling in other settings including cancer care [36,37], primary care [38] and community care [39,40]. This then suggests that nurses working in internal medicine may be missing a valuable opportunity to improve patient care and compliance with nutritional interventions.

### *5.2. Nutrition Nurse Specialist*

Specialist nurses have an important part to play in empowering ward-based nurses to deliver evidence-based care within their speciality, bridging the gap between research and bedside practice [41]. The nutrition nurse specialist (NNS) role may be known by numerous titles including 'nutrition support nurse', 'nutrition nurse practitioner/advanced practitioner' and 'nutrition support consultant nurse' [42]. Regardless of title, NNSs generally form a core part of hospital nutrition support teams, caring for patients with complex nutritional requirements. Though it is difficult to ascertain the exact value that individual members of the multidisciplinary teams bring to nutritional support, input from NNSs have been shown to reduce catheter related sepsis and other complications of parenteral nutrition [43].

However, the NNS role reaches far beyond this. The NNS may coordinate patient education on self-management of enteral or parenteral nutrition and provide training and educational programmes for other healthcare professionals [42]. Yordy et al. [44] report outcomes of a NNS-led quality improvement project. The project included a program of nutritional education for ward nurses with an audit of practice before and after education. In observations of mealtime interactions ($n = 100$), patient interruptions at mealtimes were shown to have reduced by 59% following the education program. Nursing documentation of nutritional risk factors and screening showed some improvement after education, although no statistical significance was described. The authors suggest that following targeted education, the nursing culture had changed to recognize nutrition as an essential part of the patients' treatment [35].

Some NNSs may be involved at a strategic and organisational level with the provision of nutritional services within their institution. Depending on the nature and requirements of the healthcare setting, NNSs may expand their skills to include technical procedures such as central venous catheter insertion [45] or gastrostomy insertion. Their scope is expanding further to include independent non medical prescribing [46]. However, there is a lack of evidence regarding the function of NNSs in nutritional counselling. Given the nature of the role, it is reasonable to expect that NNSs play an important part in counselling patients with complex nutritional needs and particularly those that require artificial nutrition support. For these reasons NNSs must develop effective counselling skills. Fundamentally, the overall purpose of the NNS should be an improvement in quality of nutritional care, and nutritional counselling must be a core activity in this.

Further research is required to measure the improvements that the enhanced skills of the NNS brings to nutritional care. Nevertheless, NNSs are key participants in the wider nutrition support team and have an important function in supporting and educating ward-based nurses to deliver excellent care and reinforcing multidisciplinary nutritional treatment goals.

## 6. Nutritional Counselling with the Use of Modern Technology

Nutritional counselling is usually a time- and resource-demanding procedure that requires commitment by the patient [47]. The dropout rate of up to 35% of patients enrolled in dietetic consultation interventions shows the challenge of adhering to numerous counselling sessions [1]. Modern technology, including electronic health (eHealth) and mobile health (mHealth) may help keep patients engaged in their goals [48]. According to the European Commission's definition, eHealth is the "digital health and care which refers to tools and services that use information and communication technologies (ICTs) to improve prevention, diagnosis, treatment, monitoring and management of health and lifestyle". mHealth is a subcategory of eHealth, used mainly for describing healthcare management conducted by smartphones [49].

Electronic or e-counselling, i.e., remote counselling, can reduce barriers related to patient disengagement, geographical distance, time constraints [48], socioeconomic status [50], and also low need or desire for in-person contact [47]. In addition, the integration of eHealth and mHealth technologies could render the flexibility of dietetic services administered to patients [51,52]. Smartphone applications (apps) have been used of late to improve nutrition knowledge and contribute to behavioural change (beyond weight loss) [53], while presenting positive effects on measured nutritional outcomes in chronic diseases [47]. Artificial Intelligence (AI)-based smartphone apps can provide accurate and almost real-time dietary assessments [54–59]. However, even though there is an abundance of nutrition and diet apps, the majority of them focus on diet monitoring and nutrient content estimation. There is only a limited number of studies investigating the long-term impacts of apps focusing on nutritional e-counselling [52].

E-counselling through web-based apps has also already produced some positive effects, in comparison to in-person treatment for both delivery and dissemination [60]. Weight loss of approximately 4–6 kg can be reliably achieved with web programs that involve some form of weekly human e-counselling or constant feedback from behavioural lifestyle counsellors via email, group chat, etc. [61]. The results of this study also suggest that using a hybrid approach (in-person and online) may be an effective way to reach larger and more diverse populations [61]. Weight loss targeted web applications, where participants also received e-counselling via weekly e-mails, resulted in weight loss of 4.4 kg after one year of intervention in people at risk of type 2 diabetes [62]. Providing automated, computer-tailored feedback by a weight loss targeted web application for three months was as effective as human counselling via e-mail [63]. Clinically significant weight loss could be achieved through a combination of tailored goals and the use of a mobile app, whereas people interested in lower-intensity weight loss approaches could consider stand-alone digital health treatments [64]. Furthermore, Haas et al. [50] concluded that an app which complemented the dietitians' professional skills, can provide effective support towards behavioural change and sustainable weight reduction in overweight and obese individuals. Moreover, traditional consultations delivered by dietitians were compared against remote ones delivered by eHealth technologies, using theoretical cost in weight management as the outcome measure [52]. The eHealth approach needed an initial higher investment but was less costly in the long-term than in-person counselling [52].

In a qualitative study, healthcare professionals stated that it was challenging to establish and maintain an empathetic relationship with their clients (which is one of the most crucial factors for coaching) when conducting eHealth counselling [65]. Hence, e-counselling should include specific attributes that ensure it simulates—as closely as possible—a face-to face consultation [50], tailored to the individual patient [65].

Finally, including innovative technologies into dietetic practice could assist nutritional counselling by not only enhancing the efficiency and quality of nutrition care but also increasing adherence to self-monitoring of patient-centred goals [66]. Currently there is no evidence on the most effective use of apps in a clinical setting. Thus, it is suggested that the apps are used alongside individualized dietetic support, while performance for long-term weight management is being assessed [67]. End-users (patients) should be involved in the design process concerning health advice since it increases app efficacy and usability [68]. Future research, preferably in the form of randomized controlled trials, should investigate the clinical efficacy, feasibility and cost-effectiveness of e-counselling and eHealth technologies on dietetic practice.

## 7. Conclusions

Nutritional counselling has been recognised as the first line approach in the management of numerous chronic diseases. A patient-centred approach has been identified as the best way of providing nutritional counselling. Ideally, it is carried out by dietitians and nutritionists, but other members of the medical nutrition team such as nurses and other healthcare professionals can also play an important role. Nutrition nurse specialists have a particularly key part to play in both the carrying out of nutritional counselling as well as encouraging other nurses to participate in nutritional counselling. However, research is required to fully understand the benefits that the NNS brings to nutritional counselling and care.

It is important to stress that effective counselling needs training and education, and at the same time the use of eHealth technology has the potential to improve access for some patients. However, caution is required to ensure that valuable interpersonal relationships are not lost, as these form the cornerstone of effective nutritional counselling.

**Author Contributions:** Conceptualization, M.F.V., J.F. and K.-A.P.; writing—original draft preparation, M.F.V., J.F. and K.-A.P.; writing—review and editing, M.F.V., J.F. and K.-A.P.

## Abbreviations

The following abbreviations are used in this manuscript:

| | |
|---|---|
| NNS | Nutrition nurse specialist |
| eHealth | Electronic health |
| mHealth | Mobile health |
| e-counselling | Electronic counselling |
| ICTs | Information and communication technologies |

## References


1. Mitchell, L.; Ball, L.; Ross, L.; Barnes, K.; Williams, L. Effectiveness of Dietetic Consultations in Primary Health Care: A Systematic Review of Randomized Controlled Trials. *J. Acad. Nutr. Diet.* **2017**, *117*, 1941–1962. [CrossRef] [PubMed]
2. Volkert, D.; Beck, A.M.; Cederholm, T.; Cruz-Jentoft, A.; Goisser, S.; Hooper, L.; Kiesswetter, E.; Maggio, M.; Raynaud-Simon, A.; Sieber, C.C.; et al. ESPEN guideline on clinical nutrition and hydration in geriatrics. *Clin. Nutr.* **2019**, *38*, 10–47. [CrossRef]
3. Rosal, M.; Ebbeling, C.; Lofgren, I.; Ockene, J.; Ockene, L.; Herbert, J. Facilitating dietary change: The patient centered counseling model. *J. Am. Diet. Assoc.* **2001**, *101*, 332–341. [CrossRef]
4. Ravasco, P.; Monteiro-Grillo, I.; Vidal, P.M.; Camilo, M.E. Dietary counseling improves patient outcomes: A prospective, randomized, controlled trial in colorectal cancer patients undergoing radiotherapy. *J. Clin. Oncol.* **2005**, *23*, 1431–1438. [CrossRef] [PubMed]
5. Ravasco, P.; Monteiro-Grillo, I.; Camilo, M. Individualized nutrition intervention is of major benefit to colorectal cancer patients. *Am. J. Clin. Nutr.* **2012**, *96*, 1346–1353. [CrossRef] [PubMed]
6. Orell, H.; Schwab, U.; Saarilahti, K.; Österlund, P.; Ravasco, P.; Mäkitie, A. Nutritional Counseling for Head and Neck Cancer Patients Undergoing (Chemo) Radiotherapy—A Prospective Randomized Trial. *Front. Nutr.* **2019**, *6*, 1–12. [CrossRef] [PubMed]

7. Scarlet, S. Dietary Counseling. In *Essentials of Human Nutrition*; Mann, J., Truswell, A.S., Eds.; Oxford University Press: New York, NY, USA, 1998.
8. MacLellan, D.; Berenbaum, S. Client-centred nutrition counseling: Do we know what it means? *Can. J. Diet. Pract. Res.* **2003**, *64*, 12–15. [CrossRef] [PubMed]
9. MacLellan, D.; Berenbaum, S. Dietitians' opinions and experiences of client-centred nutrition counseling. *Can. J. Diet. Pract. Res.* **2006**, *67*, 119–124. [CrossRef]
10. Lee, R.; Garvin, T. Moving from information transfer to information exchange in health and health care. *Soc. Sci. Med.* **2003**, *56*, 449–464. [CrossRef]
11. Mahan, K.; Raymond, J. *Krause's Food and Nutrition Care Process*, 14th ed.; Elsevier: St. Louis, MO, USA, 2017.
12. National Institute for Health and Care Excellence: Making Every Contact Count. Available online: https://stpsupport.nice.org.uk/mecc/index.html (accessed on 5 September 2019).
13. Rogers, C. *Client-Centered Therapy: Its Current Practice, Implications and Theory*; Houghton Mifflin: Boston, MA, USA, 1951.
14. Lu, A.; Dollahite, J. Assessment of dietitians' nutrition counselling self-efficacy and its positive relationship with reported skill usage. *J. Hum. Nutr Diet.* **2010**, *23*, 144–153. [CrossRef]
15. Academy of Nutrition and Dietetics. Nutrition Intervention. Prescription. Nutrition Care Process Model 2015. Available online: https://bit.ly/2lTiFCo (accessed on 15 May 2019).
16. Holli, B.B.; Calabrese, R.J.; Maillet, J.O.S. *Communication and Education Skills for Dietetic Professionals*; Lippincott Williams and Wilkins: Philadelphia, PA, USA, 2009.
17. Sladdin, I.; Ball, L.; Bull, C.; Chaboyer, W. Patient-centred care to improve dietetic practice: An integrative review. *J. Hum. Nutr. Diet.* **2017**, *30*, 453–470. [CrossRef] [PubMed]
18. Hall, A.M.; Ferreira, P.H.; Maher, C.G.; Latimer, J.; Ferreira, M.L. The influence of the therapist-patient relationship on treatment outcome in physical rehabilitation: A systematic review. *Phys. Ther.* **2010**, *90*, 1099–1110. [CrossRef] [PubMed]
19. Street, R.L., Jr.; Makoul, G.; Arora, N.K.; Epstein, R.M. How does communication heal? Pathways linking clinician-patient communication to health outcomes. *Patient Educ. Couns.* **2009**, *74*, 295–301. [CrossRef]
20. MacLellan, D.; Berenbaum, S. Canadian Dietitians' Understanding of the Client-Centered Approach to Nutrition Counseling. *J. Am. Diet. Assoc.* **2007**, *107*, 1414–1417. [CrossRef] [PubMed]
21. McMahon, A.-T.; Tay, P.C.; Tapsell, L.; Williams, P. Building bridges in dietary counselling: An exploratory study examining the usefulness of wellness and wellbeing concepts. *J. Hum. Nutr. Diet.* **2016**, *29*, 75–85. [CrossRef]
22. Huebner, J.; Marienfeld, S.; Abbenhardt, C.; Ulrich, C.; Muenstedt, K.; Micke, O.; Muecke, R.; Loeser, C. Counseling patients on cancer diets: A review of the literature and recommendations for clinical practice. *Anticancer. Res.* **2014**, *34*, 39–48.
23. Shofield, P.; Diggens, J.; Charleson, C.; Mariglanie, R.; Jefford, M. Effectively discussing complementary and alternative medicine in a conventional oncology setting: Communication recommendations for clinicians. *Patient Educ. Couns.* **2010**, *79*, 143–151. [CrossRef]
24. Hand, R.; Abram, J.; Brown, K.; Ziegler, P.; Scott Parrott, J.; Steiber, A. Development and Validation of the Guide for Effective Nutrition Interventions and Education (GENIE): A tool for assessing the quality of proposed nutrition education programs. *J. Nutr. Educ. Behav.* **2015**, *47*, 308–316. [CrossRef]
25. Murimi, M.; Kanyi, M.; Mupfudze, T.; Amin, M.; Mbogori, T.; Aldubayan, K. Factors Influencing Efficacy of Nutrition Education Interventions: A Systematic Review. *J. Nutr. Educ. Behav.* **2017**, *49*, 142–165. [CrossRef]
26. Rüfenacht, U.; Rühlin, M.; Wegmann, M.; Imoberdorf, R.; Ballmer, P.E. Nutritional counseling improves quality of life and nutrient intake in hospitalized undernourished patients. *Nutrition* **2010**, *26*, 53–60. [CrossRef]
27. Singh, S.; Midha, S.; Singh, N.; Joshi, Y.K.; Garg, P.K. Dietary Counseling Versus Dietary Supplements for Malnutrition in Chronic Pancreatitis: A Randomized Controlled Trial. *Clin. Gastroenterol. Hepatol.* **2008**, *6*, 353–359. [CrossRef] [PubMed]
28. Johansen, N.; Kondrup, J.; Plum, L.M.; Bak, L.; Nørregaard, P.; Bunch, E.; Bærnthsen, H.; Andersen, J.R.; Larsen, I.H.; Martinsen, A. Effect of nutritional support on clinical outcome in patients at nutritional risk. *Clin. Nutr.* **2004**, *23*, 539–550. [CrossRef]
29. Xu, X.; Parker, D.; Ferguson, C.; Hickman, L. Where is the nurse in nutritional care? *Contemp. Nurse* **2017**, *53*, 267–270. [CrossRef] [PubMed]

30. Patience, S. Advising patients on nutrition and healthy eating. *Br. J. Nurs.* **2016**, *25*, 1182–1186. [CrossRef] [PubMed]
31. Perry, L.; Hamilton, S.; Williams, J.; Jones, S. Nursing Interventions for Improving Nutritional Status and Outcomes of Stroke Patients: Descriptive Reviews of Processes and Outcomes. *Worldviews Evid. Based Nurs.* **2013**, *10*, 17–40. [CrossRef] [PubMed]
32. Tappenden, K.A.; Quatrara, B.; Parkhurst, M.L.; Malone, A.M.; Fanjiang, G.; Ziegler, T.R. Critical Role of Nutrition in Improving Quality of Care. *J. Parenter. Enter. Nutr.* **2013**, *37*, 482–497. [CrossRef] [PubMed]
33. Boaz, M.; Rychani, L.; Barami, K.; Houri, Z.; Yosef, R.; Siag, A.; Berlovitz, Y.; Leibovitz, E. Nurses and nutrition: A survey of knowledge and attitudes regarding nutrition assessment and care of hospitalized elderly patients. *J. Contin. Educ. Nurs.* **2013**, *44*, 357–364. [CrossRef]
34. Ross, L.J.; Mudge, A.M.; Young, A.M.; Banks, M. Everyone's problem but nobody's job: Staff perceptions and explanations for poor nutritional intake in older medical patients. *Nutr. Diet.* **2011**, *68*, 41–46. [CrossRef]
35. Duerksen, D.R.; Keller, H.H.; Vesnaver, E.; Laporte, M.; Jeejeebhoy, K.; Payette, H.; Gramlich, L.; Bernier, P.; Allard, J.P. Nurses' Perceptions Regarding the Prevalence, Detection, and Causes of Malnutrition in Canadian Hospitals: Results of a Canadian Malnutrition Task Force Survey. *JPEN J. Parenter. Enter. Nutr.* **2016**, *40*, 100–106. [CrossRef] [PubMed]
36. Hopkinson, J.B. Nutritional support of the elderly cancer patient: The role of the nurse. *Nutrition* **2015**, *31*, 598–602. [CrossRef] [PubMed]
37. Hopkinson, J.B.; Fenlon, D.R.; Okamoto, I.; Wright, D.N.M.; Scott, I.; Addington-Hall, J.M.; Foster, C. The Deliverability, Acceptability, and Perceived Effect of the Macmillan Approach to Weight Loss and Eating Difficulties: A Phase II, Cluster-Randomized, Exploratory Trial of a Psychosocial Intervention for Weight- and Eating-Related Distress in People with Advanced Cancer. *J. Pain Symptom Manag.* **2010**, *40*, 684–695.
38. Van Dillen, S.M.E.; Noordman, J.; van Dulmen, S.; Hiddink, G.J. Quality of weight-loss counseling by Dutch practice nurses in primary care: An observational study. *Eur. J. Clin. Nutr.* **2014**, *69*, 73. [CrossRef] [PubMed]
39. Ahn, J.-A.; Park, J.; Kim, C.-J. Effects of an individualised nutritional education and support programme on dietary habits, nutritional knowledge and nutritional status of older adults living alone. *J. Clin. Nurs.* **2018**, *27*, 2142–2151. [CrossRef] [PubMed]
40. Young, K.; Bunn, F.; Trivedi, D.; Dickinson, A. Nutritional education for community dwelling older people: A systematic review of randomised controlled trials. *Int. J. Nurs. Stud.* **2011**, *48*, 751–780. [CrossRef] [PubMed]
41. Gurzick, M.; Kesten, K.S. The impact of clinical nurse specialists on clinical pathways in the application of evidence-based practice. *J. Prof. Nurs. Off. J. Am. Assoc. Coll. Nurs.* **2010**, *26*, 42–48. [CrossRef] [PubMed]
42. Boeykens, K.; Van Hecke, A. Advanced practice nursing: Nutrition Nurse Specialist role and function. *Clin. Nutr. ESPEN* **2018**, *26*, 72–76. [CrossRef]
43. Sutton, C.D.; Garcea, G.; Pollard, C.; Berry, D.P.; Dennison, A.R. The introduction of a nutrition clinical nurse specialist results in a reduction in the rate of catheter sepsis. *Clin. Nutr.* **2005**, *24*, 220–223. [CrossRef]
44. Yordy, B.M.; Roberts, S.; Taggart, H.M. Quality Improvement in Clinical Nutrition: Screening and Mealtime Protection for the Hospitalized Patient. *Clin. Nurse Spec. CNS* **2017**, *31*, 149–156. [CrossRef]
45. Hamilton, H.C. Advantages of a nurse-led central venous vascular access service. *J. Vasc. Access.* **2004**, *5*, 109–112. [CrossRef]
46. Guenter, P.; Boullata, J.I.; Ayers, P.; Gervasio, J.; Malone, A.; Raymond, E.; Holcombe, B.; Kraft, M.; Sacks, G.; Seres, D. Standardized Competencies for Parenteral Nutrition Prescribing. *Nutr. Clin. Pract.* **2015**, *30*, 570–576. [CrossRef]
47. Fakih El Khoury, C.; Karavetian, M.; Halfens, R.; Crutzen, R.; Khoja, L.S. A systematic review of the effect of dietary mobile apps on nutritional indicators in adults with a chronic illness. *J. Acad. Nutr. Diet.* **2019**, *119*, 626–651. [CrossRef] [PubMed]
48. Stein, K. Remote Nutrition Counseling: Considerations in a New Channel for Client Communication. *J. Acad. Nutr. Diet.* **2015**, *115*, 1561–1576. [CrossRef] [PubMed]
49. European Commission. mHealth. Available online: https://ec.europa.eu/digital-single-market/en/mhealth (accessed on 24 May 2019).
50. Haas, K.; Hayoz, S.; Maurer-Wiesner, S. Effectiveness and Feasibility of a Remote Lifestyle Intervention by Dietitians for Overweight and Obese Adults: Pilot Study. *JMIR MHealth UHealth* **2019**, *7*, e12289. [CrossRef] [PubMed]

51. Rollo, M.E.; Hutchesson, M.J.; Burrows, T.L.; Krukowski, R.A.; Harvey, J.R.; Hoggle, L.B.; Collins, C.E. Video Consultations and Virtual Nutrition Care for Weight Management. *J. Acad. Nutr. Diet.* **2015**, *115*, 1213–1225. [CrossRef] [PubMed]
52. Rollo, M.E.; Burrows, T.; Vincze, L.J.; Harvey, J.; Collins, C.E.; Hutchesson, M.J. Cost evaluation of providing evidence-based dietetic services for weight management in adults: In-person versus eHealth delivery. *Nutr. Diet.* **2018**, *75*, 35–43. [CrossRef] [PubMed]
53. DiFilippo, K.N.; Huang, W.H.; Andrade, J.E.; Chapman-Novakofski, K.M. The use of mobile apps to improve nutrition outcomes: A systematic literature review. *J. Telemed. Telecare* **2015**, *21*, 243–253. [CrossRef] [PubMed]
54. Vasiloglou, M.F.; Mougiakakou, S.; Aubry, E.; Bokelmann, A.; Fricker, R.; Gomes, F.; Guntermann, C.; Meyer, A.; Studerus, D.; Stanga, Z. A Comparative Study on Carbohydrate Estimation: GoCARB vs. Dietitians. *Nutrients* **2018**, *10*, 741. [CrossRef]
55. Bally, L.; Dehais, J.; Nakas, C.T.; Anthimopoulos, M.; Laimer, M.; Rhyner, D.; Rosenberg, G.; Zueger, T.; Diem, P.; Mougiakakou, S.; et al. Carbohydrate Estimation Supported by the GoCARB System in Individuals with Type 1 Diabetes: A Randomized Prospective Pilot Study. *Diabetes Care* **2017**, *40*, e6–e7. [CrossRef]
56. Rhyner, D.; Loher, H.; Dehais, J.; Anthimopoulos, M.; Shevchik, S.; Botwey, R.H.; Duke, D.; Stettler, C.; Diem, P.; Mougiakakou, S. Carbohydrate Estimation by a Mobile Phone-Based System Versus Self-Estimations of Individuals with Type 1 Diabetes Mellitus: A Comparative Study. *J. Med. Internet Res.* **2016**, *18*, e101. [CrossRef]
57. Dehais, J.; Anthimopoulos, M.; Shevchik, S.; Mougiakakou, S. Two-view 3D reconstruction for food volume estimation. *IEEE Trans. Multimed.* **2017**, *19*, 1090–1099. [CrossRef]
58. Anthimopoulos, M.; Dehais, J.; Shevchik, S.; Ransford, B.H.; Duke, D.; Diem, P.; Mougiakakou, S. Computer vision-based carbohydrate estimation for type 1 patients with diabetes using smartphones. *J. Diabetes Sci. Technol.* **2015**, *9*, 507–515. [CrossRef] [PubMed]
59. Reber, E.; Gomes, F.; Vasiloglou, M.F.; Schuetz, P.; Stanga, Z. Nutritional Risk Screening and Assessment. *J. Clin. Med.* **2019**, *8*, 1065. [CrossRef] [PubMed]
60. Harvey-Berino, J.; West, D.; Krukowski, R.; Prewitt, E.; VanBiervliet, A.; Ashikaga, T.; Skelly, J. Internet delivered behavioral obesity treatment. *Prev. Med.* **2010**, *51*, 123–128. [CrossRef] [PubMed]
61. Tate, D.F.; Valle, C.G.; Crane, M.M.; Nezami, B.T.; Samuel-Hodge, C.D.; Hatley, K.E.; Diamond, M.; Polzien, K. Randomized trial comparing group size of periodic in-person sessions in a remotely delivered weight loss intervention. *Int. J. Behav. Nutr. Phys. Act.* **2017**, *14*, 144. [CrossRef] [PubMed]
62. Tate, D.F.; Jackvony, E.H.; Wing, R.R. Effects of Internet behavioral counseling on weight loss in adults at risk for type 2 diabetes: A randomized trial. *JAMA* **2003**, *289*, 1833–1836. [CrossRef] [PubMed]
63. Tate, D.F.; Jackvony, E.H.; Wing, R.R. A randomized trial comparing human e-mail counseling, computer-automated tailored counseling, and no counseling in an Internet weight loss program. *Arch. Intern. Med.* **2006**, *166*, 1620–1625. [CrossRef] [PubMed]
64. Patel, M.L.; Hopkins, C.M.; Brooks, T.L.; Bennett, G.G. Comparing Self-Monitoring Strategies for Weight Loss in a Smartphone App: Randomized Controlled Trial. *JMIR Mhealth Uhealth* **2019**, *7*, e12209. [CrossRef] [PubMed]
65. Brandt, C.J.; Sogaard, G.I.; Clemensen, J.; Sondergaard, J.; Nielsen, J.B. Determinants of Successful eHealth Coaching for Consumer Lifestyle Changes: Qualitative Interview Study Among Health Care Professionals. *J. Med. Internet Res.* **2018**, *20*, e237. [CrossRef]
66. Chen, J.; Gemming, L.; Hanning, R.; Allman-Farinelli, M. Smartphone apps and the nutrition care process: Current perspectives and future considerations. *Patient Educ. Couns.* **2018**, *101*, 750–757. [CrossRef]
67. Rollo, M.E.; Collins, C.E.; MacDonald-Wicks, L. Evaluation of the Introduction of an e-Health Skills Component for Dietetics Students. *Telemed. J. e-Health* **2017**, *23*, 930–933. [CrossRef]
68. Apinaniz, A.; Cobos-Campos, R.; Saez de Lafuente-Morinigo, A.; Parraza, N.; Aizpuru, F.; Pérez, I.; Goicoechea, E.; Trápaga, N.; García, L. Effectiveness of randomized controlled trial of a mobile app to promote healthy lifestyle in obese and overweight patients. *Fam. Pract.* **2019**. [CrossRef] [PubMed]

# 4

# Nutritional Challenges in Metabolic Syndrome

**Irene Hoyas** [1] **and Miguel Leon-Sanz** [2,*]

1 Department of Endocrinology and Nutrition, University Hospital Doce de Octubre, 28041 Madrid, Spain
2 Medical School, University Complutense, 28040 Madrid, Spain
* Correspondence: miguelle@ucm.es or Mlshdoc@gmail.com

**Abstract:** Metabolic Syndrome (MetS) is a combination of risk factors for the development of cardiovascular disease (CVD) and type 2 diabetes. Different diagnostic criteria were proposed, but a consensus was reached in 2009 based on values of waist circumference, blood pressure, fasting glycemia, triglycerides, and high-density lipoprotein (HDL)-cholesterol levels. The main underlying etiologic factor is insulin resistance. The quality and quantity of individual macronutrients have an influence on the development and resolution of this syndrome. However, the main treatment goal is weight loss and a decrease in insulin resistance. A controlled energy dietary recommendation, together with moderate levels of physical activity, may positively change the parameters of MetS. However, there is no single dietary or exercise prescription that works for all patients. Dietary patterns such as Mediterranean-style, dietary approaches to stop hypertension (DASH), low-carbohydrate, and low-fat diets can ameliorate insulin resistance and MetS. Long-term adherence to a healthy lifestyle is key in assuring that individuals significantly reduce the risk of CVD and diabetes mellitus.

**Keywords:** metabolic syndrome; insulin resistance; dietary pattern; carbohydrates; fat

---

## 1. Introduction

Metabolic Syndrome (MetS) is a combination of risk factors for the development of cardiovascular disease (CVD) and type 2 diabetes (T2DM). It is very common and occurs in all regions of the world in populations with reduced physical activity and excessive energy intake. Age, sex, socioeconomic status, and ethnic background may change the prevalence, but it is estimated that 25–35% of adults may have MetS. The grouping of risk factors for CVD was firstly proposed 100 years ago but was progressively developed over many decades and received different names, such as syndrome X, insulin resistance syndrome, and the deadly quartet [1].

MetS was also defined in various ways over time by different organizations and expert groups. There are four common components present in the different definitions: obesity, abdominal adiposity or indicators of insulin resistance, impaired glucose metabolism, hypertension, and atherogenic dyslipidemia. The differences among the diverse definitions depend on the cut-off points needed to fulfil the diagnostic criteria and the requirement of the obligatory presence of specific features to meet the definition of MetS [2].

In 2009, six organizations, the International Diabetes Federation, the American Heart Association, the National Heart, Liver, and Blood Institute, the World Heart Federation, the International Atherosclerosis Society, and the International Association for the Study of Obesity, reached a consensus for the definition of MetS [3]. According to the consensus, MetS can be diagnosed if the patient has any three of the following:

- Elevated waist circumference: population- and country-specific cut-off points;
- Blood pressure: systolic > 130 and/or diastolic > 85 mmHg or drug treatment;
- Fasting glucose: >100 mg/dL (5.6 mmol/L) or drug treatment;

- Triglycerides: >150 mg/dL (1.7 mmol/L) or drug treatment;
- High-density lipoprotein (HDL)-cholesterol: <40 mg/dL (1 mmol/L) (male) or <50 mg/dL (1.3 mmol/L) (female) or drug treatment.

MetS is not a disease but a cluster of individual risk factors, whose main purpose is to identify individuals with increased risk of developing CVD and diabetes mellitus. MetS facilitates the early identification of patients with excessive adipose tissue and insulin resistance, despite the fact that not every person at risk who fulfils the criteria for MetS has insulin resistance and, on the contrary, not all persons with insulin resistance have MetS [4]. The diagnosis of MetS may be helpful in convincing patients about the importance of adopting therapeutic measures to correct the different components of this syndrome. Patients who fulfil the criteria of MetS have a two-fold increased risk of CVD, 1.5-fold increased risk of all-cause mortality, and three-fold increased risk of diabetes [5,6]. These estimates may differ slightly depending on the MetS criteria set used and the population where they are applied.

However, the definition of this syndrome does not include some relevant CVD risk factors, such as family history, smoking habit, age, gender, or low-density lipoprotein (LDL)-cholesterol. That may explain why MetS is a good prognostic estimation in the long term, but other risk calculators may be more precise for prognosis at less than 10 years. MetS could also indicate risks not accounted for in other CVD risk calculators. In certain instances, it can move the CVD risk of a patient upward, from low to intermediate risk, according to traditional risk calculators, such as ATP-III, SCORE, or Framingham risk score [7].

## 2. Therapeutic Approach to Metabolic Syndrome

Among other reasons, sedentary life and the easy access to inexpensive foods contribute to the explanation of why MetS is currently so prevalent. Its treatment aims to decrease the risks of CVD and T2DM. The first and most important step is the implementation of a new lifestyle with changes in diet and physical activity, as well as the acquisition of healthier habits. Weight loss and lifestyle changes may improve individual MetS components. Behavioral interventions make it easier for individuals to incorporate and maintain these changes in their daily routines.

Weight reduction was the main goal of most intervention studies. It is associated with significant improvements in all parameters of MetS. Even moderate weight loss (around 7%) resulted in substantial reductions in blood pressure, and glucose, triglyceride, and total cholesterol concentrations [8,9]. In addition, weight reduction improves adipokines and inflammation markers, such as adiponectin and tumor necrosis factor alpha concentrations [10].

A reasonable first goal for obese patients is to aim for weight loss of approximately 10% of baseline weight in six months. If they achieve this objective, insulin resistance will improve along with risk reduction of MetS and CVD. Even a lower weight loss, between 5% and 10%, improves the sensitivity to insulin between 30 and 60%, an effect greater than that seen with insulin-sensitizing drugs [11].

Considering all the therapeutic options, caloric restriction is a very effective intervention because most persons with this syndrome are obese and sedentary. Changes in physical activity are always part of lifestyle interventions for MetS, and current scientific evidence supports the role of exercise as an effective treatment strategy for the syndrome. Along with dietary changes, a program of regular physical activity also leads to a reduction in insulin resistance and CVD risk [12].

In this review, we focus on the nutritional component of MetS therapy. We analyze the contributions of the three macronutrients to the development and treatment of MetS. We do not cover issues related to micronutrients, sweeteners, or alcohol consumption.

## 3. Influence of Dietary Macronutrients in MetS

The role of each macronutrient present in the diet in the development and treatment of MetS was extensively studied and we review the current state of knowledge of their contributions to this syndrome.

### 3.1. Carbohydrates

After oral administration, absorption, gastrointestinal and pancreatic hormone secretion, liver metabolism, and visceral and muscular uptake, carbohydrates are responsible for blood glucose and insulin levels. They should not be regarded as a homogeneous component of foods. Overall, there are three types: starch or complex carbohydrates, sugars or simple carbohydrates, and fiber, with different repercussions on the glycemic response. The metabolic effects of foods containing carbohydrates can be partially predicted by their glycemic index (GI), which ranks foods containing carbohydrates according to how they change blood glucose levels, usually by comparing 50 g of any given food with a reference food such as white bread. When the GI is low (55 or less) that particular food causes a lower and slower increase in blood glucose and, therefore, insulin levels. Related to this index is the concept of glycemic load (GL), which combines both the quantity and quality of carbohydrates. If the carbohydrate content of 100 g of potato is 14 g and the GI is 85, the GL will be $85 \times 14/100 = 12$, more than double the GL of 100 g of an apple, which is 5. The GL concept allows comparison of blood glucose response to different types and amounts of foods [13,14]. The GI depends not only on the carbohydrate composition but also on other factors (the physical form of the food, amylose or amylopectin content, complete composition of the food, presence of fiber, cooking process, etc.) [15]. Despite its conceptual appeal, the utility of GI and GL in clinical practice is not widely recognized because of lack of impact on glycemic control [16].

It is accepted that an elevated intake of carbohydrates of high GI causes insulin resistance directly and contributes to the development of T2DM in persons with MetS [17,18]. Generally, foods with low GI are also more abundant in fiber. A diet rich in fiber showed a reduction in insulinemia by 10% and insulin resistance (by HOMA index) by 13% [19]. Fiber intake increases satiety and also reduces the risk of developing T2DM, and, in patients already diagnosed with this disease, viscous fiber supplements improve conventional markers of glycemic control beyond usual care and should be considered in its management [20]. However, fiber intake through foods that are naturally high in dietary fiber is better than fiber supplements, because natural foods also provide other substances such as micronutrients and phytochemicals.

Carbohydrate and lipid contents of diets have a mutual influence on their metabolism. Diets with low GI produce lower concentrations of fasting triglycerides and LDL-cholesterol [21]. It is interesting to emphasize that, when simple carbohydrates are consumed in a proportion lower than 20–25%, they do not modify the levels of plasma triglycerides. However, in obese patients with insulin resistance, the intake of simple carbohydrates stimulates the synthesis of fatty acids and inhibits endothelial and hepatic lipoprotein lipase, and in this way promotes hypertriglyceridemia and lowers HDL-cholesterol levels [22]. In a more positive manner, the effect of carbohydrates on the increase in plasma triglyceride levels is lower if fiber intake is high. Low-glycemic-index diets are, thus, recommended for patients with MetS [23,24], contributing to decreased CVD risk, and reduced levels of glycosylated hemoglobin in type 1 and 2 DM patients [25,26].

In the last two decades, we saw a growing interest in diets with low carbohydrate content or ketogenic diets. Initially, they were discredited because it was thought that the elevated lipid content would increase the risk of CVD. However, several landmark studies showed greater weight loss during the first six months of follow-up compared to conventional low-fat hypocaloric diets [27,28]. No statistically significant differences in weight loss were seen after 12 months of follow-up. Interestingly, with these ketogenic diets, triglyceride concentrations decrease, HDL-cholesterol levels increase markedly, and insulin sensitivity and glycosylated hemoglobin (HbA1c) improve. In those cases of high HbA1c, there is a greater reduction in HbA1c levels after carbohydrate restriction rather than after protein or lipid restriction [29].

Fructose is a simple carbohydrate that deserves particular comment. When absorbed, it does not stimulate the secretion of insulin or leptin. Long-term daily consumption leads to an increase in weight and a decrease in insulin sensitivity, favoring the development of MetS and type 2 diabetes [30], both in children and in adults [31]. Soft drinks contain large amounts of high-fructose corn syrup (HFCS) and sucrose and add greater amounts of simple carbohydrates to the daily diet. It was stated that moderate fructose consumption of ≤50 g/day or 10% of energy has no deleterious effect on lipid and glucose control, and ≤100 g/day does not influence body weight. Nevertheless, a higher intake is not recommended, and the intake of sugar-sweetened beverages should be limited or avoided [32].

### 3.2. Lipids

In humans, energy intake is made up of carbohydrates and lipids. However, lipids also have functional features and play an important role in the pathogenesis of atherosclerosis. The accepted range of lipid calories in the diet is very broad and is the opposite of carbohydrates. Therefore, low-lipid or low-carbohydrate diets contain very different total amounts of lipids. For all adults, the acceptable macronutrient distribution of total fat is to be 20–35% of total calorie intake [33].

The amount of fat can influence insulin sensitivity and the risk of developing type 2 diabetes only with intakes greater than 35–40% of total energy intake [34]. A diet that contains 20–40% fat does not change insulin sensitivity, regardless of its effect on weight [35].

However, lipids in the diet are a heterogeneous group, and quality is as important as quantity. Generally, we classify lipids as saturated, monounsaturated, and polyunsaturated fats (SFAs, MUFAs, and PUFAs, respectively). The consumption of high amounts of saturated fats and *trans* fatty acids is associated with an alteration in the action of insulin, while the intake of monounsaturated fats has the opposite effect. Therefore, the ratio of monounsaturated fatty acids/saturated fat is related to insulin sensitivity (Table 1). Along with these effects on insulin, diets enriched with MUFAs improve the lipid profile, because they reduce LDL-cholesterol and triglycerides, and elevate HDL-cholesterol levels [36–38]. Polyunsaturated fats are associated with a lower relative risk of 40% for developing type 2 diabetes. In studies that included patients with type 2 diabetes, substitution of SFAs by PUFAs and carbohydrates by MUFAs caused a decrease in insulin resistance. Moreover, ω-3 PUFAs can reduce triglyceride levels, improve hypertension, reduce inflammation, and diminish cardiovascular risk in diabetic patients [39–42]. It was recently reported that the intake of 2 g of icosapent ethyl twice daily with statin therapy is associated with less CVD morbidity and mortality but with slightly higher rates of hospitalization for atrial fibrillation and serious bleeding [43].

**Table 1.** Influence of diet on insulin sensitivity.

| Diet Component | Insulin Sensitivity |
|---|---|
| Total fatty acids (>40%) | (−) |
| Polyunsaturated fatty acids | (−) |
| *trans* Fatty acids | (−) |
| Monounsaturated fatty acids | (+) |
| Fiber cereal | (+) |
| Low glycemic index | (+) |
| Alcohol | (+) |
| Salt | (−) |
| Simple sugars (>20% energy) | (−) |
| Conjugated linoleic acid | (−) |

(+): Increases insulin sensitivity. (−): Decreases insulin sensitivity.

A diet low in fat and rich in simple carbohydrates, as was used in the CARMEN study, may increase insulin resistance (measured by HOMA) and is associated with a significant increase in triglyceride levels [44]. For some time, the American Diabetic Association (ADA) recommended that the sum of carbohydrates and monounsaturated fatty acids should represent 60–70% of the total energy in the diet. Nevertheless, since the ADA 2014 position statement, there is no "first-line" approach with respect to the optimal carbohydrate quantity in the diet plan, because evidence remains inconclusive [45]. On the other hand, in overweight or obese individuals, low-fat diets are equal to but no better than other weight-reducing diets when the goal is weight reduction [46].

A healthy pattern limits saturated and *trans* fats, added sugars, and sodium. The recommendation for the general population is to consume less than 10% of calories per day as added sugars and less than 10% of calories per day as saturated fats. In the Dietary Guidelines for Americans, it is advised that individuals eat as little dietary cholesterol as possible while consuming a healthy eating pattern. The cholesterol intake in a healthy United States (US)-style diet contains approximately 100 to 300 mg of cholesterol across the 12 calorie levels [47]. European guidelines recommend that foods rich in *trans* or saturated fats (hard margarines, tropical oils, fatty or processed meat, sweets, cream, butter, and regular cheese) should be replaced with monounsaturated fats (extra virgin olive oil) and polyunsaturated fats (non-tropical vegetable oils). In this way, it is assumed that *trans* fats will be <1.0% of total energy and saturated fat <10% (<7% in the presence of high plasma cholesterol values) [48].

### 3.3. Proteins

Proteins are associated with increased satiety and the preservation of lean body mass during weight loss, but their role in the dietary recommendations for patients with MetS is less clear.

Guidelines recommend a wide range of 10–35% of energy intake as digestible protein for adults, or a minimum of 0.8 g/kg body weight per day. Within this range, ADA position statements suggest that patients with diabetes and normal renal function should consume 15–20% of their energy intake as protein. However, they recognize that there is no definitive evidence for recommending an ideal amount of protein in relation either to glycemic control or for improving CVD risk factors [49].

Protein may have an incretin role. Its consumption is associated with higher insulin secretion, equivalent to that caused by eating the same amount of glucose. Some amino acids, such as leucine, lysine, or alanine, stimulate insulin secretion. In contrast, homocysteine can inhibit it [50,51].

There are several studies that propose hyperproteic diets in the management of MetS due to the satiating effect of proteins [52–54]. These diets also contribute to the preservation of lean mass. However, these diets may favor an increase in urinary calcium excretion and bone remodeling, and their use is not totally accepted [55]. Overall, these concerns seem a little overstated. High-protein diets do not seem to lead to calcium bone loss, and have no damaging effect on the kidney unless there is a pre-existing metabolic renal dysfunction.

## 4. Dietary Patterns

The most effective intervention for metabolic intervention is caloric restriction. Nutrition change to support a 7–10% weight loss is an appropriate goal for people with prediabetes, unless additional weight loss is desired for other purposes. The contributions of different nutrients to success in the reduction have to be seen in the context of the general eating plan of the patient. There is no perfect combination of macronutrients useful for all individuals. Compliance with a healthier lifestyle and dietary intake are more important than a particular dietary pattern. This represents an advantage for patients confronting MetS. As there is no "one-size-fits-all" pattern, individuals can advance with any healthy plan that is easy for them to follow. It also opens the door to adaptations of dietary recommendations based on metabolic goals, socioeconomic factors, food availability, and personal and cultural preferences. Irrespective of the macronutrient balance in the diet, total energy intake should be appropriate to accomplish the weight management goals.

Several nutrition patterns are effective in improving diabetes control, but the optimal macronutrient composition in meal planning in persons with MetS is less well defined. As previously seen, the main concern with regard to MetS is the development of diabetes and the associated cardiovascular risk. Patients with MetS have a similar benefit to overweight/obese patients with diabetes from the adoption of several dietary patterns. As already stated, the goal in both conditions is achieving weight loss. A short description of the characteristics of the different dietary patterns and their potential benefits was recently published [49]. Multiple studies analyzed the effectiveness of different patterns and confirmed the emphasis on compliance. Table 2 summarizes the main benefits of different dietary patterns regarding weight, glucose and lipid metabolism, and blood pressure.

**Table 2.** Metabolic syndrome improvement observed with different dietary patterns. DASH—Dietary approaches to stop hypertension; CVD—Cardiovascular disease; LDL-C—Low-density lipoprotein cholesterol; HDL-C—High-density lipoprotein cholesterol.

| Dietary Patterns | Main Reported Benefits | | | | | | |
|---|---|---|---|---|---|---|---|
| | ↓ Risk of Diabetes | ↓ A1c | ↓ Triglycerides | ↓ CVD | Weight Loss | ↓ LDL-C or HDL-C | ↓ Blood Pressure |
| Low fat [1] | X | | | | X | | |
| Very low fat [2] | | | | | X | | X |
| Low carbohydrate [3] | | X | | | X | X | X |
| Very low carbohydrate [4] | | X | X | | X | X | X |
| Mediterranean-style | X | X | X | X | | | |
| DASH | X | | | | X | | X |
| Vegetarian or vegan | X | X | | | X | X | |
| Paleo diet | Lack of evidence | | | | | | |
| Zone diet (40–30–30 diet) | | Lack of evidence | | | x | Lack of evidence | |
| Healthy Nordic diet | x | | | x | x | | |

The content of the table is derived from References [56–59]. X means there is proven evidence of the benefit; x indicates hypothetical evidence. "↓" represents a decrease and improvement in risk factor. [1] Low fat = fat intake < 30% of total calories; [2] very low fat = fat intake <10% of total calories; [3] low carbohydrate = carbohydrate intake 26–45% of total calories; [4] very low carbohydrate = carbohydrate intake < 26% of total calories.

With the exception of low-carbohydrate diets, common to many of these patterns is the emphasis on no starchy vegetables, the reduction of added sugars and refined grains, and the exclusion of processed foods to favor whole foods instead. Adoption of a Mediterranean-style diet rich in whole grain cereals, fruits, vegetables, nuts, and olive oil, compared to a prudent dietary pattern (50–60% of energy as carbohydrate and <30% as fat), was associated with improvements in endothelial function and significant reductions in the markers of systemic vascular inflammation in MetS patients after two years of follow-up [60,61]. The DASH (dietary approaches to stop hypertension) diet, rich in fruits, vegetables, and low-fat dairy food and low in saturated and total fat intake, demonstrated weight reduction and a significant reduction in blood pressure [62–64]. Mediterranean-style, vegetarian, and DASH eating patterns have a lower risk of developing type 2 diabetes [59]. Overall, the lower the provision of carbohydrates is, the lower the value of A1c hemoglobin is [65]. Weight loss or A1c reductions may be statistically significant but with small differences, with, for example, vegetarian diets, of 2 kg and 0.3%, respectively [66].

Low-fat diets are used as the control or default intervention vs. other dietary patterns. Their benefits seem to derive from weight loss rather than the eating pattern itself [67]. Interestingly, when low-carbohydrate diets are used, the specific distribution of fats and, particularly, the amount of saturated fat must be taken into account because, otherwise, it may be higher than that recommended for healthy individuals [68].

If we can call intermittent fasting a dietary pattern, different forms of intermittent fasting can lead to improved beta cell responsiveness, insulin sensitivity, and blood pressure control [69].

## 5. Conclusions

MetS is a cluster of risk factors that identifies patients at risk of developing diabetes mellitus and CVD. Nutrition therapy, as part of a comprehensive lifestyle intervention, may improve obesity and insulin resistance, which play key roles in its pathogenesis.

Macronutrients may contribute to worsening or improving MetS. An elevated intake of carbohydrates of high GI causes insulin resistance directly and has an impact on the development of T2DM in persons with MetS. In contrast, low-GI diets, more abundant in fiber, increase satiety and decrease insulin resistance and the risk of developing T2DM. Low-GI diets are, thus, recommended for patients with MetS. Diets enriched with MUFAs also improve the lipid profile and increase insulin sensitivity compared with SFAs. A healthy pattern limits saturated and *trans* fats, added sugars, and sodium. Specifically, the recommendation for the general population is to consume less than 10% of calories per day as added sugars and less than 10% of calories per day as saturated fats. Proteins in the diet are associated with increased satiety, insulin secretion, and preservation of lean body mass during weight loss, and hyperproteic diets are suggested for the management of MetS.

The effects of macronutrients are important; however, we consume them combined in eating patterns. Several dietary patterns may be helpful in reversing MetS, such as Mediterranean-style, vegetarian, DASH, low-carbohydrate, or even low-fat diets. The different patterns have variable effects on each risk factor, but all of them must be compatible with caloric restriction, which is the most effective intervention for metabolic intervention.

**Author Contributions:** Both authors contributed to the literature search, summarized the information, and wrote the review.

## References

1. Eckel, R.H.; Grundy, S.M.; Zimmet, P. The metabolic syndrome. *Lancet* **2005**, *365*, 1415–1428. [CrossRef]
2. Samson, S.L.; Garber, A.J. Metabolic Syndrome. *Endocrinol. Metab. Clin. N. Am.* **2014**, *43*, 1–23. [CrossRef] [PubMed]
3. Alberti, K.G.; Eckel, R.H.; Grundy, S.M.; Zimmet, P.Z.; Cleeman, J.I.; Donato, K.A.; Fruchart, J.C.; James, W.P.; Loria, C.M.; Smith, S.C., Jr.; et al. Harmonizing the metabolic syndrome: A joint interim statement of the International Diabetes Federation Task Force on Epidemiology and Prevention; National Heart, Lung, and Blood Institute; American Heart Association; World Heart Federation; International Atherosclerosis Society; and International Association for the Study of Obesity. *Circulation* **2009**, *120*, 1642–1645.
4. Kahn, R. Metabolic syndrome: Is it a syndrome? Does it matter? *Circulation* **2007**, *115*, 1806–1810. [CrossRef] [PubMed]
5. Ford, E.S. Risk for All-Cause Mortality, Cardiovascular Disease, and Diabetes Associated with the Metabolic Syndrome. A summary of the evidence. *Diabetes Care* **2005**, *28*, 1769–1778. [CrossRef] [PubMed]
6. Mottillo, S.; Filiion, K.B.; Genest, J.; Joseph, L.; Pilote, L.; Poirier, P.; Rinfret, S.; Schiffrin, E.L.; Eisenberg, M.J. The Metabolic Syndrome and Cardiovascular Risk. A systematic review and meta-analysis. *J. Am. Coll. Cardiol.* **2010**, *56*, 1113–1132. [CrossRef] [PubMed]
7. Blaha, M.J.; Bausal, S.; Rouf, R.; Golden, S.H.; Blumenthal, R.S.; Defilippis, A.P. A practical "ABCDE" approach of the metabolic syndrome. *Mayo Clin. Proc.* **2008**, *83*, 932–941. [CrossRef]
8. Case, C.C.; Jones, P.H.; Nelson, K.; Smith, E.O.; Ballantyne, C.M. Impact of weight loss on the metabolic syndrome. *Diabetes Obes. Metab.* **2002**, *4*, 407–414. [CrossRef]
9. Phelan, S.; A Wadden, T.; I Berkowitz, R.; Sarwer, D.B.; Womble, L.G.; Cato, R.K.; Rothman, R. Impact of weight loss on the metabolic syndrome. *Int. J. Obes.* **2007**, *31*, 1442–1448. [CrossRef]
10. Xydakis, A.M.; Case, C.C.; Jones, P.H.; Hoogeveen, R.C.; Liu, M.-Y.; Smith, E.O.; Nelson, K.W.; Ballantyne, C.M. Adiponectin, Inflammation, and the Expression of the Metabolic Syndrome in Obese Individuals: The Impact of Rapid Weight Loss through Caloric Restriction. *J. Clin. Endocrinol. Metab.* **2004**, *89*, 2697–2703. [CrossRef]
11. Nestel, P. Nutritional aspects in the causation and management of the metabolic syndrome. *Endocrinol. Metab. Clin. N. Am.* **2004**, *33*, 483–492. [CrossRef] [PubMed]
12. Katzmarzyk, P.T.; Leon, A.S.; Wilmore, J.H.; Skinner, J.S.; Rao, D.C.; Rankinen, T.; Bouchard, C. Targeting the Metabolic Syndrome with Exercise: Evidence from the HERITAGE Family Study. *Med. Sci. Sports Exerc.* **2003**, *35*, 1703–1709. [CrossRef] [PubMed]
13. Liu, S.; Willett, W.C.; Stampfer, M.J.; Hu, F.B.; Franz, M.; Sampson, L.; Hennekens, C.H.; E Manson, J. A prospective study of dietary glycemic load, carbohydrate intake, and risk of coronary heart disease in US women. *Am. J. Clin. Nutr.* **2000**, *71*, 1455–1461. [CrossRef] [PubMed]
14. Burger, K.N.; Beulens, J.W.; Boer, J.M.; Spijkerman, A.M. Dietary glycemic load and glycemic index and risk of coronary heart disease and stroke in Dutch men and women: The EPIC-MORGEN study. *PLoS ONE* **2011**, *6*, e25955. [CrossRef] [PubMed]

15. Sichieri, R.; Moura, A.S.; Genelhu, V.; Hu, F.; Willett, W.C. An 18-month randomized trial of a low-glycemic-index diet and weight change in Brazilian women. *Am. J. Clin. Nutr.* **2007**, *86*, 707–713. [CrossRef] [PubMed]
16. Wheeler, M.L.; Dunbar, S.A.; Jaacks, L.M.; Karmally, W.; Mayer-Davis, E.J.; Wylie-Rosett, J.; Yancy, W.S.J. Macronutrients, food groups, and eating patterns in the management of diabetes: A systematic review of the literature, 2010. *Diabetes Care* **2012**, *35*, 434–445. [CrossRef] [PubMed]
17. Jenkins, D.J.; Jenkins, A.L.; Wolever, T.M. Low glycemic index: Lente carbohydrates and physiological effects of altered food frequency. *Am. J. Clin. Nutr.* **1994**, *59*, 706–709. [CrossRef]
18. Schulze, M.B.; Liu, S.; Rimm, E.B.; Manson, J.E.; Willett, W.C.; Hu, F.B. Glycemic index, glycemic load, and dietary fiber intake and incidence of type 2 diabetes in younger and middle-aged women. *Am. J. Clin. Nutr.* **2004**, *80*, 348–356. [CrossRef] [PubMed]
19. Pereira, M.A.; Jacobs, D.R.; Pins, J.J.; Raatz, S.K.; Gross, M.D.; Slavin, J.L.; Seaquist, E.R. Effect of whole grains on insulin sensitivity in overweight hyperinsulinemic adults. *Am. J. Clin. Nutr.* **2002**, *75*, 848–855. [CrossRef]
20. Jovanovski, E.; Khayyat, R.; Zurbau, A.; Komishon, A.; Mazhar, N.; Sievenpiper, J.L.; Mejia, S.B.; Ho, H.V.T.; Li, D.; Jenkins, A.L.; et al. Should Viscous Fiber Supplements Be Considered in Diabetes Control? Results from a Systematic Review and Meta-analysis of Randomized Controlled Trials. *Diabetes Care* **2019**, *42*, 755–766. [CrossRef]
21. Jarvi, A.E.; Karlstrom, B.E.; Granfeldt, Y.E.; Bjorck, I.E.; Asp, N.G.; Vessby, B.O. Improved glycemic control and lipid profile and normalized fibrinolytic activity on a low-glycemic index diet in type 2 diabetic patients. *Diabetes Care* **1999**, *22*, 10–18. [CrossRef] [PubMed]
22. Fried, S.K.; Rao, S.P. Sugars, hypertryglyceridemia, and cardiovascular disease. *Am. J. Clin. Nutr.* **2003**, *78*, 873–880. [CrossRef] [PubMed]
23. McMillan-Price, J.; Petocz, P.; Atkinson, F.; O'Neill, K.; Samman, S.; Caterson, I.; Brand-Miller, J. Comparison of 4 diets of varying glycemic load on weight loss and cardiovascular risk reduction in overweight and obese young adults: A randomized controlled trial. *Arch. Intern. Med.* **2006**, *166*, 1466–1475. [CrossRef] [PubMed]
24. Horton, E.S. Effects of lifestyle changes to reduce risks of diabetes and associated cardiovascular risks: Results from large-scale efficacy trials. *Obesity* **2009**, *17*, S43–S48. [CrossRef] [PubMed]
25. Buyken, A.E.; Toeller, M.; Heitkamp, G.; Karamanos, B.; Rottiers, R.; Muggeo, M.; The Eurodiab Iddm Complications Study Group. Glycemic index in the diet of European outpatients with type 1 diabetes: Relations to glycated hemoglobin and serum lipids. *Am. J. Clin. Nutr.* **2001**, *73*, 574–581. [CrossRef] [PubMed]
26. Brand-Miller, J.; Hayne, S.; Petocz, P.; Colagiuri, S. Low-glycemic index diets in the management of diabetes. A meta-analysis of randomized controlled trials. *Diabetes Care* **2003**, *26*, 2261–2267. [CrossRef] [PubMed]
27. Samaha, F.F.; Iqbal, N.; Seshadri, P.; Chicano, K.L.; Daily, D.A.; McGrory, J.; Williams, T.; Williams, M.; Gracely, E.J.; Stern, L. A Low-Carbohydrate as Compared with a Low-Fat Diet in Severe Obesity. *New Engl. J. Med.* **2003**, *348*, 2074–2081. [CrossRef]
28. Stem, L.; Iqbal, N.; Seshadri, P.; Chicano, K. The effects of low-carbohydrate versus conventional weight loss diets in severely obese adults: One-year follow-up of a randomized trial. *ACC Curr. J. Rev.* **2004**, *13*, 18. [CrossRef]
29. Saslow, L.R.; Kim, S.; Daubenmier, J.J.; Moskowitz, J.T.; Phinney, S.D.; Goldman, V.; Murphy, E.J.; Cox, R.M.; Morán, P.; Hecht, F.M. A Randomized Pilot Trial of a Moderate Carbohydrate Diet Compared to a Very Low Carbohydrate Diet in Overweight or Obese Individuals with Type 2 Diabetes Mellitus or Prediabetes. *PLoS ONE* **2014**, *9*, e91027. [CrossRef]
30. Bray, G.A.; Nielsen, S.J.; Popkin, B.M. Consumption of high-fructose corn syrup in beverages may play a role in the epidemic of obesity. *Am. J. Clin. Nutr.* **2004**, *79*, 537–543. [CrossRef]
31. Dekker, M.J.; Su, Q.; Baker, C.; Rutledge, A.C.; Adeli, K. Fructose: A highly lipogenic nutrient implicated in insulin resistance, hepatic steatosis, and the metabolic syndrome. *Am. J. Physiol. Endocrinol. Metab.* **2010**, *299*, E685–E694. [CrossRef] [PubMed]
32. Rizkalla, S.W. Health implications of fructose consumption: A review of recent data. *Nutr. Metab.* **2010**, *7*, 82. [CrossRef] [PubMed]
33. Institute of Medicine. *Dietary Reference Intakes for Energy, Carbohydrate, Fiber, Fat, Fatty Acids, Cholesterol, Protein, and Amino Acids*; The National Academies Press: Washington, DC, USA, 2005.

34. Vessby, B.; Uusitupa, M.; Hermansen, K. Substituting dietary saturated fat for monounsaturated fat impairs insulin sensitivity in healthy men and women. *Diabetologia* **2001**, *44*, 312–319. [CrossRef] [PubMed]
35. Riccardi, G.; Giaccob, R.; Rivellese, A.A. Dietary fat, insulin sensitivity and the metabolic syndrome. *Clin. Nutr.* **2004**, *23*, 447–456. [CrossRef] [PubMed]
36. Rivellese, A.; Maffettone, A.; Vessby, B.; Uusitupa, M.; Hermansen, K.; Berglund, L.; Louheranta, A.; Meyer, B.J.; Riccardi, G. Effects of dietary saturated, monounsaturated and n-3 fatty acids on fasting lipoproteins, LDL size and post-prandial lipid metabolism in healthy subjects. *Atherosclerosis* **2003**, *167*, 149–158. [CrossRef]
37. Thomsen, C.; Rasmussen, O.; Lousen, T.; Holst, J.J.; Fenselau, S.; Schrezenmeir, J.; Hermansen, K. Differential effects of saturated and monounsaturated fatty acids on postprandial lipemia and incretin responses in healthy subjects. *Am. J. Clin. Nutr.* **1999**, *69*, 1135–1143. [CrossRef] [PubMed]
38. Rasmussen, B.M.; Vessby, B.; Uusitupa, M.; Berglund, L.; Pedersen, E.; Riccardi, G.; A Rivellese, A.; Tapsell, L.; Hermansen, K.; KANWU Study Group. Effects of dietary saturated, monounsaturated, and n-3 fatty acids on blood pressure in healthy subjects. *Am. J. Clin. Nutr.* **2006**, *83*, 221–226. [PubMed]
39. Meyer, B.J.; Lane, A.E.; Mann, N.J. Comparison of Seal Oil to Tuna Oil on Plasma Lipid Levels and Blood Pressure in Hypertriglyceridaemic Subjects. *Lipids* **2009**, *44*, 827–835. [CrossRef] [PubMed]
40. Dangardt, F.; Osika, W.; Chen, Y.; Nilsson, U.; Gan, L.-M.; Gronowitz, E.; Strandvik, B.; Friberg, P. Omega-3 fatty acid supplementation improves vascular function and reduces inflammation in obese adolescents. *Atherosclerosis* **2010**, *212*, 580–585. [CrossRef]
41. McEwen, B.; Morel-Kopp, M.C.; Tofler, G.; Ward, C. Effect of omega-3 fish oil on cardiovascular risk in diabetes. *Diabetes Educ.* **2010**, *36*, 565–584. [CrossRef]
42. Summers, L.K.; Fielding, B.A.; Bradshaw, H.A.; Ilic, V.; Beysen, C.; Clark, M.L.; Moore, N.R.; Frayn, K.N. Substituting dietary saturated fat with polyunsaturated fat changes abdominal fat distribution and improves insulin sensitivity. *Diabetologia* **2002**, *45*, 369–377. [CrossRef] [PubMed]
43. Bhatt, D.L.; Steg, P.G.; Miller, M.; Brinton, E.A.; Jacobson, T.A.; Ketchum, S.B.; Doyle, R.T., Jr.; Juliano, R.A.; Jiao, L.; Granowitz, C.; et al. REDUCEIT Investigators. Cardiovascular risk reduction with icosapent ethyl for hypertriglyceridemia. *N. Engl. J. Med.* **2019**, *380*, 11–22. [CrossRef] [PubMed]
44. Saris, W.H.M.; Astrup, A.; Prentice, A.M.; Zunft, H.J.F.; Formiguera, X.; De Venne, W.P.H.G.V.-V.; Raben, A.; Poppitt, S.D.; Seppelt, B.; Johnston, S.; et al. Randomized controlled trial of changes in dietary carbohydrate/fat ratio and simple vs complex carbohydrates on body weight and blood lipids: The CARMEN study. *Int. J. Obes.* **2000**, *24*, 1310–1318. [CrossRef]
45. Evert, A.B.; Boucher, J.L.; Cypress, M.; Dunbar, S.A.; Franz, M.J.; Mayer-Davis, E.J.; Neumiller, J.J.; Nwankwo, R.; Verdi, C.L.; Urbanski, P.; et al. Nutrition therapy recommendations for the management of adults with diabetes. *Diabetes Care* **2013**, *36*, 3821–3842. [CrossRef] [PubMed]
46. Pirozzo, S.; Summerbell, C.; Cameron, C.; Glasziou, P. Should we recommend low-fat diets for obesity? *Obes. Rev.* **2003**, *4*, 83–90. [CrossRef] [PubMed]
47. U.S. Department of Health and Human Service; U.S. Department of Agriculture. 2015–2020 Dietary Guidelines for Americans, 8th ed. Available online: https://health.gov/dietaryguidelines/2015/guidelines/ (accessed on 28 June 2019).
48. Catapano, A.L.; Graham, I.; De Backer, G.; Wiklund, O.; Chapman, M.J.; Drexel, H.; Hoes, A.W.; Jennings, C.S.; Landmesser, U.; Pedersen, T.R.; et al. 2016 ESC/EAS Guidelines for the Management of Dyslipidaemias: The Task Force for the Management of Dyslipidaemias of the European Society of Cardiology (ESC) and European Atherosclerosis Society (EAS). Developed with the special contribution of the European Association for Cardiovascular Prevention & Rehabilitation (EACPR). *Eur. Heart J.* **2016**, *37*, 2999–3058. [PubMed]
49. Evert, A.B.; Dennison, M.; Gardner, C.D.; Garvey, W.T.; Lau, K.H.K.; MacLeod, J.; Mitri, J.; Pereira, R.F.; Rawlings, K.; Robinson, S.; et al. Nutrition Therapy for Adults With Diabetes or Prediabetes: A Consensus Report. *Diabetes Care* **2019**, *42*, 731–754. [CrossRef] [PubMed]
50. Gannon, M.C. Effect of Protein Ingestion on the Glucose Appearance Rate in People with Type 2 Diabetes. *J. Clin. Endocrinol. Metab.* **2001**, *86*, 1040–1047. [CrossRef] [PubMed]
51. Patterson, S.; Flatt, P.; Brennan, L.; Newsholme, P.; McClenaghan, N. Detrimental actions of metabolic syndrome risk factor, homocysteine, on pancreatic β-cell glucose metabolism and insulin secretion. *J. Endocrinol.* **2006**, *189*, 301–310. [CrossRef] [PubMed]

52. Stentz, F.B.; Brewer, A.; Wan, J.; Garber, C.; Daniels, B.; Sands, C.; Kitabchi, A.E. Remission of pre-diabetes to normal glucose tolerance in obese adults with high protein versus high carbohydrate diet: Randomized control trial. *BMJ Open Diabetes Res. Care* **2016**, *4*, e000258. [CrossRef] [PubMed]
53. Leidy, H.J.; Clifton, P.M.; Astrup, A.; Wycherley, T.P.; Westerterp-Plantenga, M.S.; Luscombe-Marsh, N.D.; Woods, S.C.; Mattes, R.D. The role of protein in weight loss and maintenance. *Am. J. Clin. Nutr.* **2015**, *101*, 1320–1329. [CrossRef] [PubMed]
54. Sluik, D.; Brouwer-Brolsma, E.M.; Berendsen, A.A.M.; Mikkilä, V.; Poppitt, S.D.; Silvestre, M.P.; Tremblay, A.; Pérusse, L.; Bouchard, C.; Raben, A.; et al. Protein intake and the incidence of pre-diabetes and diabetes in 4 population-based studies: The PREVIEW project. *Am. J. Clin. Nutr.* **2019**, *109*, 1310–1318. [CrossRef] [PubMed]
55. Calvez, J.; Poupin, N.; Chesneau, C.; Lassale, C.; Tomé, D. Protein intake, calcium balance and health consequences. *Eur. J. Clin. Nutr.* **2012**, *66*, 281–295. [CrossRef] [PubMed]
56. Mithril, C.; Dragsted, L.; Meyer, C.; Blauert, E.; Holt, M.; Astrup, A. Guidelines for the New Nordic Diet. *Public Health Nutr.* **2012**, *15*, 1941–1947. [CrossRef] [PubMed]
57. Cheuvront, S.N. The Zone Diet phenomenon: A closer look at the science behind the claims. *J. Am. Coll. Nutr.* **2003**, *22*, 9–17. [CrossRef] [PubMed]
58. Fenton, T.R.; Fenton, C.J. Paleo diet still lacks evidence. *Am. J. Clin. Nutr.* **2016**, *104*, 844. [CrossRef]
59. Uusitupa, M.; Hermansen, K.; Savolainen, M.J.; Schwab, U.; Kolehmainen, M.; Brader, L.; Mortensen, L.S.; Cloetens, L.; Johansson-Persson, A.; Onning, G.; et al. Effects of an isocaloric healthy Nordic diet on insulin sensitivity, lipid profile and inflammation markers in metabolic syndrome—A randomized study (SYSDIET). *J. Intern. Med.* **2013**, *274*, 52–66. [CrossRef]
60. Esposito, K.; Marfella, R.; Ciotola, M.; Di Palo, C.; Giugliano, F.; Giugliano, G.; D'Armiento, M.; D'Andrea, F.; Giugliano, D. Effect of a Mediterranean-Style Diet on Endothelial Dysfunction and Markers of Vascular Inflammation in the Metabolic Syndrome. *JAMA* **2004**, *292*, 1440. [CrossRef]
61. Paniagua, J.A.; De La Sacristana, A.G.; Sánchez, E.; Romero, I.; Vidal-Puig, A.; Berral, F.J.; Escribano, A.; Moyano, M.J.; Peréz-Martinez, P.; López-Miranda, J.; et al. A MUFA-rich diet improves posprandial glucose, lipid and GLP-1 responses in insulin-resistant subjects. *J. Am. Coll. Nutr.* **2007**, *26*, 434–444. [CrossRef]
62. Lien, L.F.; Brown, A.J.; Ard, J.D.; Loria, C.; Erlinger, T.P.; Feldstein, A.C.; Lin, P.-H.; Champagne, C.M.; King, A.C.; McGuire, H.L.; et al. Effects of PREMIER Lifestyle Modifications on Participants with and without the Metabolic Syndrome. *Hypertension* **2007**, *50*, 609–616. [CrossRef]
63. Sacks, F.M.; Obarzanek, E.; Windhauser, M.M.; Svetkey, L.P.; Vollmer, W.M.; McCullough, M.; Karanja, N.; Lin, P.H.; Steele, P.; Proschan, M.A. Rationale and design of the Dietary Approaches to Stop Hypertension trial (DASH). A multicenter controlled-feeding study of dietary patterns to lower blood pressure. *Ann. Epidemiology* **1995**, *5*, 108–118. [CrossRef]
64. Obarzanek, E.; Sacks, F.M.; Vollmer, W.M.; Bray, G.A.; Miller, E.R.; Lin, P.-H.; Karanja, N.M.; Most-Windhauser, M.M.; Moore, T.J.; Swain, J.F.; et al. Effects on blood lipids of a blood pressureÂ–lowering diet: The Dietary Approaches to Stop hypertension (DASH) Trial. *Am. J. Clin. Nutr.* **2001**, *74*, 80–89.
65. Sainsbury, E.; Kizirian, N.V.; Partridge, S.R.; Gill, T.; Colagiuri, S.; Gibson, A.A. Effect of dietary carbohydrate restriction on glycemic control in adults with diabetes: A systematic review and metaanalysis. *Diabetes Res. Clin. Pract.* **2018**, *139*, 239–252. [CrossRef]
66. Viguiliouk, E.; Kendall, C.W.; Kahleov'a, H.; Rahelić, D.; Salas-Salvadó, J.; Choo, V.L.; Mejia, S.B.; Stewartm, S.E.; Leiter, L.A.; Jenkins, D.J.; et al. Effect of vegetarian dietary patterns on cardiometabolic risk factors in diabetes: A systematic review and meta-analysis of randomized controlled trials. *Clin. Nutr.* **2018**, *38*, 1133–1145. [CrossRef]
67. Wing, R.R.; Bolin, P.; Brancati, F.L.; Bray, G.A.; Clark, J.M.; Coday, M.; Evans, M.; Look AHEAD Research Group. Cardiovascular effects of intensive lifestyle intervention in type 2 diabetes. *N. Engl. J. Med.* **2013**, *369*, 145–154.
68. Tay, J.; Thompson, C.H.; Luscombe-Marsh, N.D.; Thompson, C.H.; Luscombe-Marsh, N.D.; Wycherley, T.P.; Noakes, M.; Buckley, J.D.; Wittert, G.A.; Yancy, W.S., Jr.; et al. Effects of an energy-restricted low-carbohydrate, high unsaturated fat/low saturated fat diet versus a high-carbohydrate, low-fat diet in type 2 diabetes: A 2-year randomized clinical trial. *Diabetes Obes. Metab.* **2018**, *20*, 858–871. [CrossRef]
69. Sutton, E.F.; Beyl, R.; Early, K.S.; Cefalu, W.T.; Ravussin, E.; Peterson, C.M. Early time-restricted feeding improves insulin sensitivity, blood pressure, and oxidative stress even without weight loss in men with prediabetes. *Cell Metab.* **2018**, *27*, 1212–1221. [CrossRef]

# 5

# Medical Nutrition Therapy in Critically Ill Patients Treated on Intensive and Intermediate Care Units

**Andrea Kopp Lugli [1,*], Aude de Watteville [2,†], Alexa Hollinger [3,†], Nicole Goetz [4] and Claudia Heidegger [2,*]**

1 Intensive Care Unit and Intermediate Care Unit, Intensive Care Medicine and Department of Anesthesiology, University Hospital Basel, 4031 Basel, Switzerland
2 Division of Intensive Care, Department of Acute Medicine, Geneva University Hospitals, 1205 Geneva, Switzerland
3 Intensive Care Unit and Intermediate Care Unit, Intensive Care Medicine and Department of Anesthesiology, University Hospital Basel, 4031 Basel, Switzerland
4 Endocrinology, Diabetes and Metabolism, University Hospital Basel, 4031 Basel & Department of Anesthesiology, University Hospital Basel, 4031 Basel, Switzerland
* Correspondence: andrea.kopplugli@usb.ch (A.K.L.); claudia.heidegger@hcuge.ch (C.H.)
† Equally contributed.

**Abstract:** Medical nutrition therapy in critically ill patients remains challenging, not only because of the pronounced stress response with a higher risk for complications, but also due to their heterogeneity evolving from different phases of illness. The present review aims to address current knowledge and guidelines in order to summarize how they can be best implemented into daily clinical practice. Further studies are urgently needed to answer such important questions as best timing, route, dose, and composition of medical nutrition therapy for critically ill patients and to determine how to assess and to adapt to patients' individual needs.

**Keywords:** nutritional support; medical nutrition therapy; intensive care unit; intermediate care unit; critically ill patients

---

## 1. Introduction

The critical importance, complexity, and challenge of clinical nutrition for critically ill patients is best understood when recapitulating the evolution of this complex patient group and, consequently, the proposed guidelines and clinical practice strategies during the last decades, as follows: (1) Adult critically ill patients present as a heterogeneous group with regard to diagnosis, severity of illness, and the number of (pre-)existing comorbidities. (2) Critically ill patients are treated not only on intensive care units (ICU), but increasingly in smooth transition on so-called step-down or intermediate care units (IMC-U) depending on the severity of illness, the available facilities, and hospital internal regulations. Still, these patients should not be systematically divided into separate categories. From a metabolic point of view, all patients requiring intensive or intermediate care suffer from a relevant catabolic stress response, which parallels the severity of injury or illness. From an institutional point of view, IMC-Us are relatively new facilities treating patients who require less care than standard intensive care, but more than that which is available from ward care [1]. Taking these two points into account, an overlap of IMC-U and ICU treatment is owed to the organization and available facilities of each individual hospital, as follows: Patients with the same severity of illness may be treated in one hospital on the ICU and in another hospital on the IMC-U. Since IMC-Us are an emerging type of treatment facility, IMC-U specific randomized clinical trials (RCTs) and guidelines are still missing and should be a field of future research. Therefore, patients in both of these groups are considered to be critically ill patients throughout this review article as their nutritional needs, first and foremost, parallel the course of illness and are not defined by the treating facility per se. (3) The ICU population suffers from a high prevalence of malnutrition when admitted to hospital (up to 60%) and during the intensive care treatment phase [2–5]. (4) The diagnosis of malnutrition and the assessment of nutritional needs are complex and ask for systematic re-evaluation and adaptation. (5) Some study data from recent years have highlighted the association between protein and caloric deficiency and higher morbidity and mortality rates [2,6–9]. These findings have introduced the conversion from "nutritional support" as an adjunctive care to "nutrition therapy", which not only covers micro- and macronutrient needs, but also intends to blunt the metabolic response, cellular injury, and immunological alteration. However, several further studies showed no clinical benefit [10–13] for higher protein and calorie administration in the ICU or reported harmful results, such as increased adjusted mortality at 6 months for mechanically ventilated patients [10] and less gastrointestinal tolerance in patients with acute lung injury [13]. Additionally, the idea of pharmaco-nutrition was abandoned after several neutral and one lethal trial [14–16]. On these grounds, the current European Society for Clinical Nutrition and Metabolism (ESPEN) guideline defines the term "medical nutrition therapy" (MNT), which encompasses oral nutritional supplements, enteral, and parenteral nutrition. Furthermore, ESPEN underlines the need for well conducted trials on optimal protein intake since currently available studies are not comparable in terms of patient selection and calorie and protein intake, as well as timing and route of administration. Yet, ESPEN evokes the possibility that it is possible that, similar to caloric targets, optimal protein targets change over time in the ICU and that a high protein intake is only beneficial if not associated with overfeeding [17]. However, so far this hypothesis is not yet confirmed by RCTs.

To date, nutritional practices are widely diverse [18] and many studies, reviews, and guidelines address only one or some of the relevant aspects of MNT [7,17,19–47]. The ESPEN guidelines [17] and those of the American Society on Parenteral and Enteral Nutrition (ASPEN) [27], as well as the Canadian Critical Care Practice Guidelines (CCPG) [48], are among the most regularly updated evidence-based guidelines. All three underline the relevance of the points stated above and the need for further carefully planned randomized trials. The present review aims to address current knowledge and guidelines in order to summarize how they can best be implemented into daily clinical practice. We specified the different guidelines' recommendation grades. The ESPEN guidelines use standard operation procedure (grade A, B, 0, or good practice point (GPP)) [49] and the ASPEN guidelines grade the study evidence level, from high to very low for RCTs and low to very low for observational studies; the good practice statement is ungraded [50].

## 2. Screening

A high prevalence of malnutrition is observed at ICU admission [5], with a further energy and protein deficit (50% and 60%, respectively) occurring during ICU stay [51,52]. Indeed, an international multicenter observational study revealed an association between the increase of energy and protein intake and the decrease of mortality in patients with a body mass index (BMI) <25 or >35 kg/m$^2$ [6]. The same research group failed to validate this concept in the TOP-UP trial [53]. More generally, no nutritional intervention reduced mortality in critically ill patients, except withholding early glutamine in patients with multiorgan failure [14].

On the other hand, some recent RCTs investigating the timing of initiation as well as the quantity and the route of MNT showed contradictory results [7,54–57]. Waiting for more conclusive studies, actual guidelines suggest that all critically ill patients should be routinely screened with the aim of preventing malnutrition [17,27].

Many different screening tools to identify the malnutrition risk are available. Some scores are widely used, such as (1) the Nutrition Risk Screening (NRS) 2002 [58], focusing on nutritional state, illness severity, and age; (2) the Nutrition Risk in the Critically Ill (NUTRIC) score [59], including a severity score, comorbidities, and the number of hospital days; (3) the Subjective Global Assessment (SGA), combining historical data and a clinical examination [60]; and (4) the Mini-Nutrition Assessment (MNA) [61], which is specific for the elderly population. Despite the large number of existing scores, none has been validated for the critically ill thus far [62] and none have been able to identify patients who improve with enhanced feeding.

Laboratory data, such as albumin and pre-albumin, are frequently used as markers of nutritional status, but cannot be clearly interpreted during critical illness, as low albumin and prealbumin levels occur as a response to increased inflammation [63].

Weight changes are also difficult to interpret considering the relevant amounts of fluid administration and depletion during the ICU and IMC-U stay. Thus, weight loss does not reflect loss of lean body mass. Nevertheless, this aspect is an important issue for the detection of malnutrition, as the loss of lean body mass has been associated with longer hospitalization and reduced quality of life and functional abilities [60]. Some methods, such as ultrasound [64] or computerized tomography (CT) scan [65], are promising tools that can help to determine the extent of lean body mass loss. However, these methods still need to be validated in clinical practice. Moreover, the way in which they influence therapy is not yet clear. Bioelectrical impedance to assess body composition and lean body mass may be useful, but its interpretation is complicated by important fluid changes that occur in the critically ill [66].

Concerning these screening tools, ASPEN [27] and ESPEN [17] have taken different positions. While the current ASPEN guidelines recommend using either the NRS 2002 or the NUTRIC-Score for nutritional risk determination [27], the new ESPEN guidelines propose a more general clinical assessment including anamnesis, evaluation of muscle mass and strength, unintentional weight loss, and body composition (GPP). Furthermore, all critically ill patients with a length of stay of more than 48 h should be considered at risk for malnutrition (GPP) [17].

## 3. Assessment of Medical Nutrition Therapy

### 3.1. *Energy Needs*

It is extremely challenging to assess energy requirements of the critically ill, as the requirements depend on many factors and may be dynamic over time [67].

Initially, critical illness provokes an acute early phase [17] characterized by a major metabolic instability with hypermetabolism, insulin resistance, glycemia perturbation, and increased catabolism with the production of endogenous substrates [68]. This is followed by an acute late period with a certain degree of stabilization but persistent catabolism. Finally, when the inflammatory state and critical conditions decrease, the late phase or chronic phase sets in, with the beginning of anabolism and rehabilitation [43]. Moreover, energy expenditure (EE) is also modulated by many other conditions such as underlying illness, inflammatory state, medications, body composition, and nutritional status prior to admission [67].

While predictive formulas to estimate EE are widely used for MNT, many studies have shown them to be inaccurate and imprecise [69–72]. Up to now, no predictive equation has been validated for the critically ill [17,27]. If predictive formulas are used, hypocaloric MNT (<70% of the estimated EE) should be preferred over isocaloric nutrition during the first week of the ICU and IMC-U stay in order to avoid overnutrition [17].

For some time, the ESPEN guidelines have recommended the use of indirect calorimetry (IC) to determine EE as the best standard practice [73,74]. This attitude is reiterated in the current ASPEN (grade very low) and ESPEN guidelines (grade B) [17,27]. Furthermore, the ESPEN guidelines suggest that if IC is used, an isocaloric nutrition can be progressively implemented after the early phase of acute illness (grade 0). However, during the early phase of acute illness, hypocaloric nutrition (not exceeding 70% of EE) should be administered (grade B). Still, the exact way to use IC measurements to guide MNT needs to be validated by further studies.

The IC measurement is based on $O_2$ and $CO_2$ concentrations as well as the volume of expired gas/minute [67]. The EE is then calculated directly by the calorimeter according to the Weir's equation [75]. This measurement can be performed either in mechanically ventilated or spontaneously breathing patients. Measurements are influenced by several factors such as medications, stress, body temperature, mechanical ventilation, agitation, etc. [76,77]. The currently available IC devices are expensive, time consuming, and not always accurate; thus, IC measurements cannot be performed regularly. The International Multicentric Study Group for Indirect Calorimetry (ICALIC) recently developed a new IC aimed at meeting clinical needs [67].

The ICALIC study group suggests IC measurements on day 3 to 4 after admission [67], which should be repeated as soon as clinical conditions change. They suggest adapting energy targets to the result of the last IC measurement with the aim of optimizing nutritional management [67].

If IC is not available, energy expenditure calculated from the carbon dioxide production (VCO2) extracted from the ventilator or oxygen consumption (VO2) from pulmonary arterial catheter are recommended by the new ESPEN guidelines [17]. However, these methods were not shown to be accurate compared to IC measurements [78–80] and can only be obtained with invasive monitoring.

*3.2. Protein Needs*

Although the coverage of energy needs is an area that has been studied for several years, the importance of the protein needs has only recently become a subject of focus. Indeed, critical illness causes protein catabolism resulting in important muscle loss, which influences a patient's survival and clinical outcome [81]. Current recommendations on protein intake for critically ill patients are based mainly on observational data and only a few RCTs having different designs. Thus, it is difficult to draw definitive conclusions.

Various recent observational studies have focused on the association between protein intake and patients' clinical outcomes, suggesting an association between mortality reduction and protein intake [82–84]. For instance, decreased mortality has been related to protein intake ≥1.2 g/kg/day in non-septic and non-overfeed critically ill patients [84] by achieving ≥80% of the prescribed protein intake [82] and to a protein intake of >1 g/kg/day [83].

Conversely, recent RCTs on protein needs have shown contradictory results and up-to-date no mortality benefit with higher amino acid intake could be shown by RCTs. In the Ferrie study ($n$ = 120), the administration of 1.2 g/kg parenteral amino acids (AA) compared to 0.8 g/kg was associated with attenuated muscle wasting, less fatigue, and better nitrogen balance, but no difference in mortality or length of stay was observed [85].

The Nephro-Protective trial ($n$ = 474), with higher AA administration in the intervention group, did not affect the duration of renal dysfunction but only showed an improved estimated glomerular filtration rate (eGFR) and daily urinary output. Furthermore, serum urea was significantly higher, with a trend toward increased renal replacement therapy (RTT) in patients receiving AA therapy, which was not present after controlling for baseline imbalance in terms of renal failure at the time of study enrollment [86].

Other recent RCTs, such as the EAT-ICU ($n$ = 203) and the TOP-UP trial ($n$ = 125) on protein needs, have confirmed no differences on clinical outcomes including mortality, hospital stay, days of ventilation, nosocomial infections, or organ failure rates [53,56]. However, the EAT-ICU trial also showed a prolonged ICU length of stay (post-hoc analysis) as well as a trend to increased plasma urea levels in the Early Goal-directed Nutrition group [56].

The EPaNIC trial ($n$ = 4640) showed that early initiation of parenteral nutrition (PN) was associated with a longer course of RTT and a longer ICU stay. Similar functional status was observed in the early and late PN group [54]. A prospectively planned subanalysis of the EPaNIC trial found an increased incidence of ICU-acquired muscle weakness with slower recovery in the early-PN group [87]. Apart from this, in another post hoc analysis of the EPaNIC trial, delayed recovery was also attributed to the early administration of amino acids by PN [88].

The results of the recent RCTs underline the urgent need for further studies to provide answers to questions still outstanding, such as the right amount of protein to administer and the best timing.

Based on the available results and without the possibility to assess individual protein needs during a protein-loss phase, ESPEN guidelines [17] suggest a progressive provision of 1.3 g/kg/day of protein equivalent during critical illness (grade 0). In contrast, the ASPEN guidelines [27] propose a protein intake of 1.2–2.0 g/kg/day (grade very low).

Exercise in combination with achieving protein targets has also been suggested to maximally maintain muscle mass [17,89,90].

## 4. Practical Implementation

### 4.1. Special Risk Groups

A few distinct patient subgroups, consisting of critically ill surgical and medical patients at particular risk for malnutrition, are defined and discussed below.

#### 4.1.1. Obese and Bariatric Patients

One steadily growing sub-population consists of patients who are already metabolically challenged (i.e., diabetic, severely obese, and post-bariatric/obese surgery patients) [91].

As the number of bariatric operations increases, one must keep in mind that approximately 30% of bariatric patients develop nutritional complications [91]. Furthermore, the proportion of obese critically ill patients is growing parallel to the increasing prevalence in the general population [92]. The ASPEN guidelines suggest to additionally focus the nutritional assessment of these patients on biomarkers of metabolic syndrome, evaluation of comorbidities, and the level of inflammation [27].

In order to estimate patient nutritional needs, resting EE is best assessed by IC [20]. If not available, energy intake can be guided by adjusted body weight (BW) and protein delivery by urinary nitrogen losses or lean body mass determination (using CT or other tools), according to the ESPEN guidelines [17].

Several existing predictive scores, such as the Mifflin-St Jeor (MSJ) and the Harris–Benedict equations [93,94], can be applied if IC is not available in the case of complicated bariatric patients [20,94]. However, it is important to consider that these scores are not specifically validated for post-bariatric patients and IC is recommended in the first place [17].

The ESPEN guidelines recommend an isocaloric high protein diet including a protein intake of 1.3 g/kg adjusted BW/day (GPP) [17]. On the other hand, the ASPEN guidelines [27] suggest a hypocaloric high-protein feeding protocol, with 65%–70% of measured energy requirements using IC or weight-based equations (calories: BMI 30–50 kg/m$^2$ = 11–14 kcal/kg actual BW/day, BMI > 50 kg/m$^2$ = 22–25 kcal/kg ideal BW/day; protein: BMI 30–40 kg/m$^2$ = 2 g/kg ideal BW/day, BMI ≥ 40 kg/m$^2$ = 2.5/kg ideal BW/day), for all classes of obesity.

In order to avoid micronutrient (iron, calcium, vitamin D, vitamin $B_{12}$, folate) deficiency after bariatric surgery, life-long multivitamin supplementation is necessary for post-bariatric patients. Since many patients show malabsorption for iron, a documented deficiency is best supplemented intravenously [91].

#### 4.1.2. Geriatric Patients

Patients aged ≥65 years comprise a large portion of the critically ill population and often struggle with nutritional intake and risk of malnutrition. In the ICU and IMC-U setting, additional acute illness on top of an already frail state often leads to poor outcomes [95]. The assessment of the frailty score in this subgroup might be a valuable addition to malnutrition screening [21].

A state of sarcopenia in acutely ill elderly patients is associated with increased short-term mortality [22]. The course of elderly patients according to their nutritional status (BMI and albumin levels) was evaluated and resulted in a higher prognostic value than their absolute age [23].

However, a recent review emphasized the importance of additional parameters such as energy intake, weight loss, and grip strength, whereas biochemical markers were susceptible to the underlying disease process and were not always reliable [96].

Swallowing and chewing problems may be an important issue affecting oral intake in geriatric patients. Therefore, smaller and more frequent meals completed by oral nutritional supplements (ONS) are suggested [96]. Evaluation of swallowing, dental status, oral health, and potential drug side effects that might impair oral feeding should be conducted systematically [95].

About 20% of older critically ill patients have sarcopenia before hospitalization [22,97] and are subjected to various antianabolic and procatabolic factors during critical illness. An ESPEN expert working group recommends 1.2–1.5 g protein/kg/day in elderly patients suffering or at risk for malnutrition, since they have acute or chronic illness. Even higher protein intakes are recommended for this patient population in case of severe illness or injury [98]. In a recent review of older ICU patients, besides the provision of at least 1.2–1.5 g protein/kg usual BW/day, a combination including regular and early ambulation (if possible) and/or physical therapy and follow-up rehabilitation are prudently recommended to counteract muscle loss [97]. These recommendations are based on observational data or studies in non-critically ill patients [99,100]. Therefore, this review acknowledges the need of further research to consolidate the most efficacious in-unit and post-discharge nutrition and physical activity strategies with well conducted clinical trials [97].

Vitamin D deficiency is common in the elderly and the critically ill and is associated with increased mortality. According to the 2019 ESPEN guidelines, vitamin D can be supplemented (GPP) with a single dose of 500,000 IU vitamin D3 within one week after admission (grade 0) in case of measured low plasma levels (25-hydroxy vitamin D <12.5 ng/mL, or <50 nmol/L) [17].

#### 4.1.3. Other Risk Groups

With the development of advanced medicine, the new patient group of so-called chronic critically ill patients has emerged and is often treated in the step-down unit. A recent review provides a thorough discussion of the nutritional approach for these patients [101]. The ASPEN guidelines, based on expert consensus, define chronic critically ill patients as having persistent organ dysfunction requiring ICU treatment >21 days and suggest management with aggressive high-protein EN therapy and, when feasible, use of a resistance exercise program [27].

Patients with renal failure can be placed on a standard enteral formula following the recent ICU recommendations for protein administration [17,27]. According to the ASPEN guidelines, a special formula might be indicated in case of significant electrolyte or volume abnormalities. Renal replacement therapy may require increased protein support (≤2.5 g/kg/day) (grade very low) and adapted micronutrient support [17,27]. Importantly, protein support should not be restricted in order to avoid or delay initiation of dialysis therapy [27].

The ESPEN Society provides separate nutritional management recommendations for severe burn patients [102] and for patients with acute or chronic liver failure [103].

Patients with alcohol abuse are particularly at risk for thiamine deficiency, as are patients with severe sepsis, congestive heart failure, or burn injuries [104]. Recommended daily doses for alcoholic patients are substantially higher than for non-alcoholic patients, reaching up to 500 mg thiamine three times daily [105]. Another review underlines the importance of additive therapies such as correction of electrolyte disturbances and malnourishment [106].

### *4.2. International Guidelines on Nutrition in Critically Ill Patients*

In this review on most recent practices to provide adequate nutrition in the critically ill, we concentrated on three widely used and regularly updated international guidelines issued by the Canadian Critical Care Society/Canadian Critical Care Trials Group (CCCS/CCCTG) [48] in 2015, by ASPEN [27] in 2016, and, most recently, by ESPEN [17]. These three guidelines discuss main and subtopics of critical care nutrition in which most recommendations are based on expert consensus

(Table S1). As such, ESPEN guidelines include the most recent studies and meta-analyses from robust RCTs. Moreover, recommendations have been well separated into grade A, B, level 0, or GPP, according to the strength of the evidence [107]. The ASPEN guidelines include the largest number of recommendations, whereas certain aspects of the guidelines are not exclusively covered by the European and Canadian societies (ESPEN; CCCS/CCTG) (e.g., non-intubated patients (ESPEN), ornithine ketoglutarate in burn patients or specific mentioning of vitamin C supplementation (CCCS/CCTG), or recommendation on insulin administration (ESPEN; CCCS/CCTG). Many recommendations in the ASPEN guidelines target a certain group of critically ill, whereas the ESPEN and CCCS/CCCTG guidelines address the critically ill in general (e.g., vitamin D supplementation). Notably, ASPEN proposes a higher number of recommendations for subgroups of critically ill patients by labelling with a grade of expert consensus due to the lack of solid evidence. Moreover, the concept of ALI (acute lung injury), not part of the 2013 Berlin definition of acute respiratory distress syndrome (ARDS), is not mentioned in the ESPEN guidelines [28]. ASPEN and ESPEN offer recommendations for frequent diseases seen in critical care, such as sepsis and acute pancreatitis and statements for trauma and burn patients. In addition, the American society includes a chapter on end-of-life care.

### *4.3. Medical Nutrition Therapy: EN, PN, ONS, and Combinations*

Routes, quantity, and timing of nutritional delivery have been widely discussed over recent decades. With the increasing administration of parenteral nutrition (PN) to the critically ill, some studies have shown more infectious complications in comparison to enteral nutrition (EN) [29,30]. Enteral feeding was subsequently used in first line with an important reduction in the use of PN [108]. However, achieving energy and protein targets with EN alone is difficult during the ICU and IMC-U stay and may result in undernutrition in most patients [31,32]. Recent RCTs have shown no increase in the rate of complications independent of the chosen route of nutrition [57,109]. Avoiding under- or overnutrition is more important than the feeding route [108].

The SPN study ($n = 305$) showed that the use of supplemental parenteral nutrition (SPN) (when EN was insufficient to match the energy targets at day 4 after ICU admission) could reduce nosocomial infections after the end of the intervention and until the end of the observation period (days 9 to 28), as well as antibiotic use during the ICU stay [7]. However, no impact on infections was shown when counting the infection rate from the randomization day onward. The TICACOS pilot study ($n = 130$) [55] showed, based on prospective intention to treat analysis of the data, that IC-guided nutrition therapy provoked an increase in complications with more infections, longer duration of ventilation, and prolonged ICU stays. A per protocol analysis, on the contrary, suggested a short-lived survival benefit [55].

Some other studies (e.g., EAT-ICU ($n = 203$) [56], TARGET ($n = 3957$) [11], EDEN ($n = 1000$) [13]) showed no difference between the early versus standard initiation groups in primary clinical outcomes, but secondary outcomes revealed hyperglycemia [13,56] and decreased gastric tolerance [11,13] in the early nutrition intervention group. The PermiT trial ($n = 894$) group studied permissive underfeeding (40–60% of calculated caloric requirements) compared to standard enteral feeding (70–100%) with similar protein intake. The results showed no difference in 90-day mortality and no differences in other significant outcomes between the groups [12]. The results of the EPaNIC trial ($n = 4640$) revealed no difference in 90-day mortality but an increased complication rate with early initiation of parenteral support (i.e., infections, longer mechanical ventilation, and length of stay) [54].

The divergence of results may be related to the heterogeneous patient population and highly variable study designs with differences such as the amount of calories administered, the timing of EN or PN initiation, and the use of IC or predictive formulas.

Considering these contradictory findings, expert guidelines agree on the following indications for MNT [17,27]: (1) Oral nutrition should be preferred over EN or PN in patients able to eat voluntarily (GPP). (2) If needed, oral nutritional supplements (ONS) can be given with the aim to achieve energy and protein needs [34]. (3) Early EN (within 48 h) is suggested for all patients with a functional digestive tract who cannot eat voluntarily (grade B). Enteral feeding can be performed progressively after the early phase of the critical illness and, after 3 days, caloric delivery can be increased up to 80–100% of the measured EE (grade 0). (4) In patients who do not tolerate full EN during the first week, initiation of SPN should be considered on a case-by-case basis and should only be started after all strategies to maximize EN tolerance have been attempted (GPP). (5) In case of impossible oral feeding and EN contraindications, PN must also be started progressively during the first week of the ICU stay.

The timing of PN initiation is a highly debated topic. ESPEN experts propose an early implementation of PN within 3–7 days in case of contraindications to oral feeding or EN (grade B). SPN should be considered for patients who do not tolerate full-dose EN during the first week of ICU or IMC-U stay (GPP). In contrast, the ASPEN guidelines recommend SPN in case of insufficient early EN (<60% of energy and protein requirements) only after 7–10 days. Further, the ESICM guidelines extensively discuss clinical states and medications that warrant delayed EN initiation [17,27,110].

### 4.4. *Adaptation/Reassessment and Monitoring*

Monitoring is an essential part of nutritional management and is central to achieving high-quality nutritional care. The quantity of prescribed and received nutrition in terms of volume, energy, and protein must be assessed including non-nutritional calories (e.g., Propofol®, citrate) [35] in order to avoid under- or overfeeding. Gastric tolerance must be monitored, including clinical abdominal examination and evaluation of stools, gastric residual volume, or vomit [111]. Laboratory monitoring of glycemia, electrolytes, liver parameters, and triglycerides is necessary to assess MNT tolerance [35]; prealbumin can be helpful to assess the efficacy of the MNT [36].

### 4.5. *Role of the Intensive Care Unit Dietician*

Even if nutritional guidelines and local protocols have been shown to be helpful in standardizing and improving the quality of MNT in ICUs [37,38], physicians and nurses have reported a lack of knowledge, training, and time in nutrition management [39,40]. Dieticians, specialized in ICU nutrition, can provide valuable help concerning nutrition management for the ICU teams. It was suggested that the presence of dieticians in the ICU team was helpful to achieve the desired daily energy and protein targets during the ICU stay [39]. Their role should also include detection of too early aggressive nutrition support with the aim to prevent refeeding and overfeeding. To increase the quality of the care, we recommend working in a multidisciplinary team including intensivists, ICU nutritional specialists, dieticians, nurses, physiotherapists, and others if necessary. In addition, regular adaptation of local protocols to the current guidelines and facilitating protocol adherence is necessary [41]. These efforts should be extended to patients on the IMC-U.

### 4.6. *Continuation of Medical Nutrition Therapy After Transfer or Discharge to Home*

MNT is not only important during ICU/IMC-U stay, it is an essential part of both the post-ICU/IMC-U recovery phase and after hospital discharge [43]. While advances in medicine and improvements in the quality of care have reduced ICU mortality in recent years, the number of post-critically ill patients in rehabilitation has consequently increased [112]. Low oral intake (e.g., only 700 kcal/day for one week after extubation) has been reported to be an amount insufficient to cover the energy needs of 97% of patients [42,76]. In this context, most critically ill patients would need continuous medium-length or long-term MNT (ONS, EN, PN, and SPN) coupled with exercise for rehabilitation. MNT can also be continued at home after hospital discharge. However, it is also important to consider the physical and mental abilities of patients and their relatives, in addition to the patient's living conditions, with the aim of achieving a supportive environment [44]. Educating the patient and his/her close relatives should be proposed to achieve the highest level of independence possible [44]. Follow up involving a multidisciplinary nutrition team helps to increase the quality of care, facilitating the adaptation of the therapy and the support in case of possible complications [44].

## 5. Complications

### 5.1. Over- and Underfeeding

Over- and underfeeding frequently occur in critical care patients as nutritional substrates, whether given parenterally or enterally, do not have the same metabolic consequences in the critically ill. While overfeeding occurs more often with PN, underfeeding is more common in enterally fed patients. Patients most at risk for energy excess or nutritional deficits are those with low caloric targets (e.g., due to small body size, non-nutritional energy (e.g., Propofol® for sedation) or geriatric patients) [113].

Overfeeding is defined as the administration of excess energy in relation to the body's need to maintain metabolic homeostasis when exceeding >110% of the EE [17] and can lead to a multitude of complications and increased mortality. Depending on the macro-nutrients delivered in excess, these complications include hypercapnia, refeeding syndrome (RFS) and liver disturbances, hyperglycemia and hypertriglyceridemia, as well as azotemia, hypertonic dehydration, and metabolic acidosis [114]. Therefore, higher protein amounts (1.3 g/kg/day) can be delivered progressively as long as these amounts are not associated with overfeeding (grade 0) [17].

The lower limit of optimal energy supplementation to the critically ill is not yet clearly defined and may vary depending on the underlying disease and nutritional status of the patient. Underfeeding (<70% of the defined target) [17] often occurs during EN due to feeding intolerance, airway management, or disruption of feeding due to elective procedures [115].

### 5.2. Refeeding Syndrome

RFS is recognized as a life-threatening cause-independent complication in severely malnourished patients. These patients may show severe adverse reactions involving the cardiac, respiratory, hematological, hepatic, and neuromuscular systems when refed too rapidly, especially with carbohydrates [46]. The difficulty to precisely define RFS limits screening and estimated numbers of unreported cases are presumably high. Therefore, assessing the risk of RFS before starting MNT in high-risk patients [46,47], including those with anorexia nervosa, chronic alcoholics, elderly patients with multiple comorbidities, patients with signs of chronic malnutrition (e.g., marasmus, severe inflammatory bowel disease, short bowel syndrome), the morbidly obese, and patients receiving PN, has been suggested [47]. Furthermore, an algorithm for RFS management has been proposed, including an initial risk assessment and recommendations for electrolyte and fluid repletion [116,117]. However, a more recent retrospective study [118] in critically ill patients with prolonged ventilation found no baseline characteristics predicting RFS. Patients developing RFS had a reduced 6-month mortality risk when receiving low caloric intake. These results confirm those of a previous trial proposing a caloric restriction in the context of RFS [119] as follows: (1) Reduced energy intake of 20 kcal/h for at least 2 days, (2) if serum phosphate concentrations did not need to be supplemented, as determined per protocol (as described in the Appendix S3 of [119]), energy intake should be returned to normal during 2–3 days, (3) a gradual return to 40 kcal/h for 24 h, then increased goals to 60 kcal/h for 24 h, followed by 80% of calculated energy goals for another 24 h, with 100% of goals achieved by day 4 [119].

According to the National Institute for Health and Care Excellence (NICE) guidelines, patients at risk should be nourished with regular control of electrolytes as follows: (1) Feeding starting at 10 kcal/kg/day, (2) increasing to full need over ≥4 days, and (3) supplementation of thiamine (vitamin B1, 200–300 mg/day) for the first 10 days [47,120].

### 5.3. Parenteral Nutrition

Complications attributed to the use of PN include mechanical complications with catheter obstruction, catheter infections, venous thrombosis, or pneumothorax [121]. Short-term metabolic complications can occur as well as fluid imbalance (overload or dehydration), electrolyte disturbances, glycemic abnormalities, and dyslipidemia [122]. These complications can be avoided by systematic and precise monitoring [122]. Major long-term metabolic complications include metabolic bone diseases and hepatobiliary disorders. It was shown that the frequency of osteoporosis and osteomalacia increases in patients with long-term PN [123]. In addition, intestinal failure-associated liver disease can occur during parenteral feeding, and cholestasis and hepatic steatosis in those with long-term PN. Hepatobiliary disorders have been attributed to overfeeding during PN [121,124].

Some recent studies suggest that, if provided in isocaloric doses, PN and EN result in similar clinical outcomes [7,57,109]. Therefore, PN is not in opposition to EN but can be used as an additional therapy as soon as a close monitoring of the MNT is assured [39,108]. However, PN should not be started before all strategies to maximize EN tolerance have been attempted (GPP) [17].

### *5.4. Enteral Nutrition*

Two large randomized trials specifically designed to investigate the feeding route in critically ill patients [57,109] found more episodes of both hypoglycemia and vomiting with EN compared to PN. Furthermore, the NUTRIREA-2 trial assessing severely ill ICU patients under mechanical ventilation and on vasopressors detected a pronounced difficulty to reach protein and calorie targets and an increased risk for gastrointestinal complications (e.g., diarrhea, bowel ischemia, acute colonic pseudo-obstruction) with early EN [57].

#### Enteral Nutrition and Dysphagia: Risk of Aspiration, Swallowing Screening

Dysphagia occurs in 50–70% of the critically ill [125]. Risk factors include older age, congestive heart failure, sepsis, perioperative stroke, non-coronary bypass surgical procedures, transesophageal echocardiography, and previous stroke [125]. Patients suffering from dysphagia are at major risk for aspiration. Several high-quality swallowing tests (e.g., DePippo, Horner, Kidd) developed to thoroughly assess aspiration risk have been summarized in a recent review [126] in which the authors report the swallowing screening published by Daniels et al. in 1998 to be the most convenient. This assessment is also applicable for intubated patients for a certain period of time. Moreover, it is considered by non-speech therapists (i.e., nurses specialized in intensive care) to be the most suitable assessment.

In case of aspiration risk, feeding tubes are used to nourish the patient. Tube selection depends on the expected duration of feeding. Furthermore, the selection of a large bore tube (≥14 French) ensures gastric suctioning and decompression in case of gastroparesis and paralytic ileus, which are usually present during the early postoperative period.

The measurement of gastric residual volume (GRV) for the assessment of gastrointestinal function is commonly used and may help to detect intolerance to EN during initiation and progression of EN, especially in patients who underwent abdominal procedures or major surgery. However, monitoring of GRV in case of established EN may not be necessary. The ESPEN guidelines suggest that EN should be delayed when GRV is >500 mL/6 h, and prokinetic treatment should be considered if acute abdominal complications are excluded [17]. ASPEN and the Surviving Sepsis Initiative support the use of prokinetics (e.g., metoclopramide (three times 10 mg/day) and erythromycin (3–7 mg/kg/day)) in the case of feeding intolerance [27,127].

## 6. Financial Aspects

Disease-related malnutrition has relevant consequences on patient outcome, especially in the most severely ill patients treated on ICUs and IMC-Us. However, for several reasons it remains difficult to demonstrate the economic benefit related to improved outcome rooted in MNT. The comparison of different clinical practices in hospitals and countries, variable costs for hospital staff and MNT products, and heterogeneous accounting systems complicate any reliable comparison of cost and benefit. Furthermore, the acquisition of nationwide and international data is limited and explains why study data are scarce [128] and why cost-economic analyses show discrepancies in this important field of interest.

Relevant data for the critically ill exist concerning the potentially cost-saving introduction of the pre-mixed multi-chamber bag compared to compound PN. In a real-world analysis of PN use, potential savings of up to $1545 USD per patient using a multi-chamber bag could be achieved according to US data from the Premier Perspective™ database [129]. Patients on PN also benefit from a nutritional care team in order to assure adequate indication, application, and adaptation of PN, resulting in savings of 245,000 € EUR in one year per 100 treated patients in a Swiss university hospital [130]. A meta-analysis involving six clinical trials evaluating early EN in the ICU setting found a statistically significant reduction in mortality compared to standard timing of EN [131]. A cost-effectiveness analysis of these data showed a $14,462 USD reduction in total costs per patient for acute hospital care of patients receiving EN within 24 h after admission. These results were robust also when including sensitivity analysis with European cost data [132].

The Swiss SPN study added PN on days 4–8, whenever >60% of the caloric needs where not covered by EN on day 3. Based on the Swiss accounting system (Swiss DRG), a simulated calculation revealed a risk reduction for infection of 10%, resulting in savings of 63,048 CHF per infection [7,133]. The cost-analysis of the EPaNIC trial showed increased expenses with early-PN, mainly due to pharmacy-related costs and higher expenditures for PN and anti-infectious agents when compared to late PN patients who only received PN when EN remained insufficient after the first week of ICU treatment. Withholding early PN resulted in a net cost saving of 1210 Euro per patient [134].

The pronounced loss of lean body tissue, lack of mobilization, and increased protein energy needs all lead to higher complication rates with increased morbidity and mortality in this most fragile group of critically ill patients. Further studies, such as the recently published EFFORT study [135], should describe the effect of MNT not only in terms of clinical benefit but also with regard to monetary equivalent. Such data are of utmost interest to support and spread the relevance of MNT and linked-care teams.

## 7. Conclusions

MNT in all categories of critically ill patients remains a challenge, not only because these patients suffer from a pronounced stress response and are at higher risk for complications, but also due to their heterogeneity and their different illness phases (acute, subacute, chronic critically ill; pre- or post-resuscitation). Further studies are urgently needed to answer important questions such as the best timing, route, dose, and composition of MNT for the critically ill and to determine how to assess and to adapt to each patient's individual needs.

Current guidelines, as presented and discussed in this review, integrate actual knowledge and best clinical practice. Further steps would be to introduce them into (pre-existing) local feeding protocols. A MNT team offers an important additional value to optimize both patient care and education of hospital staff.

**Author Contributions:** Conceptualization: A.K.L. and C.H. Writing, original draft preparation, review, and editing: A.K.L., A.d.W., A.H., N.G. and C.H.

**Acknowledgments:** The authors would like to thank Allison Dwileski, BSc (Department of Anesthesiology, University Hospital Basel, Switzerland) for her editorial support.

## References

1. Nasraway, S.A.; Cohen, I.L.; Dennis, R.C.; Howenstein, M.A.; Nikas, D.K.; Warren, J.; Wedel, S.K. Guidelines on admission and discharge for adult intermediate care units. American College of Critical Care Medicine of the Society of Critical Care Medicine. *Crit. Care Med.* **1998**, *26*, 607–610. [CrossRef]

2. Havens, J.M.; Columbus, A.B.; Seshadri, A.J.; Olufajo, O.A.; Mogensen, K.M.; Rawn, J.D.; Salim, A.; Christopher, K.B. Malnutrition at Intensive Care Unit Admission Predicts Mortality in Emergency General Surgery Patients. *JPEN J. Parenter. Enter. Nutr.* **2018**, *42*, 156–163. [CrossRef]
3. Imoberdorf, R.; Meier, R.; Krebs, P.; Hangartner, P.J.; Hess, B.; Stäubli, M.; Wegmann, D.; Rühlin, M.; Ballmer, P.E. Prevalence of undernutrition on admission to Swiss hospitals. *Clin. Nutr.* **2010**, *29*, 38–41. [CrossRef]
4. Kyle, U.G.; Genton, L.; Pichard, C. Hospital length of stay and nutritional status. *Curr. Opin. Clin. Nutr. Metab. Care* **2005**, *8*, 397–402. [CrossRef]
5. Mogensen, K.M.; Robinson, M.K.; Casey, J.D.; Gunasekera, N.S.; Moromizato, T.; Rawn, J.D.; Christopher, K.B. Nutritional Status and Mortality in the Critically Ill. *Crit. Care Med.* **2015**, *43*, 2605–2615. [CrossRef]
6. Alberda, C.; Gramlich, L.; Jones, N.; Jeejeebhoy, K.; Day, A.G.; Dhaliwal, R.; Heyland, D.K. The relationship between nutritional intake and clinical outcomes in critically ill patients: Results of an international multicenter observational study. *Intensiv. Care Med.* **2009**, *35*, 1728–1737. [CrossRef]
7. Heidegger, C.P.; Berger, M.M.; Graf, S.; Zingg, W.; Darmon, P.; Costanza, M.C.; Thibault, R.; Pichard, C. Optimisation of energy provision with supplemental parenteral nutrition in critically ill patients: A randomised controlled clinical trial. *Lancet* **2013**, *381*, 385–393. [CrossRef]
8. Rubinson, L.; Diette, G.B.; Song, X.; Brower, R.G.; Krishnan, J.A. Low caloric intake is associated with nosocomial bloodstream infections in patients in the medical intensive care unit. *Crit. Care Med.* **2004**, *32*, 350–357. [CrossRef]
9. Villet, S.; Chiolero, R.L.; Bollmann, M.D.; Revelly, J.-P.; Rn, M.-C.C.; Delarue, J.; Berger, M.M. Negative impact of hypocaloric feeding and energy balance on clinical outcome in ICU patients. *Clin. Nutr.* **2005**, *24*, 502–509. [CrossRef]
10. Van Zanten, A.R.; Sztark, F.; Kaisers, U.X.; Zielmann, S.; Felbinger, T.W.; Sablotzki, A.R.; De Waele, J.J.; Timsit, J.F.; Honing, M.L.; Keh, D.; et al. High-protein enteral nutrition enriched with immune-modulating nutrients vs. standard high-protein enteral nutrition and nosocomial infections in the ICU: A randomized clinical trial. *JAMA* **2014**, *312*, 514–524. [CrossRef]
11. Chapman, M.; Peake, S.L.; Bellomo, R.; Davies, A.; Deane, A.; Horowitz, M.; Hurford, S.; Lange, K.; Little, L.; Mackle, D.; et al. Energy-Dense versus Routine Enteral Nutrition in the Critically Ill. *N. Engl. J. Med.* **2018**, *379*, 1823–1834.
12. Arabi, Y.M.; Aldawood, A.S.; Haddad, S.H.; Al-Dorzi, H.M.; Tamim, H.M.; Jones, G.; Mehta, S.; McIntyre, L.; Solaiman, O.; Sakkijha, M.H.; et al. Permissive Underfeeding or Standard Enteral Feeding in Critically Ill Adults. *N. Engl. J. Med.* **2015**, *372*, 2398–2408. [CrossRef]
13. National Heart, Lung, and Blood Institute Acute Respiratory Distress Syndrome (ARDS) Clinical Trials Network; Rice, T.W.; Wheeler, A.P.; Thompson, B.T.; Steingrub, J.; Hite, R.D.; Moss, M.; Morris, A.; Dong, N.; Rock, P. Initial trophic vs. full enteral feeding in patients with acute lung injury: The EDEN randomized trial. *JAMA* **2012**, *307*, 795–803.
14. Heyland, D.; Muscedere, J.; Wischmeyer, P.E.; Cook, D.; Jones, G.; Albert, M.; Elke, G.; Berger, M.M.; Day, A.G.; Canadian Critical Care Trials Group. A randomized trial of glutamine and antioxidants in critically ill patients. *N. Engl. J. Med.* **2013**, *368*, 1489–1497. [CrossRef]
15. Andrews, P.J.; Avenell, A.; Noble, D.W.; Campbell, M.K.; Croal, B.L.; Simpson, W.G.; Vale, L.D.; Battison, C.G.; Jenkinson, D.J.; Cook, J.A.; et al. Randomised trial of glutamine, selenium, or both, to supplement parenteral nutrition for critically ill patients. *BMJ* **2011**, *342*, 1542. [CrossRef]
16. Wernerman, J.; Kirketeig, T.; Andersson, B.; Berthelson, H.; Ersson, A.; Friberg, H.; Guttormsen, A.B.; Hendrikx, S.; Pettilä, V.; Rossi, P.; et al. Scandinavian glutamine trial: A pragmatic multi-centre randomised clinical trial of intensive care unit patients. *Acta Anaesthesiol. Scand.* **2011**, *55*, 812–818. [CrossRef]
17. Singer, P.; Blaser, A.R.; Berger, M.M.; Alhazzani, W.; Calder, P.C.; Casaer, M.P.; Hiesmayr, M.; Mayer, K.; Montejo, J.C.; Pichard, C.; et al. ESPEN guideline on clinical nutrition in the intensive care unit. *Clin. Nutr.* **2019**, *38*, 48–79. [CrossRef]
18. Bendavid, I.; Singer, P.; Theilla, M.; Themessl-Huber, M.; Sulz, I.; Mouhieddine, M.; Schuh, C.; Mora, B.; Hiesmayr, M. NutritionDay ICU: A 7 year worldwide prevalence study of nutrition practice in intensive care. *Clin. Nutr.* **2017**, *36*, 1122–1129. [CrossRef]

19. Looijaard, W.; Denneman, N.; Broens, B.; Girbes, A.R.J.; Weijs, P.J.M.; Oudemans-van Straaten, H.M. Achieving protein targets without energy overfeeding in critically ill patients: A prospective feasibility study. *Clin. Nutr.* **2018**. [CrossRef]
20. Pompilio, C.E.; Pelosi, P.; Castro, M.G. The Bariatric Patient in the Intensive Care Unit: Pitfalls and Management. *Curr. Atheroscler. Rep.* **2016**, *18*, 55. [CrossRef]
21. Lorenzo-López, L.; Maseda, A.; De Labra, C.; Regueiro-Folgueira, L.; Rodríguez-Villamil, J.L.; Millán-Calenti, J.C. Nutritional determinants of frailty in older adults: A systematic review. *BMC Geriatr.* **2017**, *17*, 108. [CrossRef]
22. Cerri, A.P.; Bellelli, G.; Mazzone, A.; Pittella, F.; Landi, F.; Zambon, A.; Annoni, G. Sarcopenia and malnutrition in acutely ill hospitalized elderly: Prevalence and outcomes. *Clin. Nutr.* **2015**, *34*, 745–751. [CrossRef]
23. Onal, O.; Ozgun, G. Comparison of the Course and Prognosis of Geriatric Patients Admitted to the Intensive Care Unit According to BMI and Albumin Values. *Anesth. Pain Med.* **2016**, *6*, e32509. [CrossRef]
24. Grigoryan, K.V.; Javedan, H.; Rudolph, J.L. Ortho-Geriatric Care Models and Outcomes in Hip Fracture Patients: A Systematic Review and Meta-Analysis. *J. Orthop. Trauma* **2014**, *28*, e49–e55. [CrossRef]
25. Manzanares, W.; Hardy, G. Thiamine supplementation in the critically ill. *Curr. Opin. Clin. Nutr. Metab. Care* **2011**, *14*, 610–617. [CrossRef]
26. Nishimoto, A.; Usery, J.; Winton, J.C.; Twilla, J. High-dose Parenteral Thiamine in Treatment of Wernicke's Encephalopathy: Case Series and Review of the Literature. *In Vivo* **2017**, *31*, 121–124. [CrossRef]
27. McClave, S.A.; Taylor, B.E.; Martindale, R.G.; Warren, M.M.; Johnson, D.R.; Braunschweig, C.; McCarthy, M.S.; Davanos, E.; Rice, T.W.; Cresci, G.A.; et al. Guidelines for the Provision and Assessment of Nutrition Support Therapy in the Adult Critically Ill Patient: Society of Critical Care Medicine (SCCM) and American Society for Parenteral and Enteral Nutrition (A.S.P.E.N.). *JPEN J. Parenter. Enter. Nutr.* **2016**, *40*, 159–211. [CrossRef]
28. Fanelli, V.; Vlachou, A.; Ghannadian, S.; Simonetti, U.; Slutsky, A.S.; Zhang, H. Acute respiratory distress syndrome: New definition, current and future therapeutic options. *J. Thorac. Dis.* **2013**, *5*, 326–334.
29. Fong, Y.; Marano, M.A.; Barber, A.; He, W.; Moldawer, L.L.; Bushman, E.D.; Coyle, S.M.; Shires, G.T.; Lowry, S.F. Total Parenteral Nutrition and Bowel Rest Modify the Metabolic Response to Endotoxin in Humans. *Ann. Surg.* **1989**, *210*, 449–457. [CrossRef]
30. The Veterans Affairs Total Parenteral Nutrition Cooperative Study Group. Perioperative total parenteral nutrition in surgical patients. *N. Engl. J. Med.* **1991**, *325*, 525–532. [CrossRef]
31. Genton, L.; Dupertuis, Y.M.; Romand, J.-A.; Simonet, M.L.; Jolliet, P.; Huber, O.; Kudsk, K.A.; Pichard, C. Higher calorie prescription improves nutrient delivery during the first 5 days of enteral nutrition. *Clin. Nutr.* **2004**, *23*, 307–315. [CrossRef]
32. Spain, D.A.; McClave, S.A.; Sexton, L.K.; Adams, J.L.; Blanford, B.S.; Sullins, M.E.; Owens, N.A.; Snider, H.L. Infusion Protocol Improves Delivery of Enteral Tube Feeding in the Critical Care Unit. *J. Parenter. Enter. Nutr.* **1999**, *23*, 288–292. [CrossRef]
33. Simpson, F.; Doig, G.S. Parenteral vs. enteral nutrition in the critically ill patient: A meta-analysis of trials using the intention to treat principle. *Intensive Care Med.* **2005**, *31*, 12–23. [CrossRef]
34. Cawood, A.L.; Elia, M.; Stratton, R.J. Systematic review and meta-analysis of the effects of high protein oral nutritional supplements. *Ageing Res. Rev.* **2012**, *11*, 278–296. [CrossRef]
35. Berger, M.M.; Reintam-Blaser, A.; Calder, P.C.; Casaer, M.; Hiesmayr, M.J.; Mayer, K.; Montejo, J.C.; Pichard, C.; Preiser, J.C.; van Zanten, A.R.H.; et al. Monitoring nutrition in the ICU. *Clin. Nutr.* **2019**, *38*, 584–593. [CrossRef]
36. Delliere, S.; Cynober, L. Is transthyretin a good marker of nutritional status? *Clin. Nutr.* **2017**, *36*, 364–370. [CrossRef]
37. Barr, J.; Hecht, M.; Flavin, K.E.; Khorana, A.; Gould, M.K. Outcomes in critically ill patients before and after the implementation of an evidence-based nutritional management protocol. *Chest* **2004**, *125*, 1446–1457. [CrossRef]
38. Wøien, H.; Bjørk, I.T. Nutrition of the critically ill patient and effects of implementing a nutritional support algorithm in ICU. *J. Clin. Nurs.* **2006**, *15*, 168–177. [CrossRef]
39. Soguel, L.; Revelly, J.P.; Schaller, M.D.; Longchamp, C.; Berger, M.M. Energy deficit and length of hospital stay can be reduced by a two-step quality improvement of nutrition therapy: The intensive care unit dietitian can make the difference. *Crit. Care Med.* **2012**, *40*, 412–419. [CrossRef]

40. Mowe, M.; Bosaeus, I.; Rasmussen, H.H.; Kondrup, J.; Unosson, M.; Rothenberg, E.; Irtun, O.; Scandinavian Nutrition Group. Insufficient nutritional knowledge among health care workers? *Clin. Nutr.* **2008**, *27*, 196–202. [CrossRef]
41. Jones, N.E.; Suurdt, J.; Ouelette-Kuntz, H.; Heyland, D.K. Implementation of the Canadian Clinical Practice Guidelines for Nutrition Support: a multiple case study of barriers and enablers. *Nutr. Clin. Pract.* **2007**, *22*, 449–457. [CrossRef]
42. Wischmeyer, P.E. Are we creating survivors … or victims in critical care? Delivering targeted nutrition to improve outcomes. *Curr. Opin. Crit. Care* **2016**, *22*, 279–284. [CrossRef]
43. Wischmeyer, P.E. Tailoring nutrition therapy to illness and recovery. *Crit. Care* **2017**, *21* (Suppl. 3), 316. [CrossRef]
44. Staun, M.; Pironi, L.; Bozzetti, F.; Baxter, J.; Forbes, A.; Joly, F.; Jeppesen, P.; Moreno, J.; Hebuterne, X.; Pertkiewicz, M.; et al. ESPEN Guidelines on Parenteral Nutrition: Home parenteral nutrition (HPN) in adult patients. *Clin. Nutr.* **2009**, *28*, 467–479. [CrossRef]
45. Reintam Blaser, A.; Berger, M.M. Early or Late Feeding after ICU Admission? *Nutrients* **2017**, *9*, 1278. [CrossRef]
46. Stanga, Z.; Brunner, A.; Leuenberger, M.; Grimble, R.F.; Shenkin, A.; Allison, S.P.; Lobo, D.N. Nutrition in clinical practice-the refeeding syndrome: Illustrative cases and guidelines for prevention and treatment. *Eur. J. Clin. Nutr.* **2008**, *62*, 687–694. [CrossRef]
47. Walmsley, R.S. Refeeding syndrome: Screening, incidence, and treatment during parenteral nutrition. *J. Gastroenterol. Hepatol.* **2013**, *28*, 113–117. [CrossRef]
48. The Canadian Critical Care Society (CCCS) and the Canadian Critical Care Trials Group (CCCTG). The 2015 Clinical Practice Guidelines on Critical Care Nutrition. Available online: https://www.criticalcarenutrition.com/resources/cpgs/past-guidelines/2015 (accessed on 31 May 2019).
49. Bischoff, S.C.; Singer, P.; Koller, M.; Barazzoni, R.; Cederholm, T.; Van Gossum, A. Standard operating procedures for ESPEN guidelines and consensus papers. *Clin. Nutr.* **2015**, *34*, 1043–1051. [CrossRef]
50. Atkins, D.; Best, D.; Briss, P.A.; Eccles, M.; Falck-Ytter, Y.; Flottorp, S.; Guyatt, G.H.; Harbour, R.T.; Haugh, M.C.; Henry, D.; et al. Grading quality of evidence and strength of recommendations. *BMJ* **2004**, *328*, 1490.
51. Cahill, N.E.; Dhaliwal, R.; Day, A.G.; Jiang, X.; Heyland, D.K. Nutrition therapy in the critical care setting: What is "best achievable" practice? An international multicenter observational study. *Crit. Care Med.* **2010**, *38*, 395–401. [CrossRef]
52. Kyle, U.G.; Genton, L.; Heidegger, C.P.; Maisonneuve, N.; Karsegard, V.L.; Huber, O.; Mensi, N.; Romand, J.A.; Jolliet, P.; Pichard, C. Hospitalized mechanically ventilated patients are at higher risk of enteral underfeeding than non-ventilated patients. *Clin. Nutr.* **2006**, *25*, 727–735. [CrossRef]
53. Wischmeyer, P.E.; Hasselmann, M.; Kummerlen, C.; Kozar, R.; Kutsogiannis, D.J.; Karvellas, C.J.; Besecker, B.; Evans, D.K.; Preiser, J.-C.; Gramlich, L.; et al. A randomized trial of supplemental parenteral nutrition in underweight and overweight critically ill patients: The TOP-UP pilot trial. *Crit. Care* **2017**, *21*, 142. [CrossRef]
54. Casaer, M.P.; Mesotten, D.; Hermans, G.; Wouters, P.J.; Schetz, M.; Meyfroidt, G.; Van Cromphaut, S.; Ingels, C.; Meersseman, P.; Müller, J.; et al. Early versus Late Parenteral Nutrition in Critically Ill Adults. *N. Engl. J. Med.* **2011**, *365*, 506–517. [CrossRef]
55. Singer, P.; Anbar, R.; Cohen, J.; Shapiro, H.; Shalita-Chesner, M.; Lev, S.; Grozovski, E.; Theilla, M.; Frishman, S.; Madar, Z. The tight calorie control study (TICACOS): A prospective, randomized, controlled pilot study of nutritional support in critically ill patients. *Intensiv. Care Med.* **2011**, *37*, 601–609. [CrossRef]
56. Allingstrup, M.J.; Kondrup, J.; Wiis, J.; Claudius, C.; Pedersen, U.G.; Hein-Rasmussen, R.; Bjerregaard, M.R.; Steensen, M.; Jensen, T.H.; Lange, T.; et al. Early goal-directed nutrition versus standard of care in adult intensive care patients: The single-centre, randomised, outcome assessor-blinded EAT-ICU trial. *Intensiv. Care Med.* **2017**, *43*, 1637–1647. [CrossRef]
57. Reignier, J.; Boisrame-Helms, J.; Brisard, L.; Lascarrou, J.B.; Ait Hssain, A.; Anguel, N.; Argaud, L.; Asehnoune, K.; Asfar, P.; Bellec, F.; et al. Enteral versus parenteral early nutrition in ventilated adults with shock: A randomised, controlled, multicentre, open-label, parallel-group study (NUTRIREA-2). *Lancet* **2018**, *391*, 133–143. [CrossRef]
58. Kondrup, J.; Rasmussen, H.H.; Hamberg, O.; Stanga, Z.; Ad Hoc, E.W.G. Nutritional risk screening (NRS 2002): A new method based on an analysis of controlled clinical trials. *Clin. Nutr.* **2003**, *22*, 321–336. [CrossRef]

59. De Vries, M.C.; Koekkoek, W.K.; Opdam, M.H.; van Blokland, D.; van Zanten, A.R. Nutritional assessment of critically ill patients: Validation of the modified NUTRIC score. *Eur. J. Clin. Nutr.* **2018**, *72*, 428–435. [CrossRef]
60. Detsky, A.S.; Baker, J.P.; Mendelson, R.A.; Wolman, S.L.; Wesson, D.E.; Jeejeebhoy, K.N. Evaluating the Accuracy of Nutritional Assessment Techniques Applied To Hospitalized Patients: Methodology and Comparisons. *J. Parenter. Enter. Nutr.* **1984**, *8*, 153–159. [CrossRef]
61. Vellas, B.; Guigoz, Y.; Garry, P.J.; Nourhashemi, F.; Bennahum, D.; Lauque, S.; Albarède, J.-L. The mini nutritional assessment (MNA) and its use in grading the nutritional state of elderly patients. *Nutrition* **1999**, *15*, 116–122. [CrossRef]
62. Kondrup, J. Nutrition risk screening in the ICU. *Curr. Opin. Clin. Nutr. Metab. Care* **2019**, *22*, 159–161. [CrossRef]
63. Shenkin, A. Serum prealbumin: Is it a marker of nutritional status or of risk of malnutrition? *Clin. Chem.* **2006**, *52*, 2177–2179. [CrossRef]
64. Wischmeyer, P.E.; San-Millan, I. Winning the war against ICU-acquired weakness: New innovations in nutrition and exercise physiology. *Crit. Care* **2015**, *19* (Suppl. 3), S6.
65. Looijaard, W.G.; Dekker, I.M.; Stapel, S.N.; Girbes, A.R.; Twisk, J.W.; Oudemans-van Straaten, H.M.; Weijs, P.J. Skeletal muscle quality as assessed by CT-derived skeletal muscle density is associated with 6-month mortality in mechanically ventilated critically ill patients. *Crit. Care* **2016**, *20*, 386. [CrossRef]
66. Lee, J.E. Increased intra-abdominal pressure in acute kidney injury: A cause or an effect? *Kidney Res. Clin. Pract.* **2015**, *34*, 67–68. [CrossRef]
67. Oshima, T.; Berger, M.M.; De Waele, E.; Guttormsen, A.B.; Heidegger, C.-P.; Hiesmayr, M.; Singer, P.; Wernerman, J.; Pichard, C. Indirect calorimetry in nutritional therapy. A position paper by the ICALIC study group. *Clin. Nutr.* **2017**, *36*, 651–662. [CrossRef]
68. Singh, R.; Cuervo, A.M. Autophagy in the Cellular Energetic Balance. *Cell Metab.* **2011**, *13*, 495–504. [CrossRef]
69. Anderegg, B.A.; Worrall, C.; Barbour, E.; Simpson, K.N.; DeLegge, M. Comparison of Resting Energy Expenditure Prediction Methods with Measured Resting Energy Expenditure in Obese, Hospitalized Adults. *J. Parenter. Enter. Nutr.* **2009**, *33*, 168–175. [CrossRef]
70. Boullata, J.; Williams, J.; Cottrell, F.; Hudson, L.; Compher, C. Accurate Determination of Energy Needs in Hospitalized Patients. *J. Am. Diet. Assoc.* **2007**, *107*, 393–401. [CrossRef]
71. Graf, S.; Pichard, C.; Genton, L.; Oshima, T.; Heidegger, C.P. Energy expenditure in mechanically ventilated patients: The weight of body weight! *Clin. Nutr.* **2017**, *36*, 224–228. [CrossRef]
72. Kross, E.K.; Sena, M.; Schmidt, K.; Stapleton, R.D. A Comparison of Predictive Equations of Energy Expenditure and Measured Energy Expenditure in Critically Ill Patients. *J. Crit. Care* **2012**, *27*, 321.e5–321.e12. [CrossRef]
73. Kreymann, K.G.; Berger, M.M.; Deutz, N.E.; Hiesmayr, M.; Jolliet, P.; Kazandjiev, G.; Nitenberg, G.; van den Berghe, G.; Wernerman, J.; Ebner, C.; et al. ESPEN Guidelines on Enteral Nutrition: Intensive care. *Clin. Nutr.* **2006**, *25*, 210–223. [CrossRef]
74. Singer, P.; Berger, M.M.; Berghe, G.V.D.; Biolo, G.; Calder, P.; Forbes, A.; Griffiths, R.; Kreyman, G.; Leverve, X.; Pichard, C. ESPEN Guidelines on Parenteral Nutrition: Intensive care. *Clin. Nutr.* **2009**, *28*, 387–400. [CrossRef]
75. Weir, J.B.D.V. New methods for calculating metabolic rate with special reference to protein metabolism. *J. Physiol.* **1949**, *109*, 1–9. [CrossRef]
76. Frankenfield, D.C.; Ashcraft, C.M. Estimating Energy Needs in Nutrition Support Patients. *J. Parenter. Enter. Nutr.* **2011**, *35*, 563–570. [CrossRef]
77. Psota, T.; Chen, K.Y. Measuring energy expenditure in clinical populations: Rewards and challenges. *Eur. J. Clin. Nutr.* **2013**, *67*, 436–442. [CrossRef]
78. Kagan, I.; Zusman, O.; Bendavid, I.; Theilla, M.; Cohen, J.; Singer, P. Validation of carbon dioxide production (VCO2) as a tool to calculate resting energy expenditure (REE) in mechanically ventilated critically ill patients: A retrospective observational study. *Crit. Care* **2018**, *22*, 186. [CrossRef]
79. Soussi, S.; Vallee, F.; Roquet, F.; Bevilacqua, V.; Benyamina, M.; Ferry, A.; Cupaciu, A.; Chaussard, M.; De Tymowski, C.; Boccara, D.; et al. Measurement of Oxygen Consumption Variations in Critically Ill Burns Patients: Are the Fick Method and Indirect Calorimetry Interchangeable? *Shock* **2017**, *48*, 532–538. [CrossRef]

80. Oshima, T.; Graf, S.; Heidegger, C.-P.; Genton, L.; Pugin, J.; Pichard, C. Can calculation of energy expenditure based on $CO_2$ measurements replace indirect calorimetry? *Crit. Care* **2017**, *21*, 13. [CrossRef]
81. Weijs, P.J.M. Route, early or energy? Protein improves protein balance in critically ill patients. *Crit. Care* **2018**, *22*, 91. [CrossRef]
82. Nicolo, M.; Heyland, D.K.; Chittams, J.; Sammarco, T.; Compher, C. Clinical Outcomes Related to Protein Delivery in a Critically Ill Population: A Multicenter, Multinational Observation Study. *JPEN J. Parenter. Enter. Nutr.* **2016**, *40*, 45–51. [CrossRef]
83. Weijs, P.J.; Mogensen, K.M.; Rawn, J.D.; Christopher, K.B. Protein Intake, Nutritional Status and Outcomes in ICU Survivors: A Single Center Cohort Study. *J. Clin. Med.* **2019**, *8*, 43. [CrossRef]
84. Weijs, P.J.; Looijaard, W.G.; Beishuizen, A.; Girbes, A.R.; Oudemans-van Straaten, H.M. Early high protein intake is associated with low mortality and energy overfeeding with high mortality in non-septic mechanically ventilated critically ill patients. *Crit. Care* **2014**, *18*, 701. [CrossRef]
85. Ferrie, S.; Allman-Farinelli, M.; Daley, M.; Smith, K. Protein Requirements in the Critically Ill: A Randomized Controlled Trial Using Parenteral Nutrition. *JPEN J. Parenter. Enter. Nutr.* **2016**, *40*, 795–805. [CrossRef]
86. Doig, G.S.; Simpson, F.; Bellomo, R.; Heighes, P.T.; Sweetman, E.A.; Chesher, D.; Pollock, C.; Davies, A.; Botha, J.; Harrigan, P.; et al. Intravenous amino acid therapy for kidney function in critically ill patients: A randomized controlled trial. *Intensiv. Care Med.* **2015**, *41*, 1197–1208. [CrossRef]
87. Hermans, G.; Casaer, M.P.; Clerckx, B.; Guiza, F.; Vanhullebusch, T.; Derde, S.; Meersseman, P.; Derese, I.; Mesotten, D.; Wouters, P.J.; et al. Effect of tolerating macronutrient deficit on the development of intensive-care unit acquired weakness: A subanalysis of the EPaNIC trial. *Lancet Respir. Med.* **2013**, *1*, 621–629. [CrossRef]
88. Casaer, M.P.; Wilmer, A.; Hermans, G.; Wouters, P.J.; Mesotten, D.; Van den Berghe, G. Role of disease and macronutrient dose in the randomized controlled EPaNIC trial: A post hoc analysis. *Am. J. Respir. Crit. Care Med.* **2013**, *187*, 247–255. [CrossRef]
89. Burtin, C.; Clerckx, B.; Robbeets, C.; Ferdinande, P.; Langer, D.; Troosters, T.; Hermans, G.; Decramer, M.; Gosselink, R. Early exercise in critically ill patients enhances short-term functional recovery. *Crit. Care Med.* **2009**, *37*, 2499–2505. [CrossRef]
90. Schaller, S.J.; Anstey, M.; Blobner, M.; Edrich, T.; Grabitz, S.D.; Gradwohl-Matis, I.; Heim, M.; Houle, T.; Kurth, T.; Latronico, N.; et al. Early, goal-directed mobilisation in the surgical intensive care unit: A randomised controlled trial. *Lancet* **2016**, *388*, 1377–1388. [CrossRef]
91. Fujioka, K.; DiBaise, J.K.; Martindale, R.G. Nutrition and metabolic complications after bariatric surgery and their treatment. *JPEN J. Parenter. Enter. Nutr.* **2011**, *35* (Suppl. 5), 52S–59S. [CrossRef]
92. Schindler, K.; Themessl-Huber, M.; Hiesmayr, M.; Kosak, S.; Lainscak, M.; Laviano, A.; Ljungqvist, O.; Mouhieddine, M.; Schneider, S.; De Van Der Schueren, M.; et al. To eat or not to eat? Indicators for reduced food intake in 91,245 patients hospitalized on nutritionDays 2006–2014 in 56 countries worldwide: A descriptive analysis. *Am. J. Clin. Nutr.* **2016**, *104*, 1393–1402. [CrossRef]
93. Amirkalali, B.; Hosseini, S.; Heshmat, R.; Larijani, B. Comparison of Harris Benedict and Mifflin-ST Jeor equations with indirect calorimetry in evaluating resting energy expenditure. *Indian J. Med. Sci.* **2008**, *62*, 283–290.
94. Beebe, M.L.; Crowley, N. Can Hypocaloric, High Protein Nutrition Support Be Used in Complicated Bariatric Patients to Promote Weight Loss? *Nutr. Clin. Pract.* **2015**, *30*, 522–529. [CrossRef]
95. Volkert, D.; Beck, A.M.; Cederholm, T.; Cruz-Jentoft, A.; Goisser, S.; Hooper, L.; Kiesswetter, E.; Maggio, M.; Raynaud-Simon, A.; Sieber, C.C.; et al. ESPEN guideline on clinical nutrition and hydration in geriatrics. *Clin. Nutr.* **2019**, *38*, 10–47. [CrossRef]
96. Wade, C.E.; Kozar, R.A.; Dyer, C.B.; Bulger, E.M.; Mourtzakis, M.; Heyland, D.K. Evaluation of nutrition deficits in adult and elderly trauma patients. *JPEN J. Parenter. Enter. Nutr.* **2015**, *39*, 449–455. [CrossRef]
97. Phillips, S.M.; Dickerson, R.N.; Moore, F.A.; Paddon-Jones, D.; Weijs, P.J.M. Protein Turnover and Metabolism in the Elderly Intensive Care Unit Patient. *Nutr. Clin. Pract.* **2017**, *32*, 112S–120S. [CrossRef]
98. Deutz, N.E.P.; Bauer, J.M.; Barazzoni, R.; Biolo, G.; Boirie, Y.; Bosy-Westphal, A.; Cederholm, T.; Cruz-Jentoft, A.J.; Krznaric, Z.; Nair, K.S.; et al. Protein intake and exercise for optimal muscle function with aging: Recommendations from the ESPEN Expert Group. *Clin. Nutr.* **2014**, *33*, 929–936. [CrossRef]
99. Dickerson, R.N.; Maish, G.O., 3rd; Croce, M.A.; Minard, G.; Brown, R.O. Influence of aging on nitrogen accretion during critical illness. *JPEN J. Parenter. Enter. Nutr.* **2015**, *39*, 282–290. [CrossRef]

100. Loenneke, J.P.; Loprinzi, P.D.; Murphy, C.H.; Phillips, S.M. Per meal dose and frequency of protein consumption is associated with lean mass and muscle performance. *Clin. Nutr.* **2016**, *35*, 1506–1511. [CrossRef]
101. Schulman, R.C.; Mechanick, J.I. Metabolic and nutrition support in the chronic critical illness syndrome. *Respir. Care* **2012**, *57*, 958–977. [CrossRef]
102. Rousseau, A.-F.; Losser, M.-R.; Ichai, C.; Berger, M.M. ESPEN endorsed recommendations: Nutritional therapy in major burns. *Clin. Nutr.* **2013**, *32*, 497–502. [CrossRef]
103. Plauth, M.; Bernal, W.; Dasarathy, S.; Merli, M.; Plank, L.D.; Schütz, T.; Bischoff, S.C. ESPEN guideline on clinical nutrition in liver disease. *Clin. Nutr.* **2019**, *38*, 485–521. [CrossRef]
104. Dixit, D.; Endicott, J.; Burry, L.; Ramos, L.; Yeung, S.Y.A.; Devabhakthuni, S.; Chan, C.; Tobia, A.; Bulloch, M.N. Management of Acute Alcohol Withdrawal Syndrome in Critically Ill Patients. *Pharmacother. J. Hum. Pharmacol. Drug Ther.* **2016**, *36*, 797–822. [CrossRef]
105. Finocchiaro, D.; Hook, J. Enteral Nutritional Support of the Critically Ill Older Adult. *Crit. Care Nurs. Q.* **2015**, *38*, 253–258. [CrossRef]
106. Vargas, N.; Tibullo, L.; Landi, E.; Carifi, G.; Pirone, A.; Pippo, A.; Alviggi, I.; Tizzano, R.; Salsano, E.; Di Grezia, F.; et al. Caring for critically ill oldest old patients: a clinical review. *Aging Clin. Exp. Res.* **2017**, *29*, 833–845. [CrossRef]
107. McClave, S.A.; Patel, J.J.; Weijs, P.J.M. Editorial: Introduction to the 2018 ESPEN guidelines on clinical nutrition in the intensive care unit: Food for thought and valuable directives for clinicians! *Curr. Opin. Clin. Nutr. Metab. Care* **2019**, *22*, 141–145. [CrossRef]
108. Berger, M.M.; Pichard, C. Parenteral nutrition in the ICU: Lessons learned over the past few years. *Nutrition* **2019**, *59*, 188–194. [CrossRef]
109. Harvey, S.E.; Parrott, F.; Harrison, D.A.; Bear, D.E.; Segaran, E.; Beale, R.; Bellingan, G.; Leonard, R.; Mythen, M.G.; Rowan, K.M.; et al. Trial of the route of early nutritional support in critically ill adults. *N. Engl. J. Med.* **2014**, *371*, 1673–1684. [CrossRef]
110. Reintam Blaser, A.; Starkopf, J.; Alhazzani, W.; Berger, M.M.; Casaer, M.P.; Deane, A.M.; Fruhwald, S.; Hiesmayr, M.; Ichai, C.; Jakob, S.M.; et al. Early enteral nutrition in critically ill patients: ESICM clinical practice guidelines. *Intensive Care Med.* **2017**, *43*, 380–398. [CrossRef]
111. Reintam Blaser, A.; Malbrain, M.L.; Starkopf, J.; Fruhwald, S.; Jakob, S.M.; De Waele, J.; Braun, J.P.; Poeze, M.; Spies, C. Gastrointestinal function in intensive care patients: Terminology, definitions and management. Recommendations of the ESICM Working Group on Abdominal Problems. *Intensive Care Med.* **2012**, *38*, 384–394. [CrossRef]
112. Wischmeyer, P.E.; Puthucheary, Z.; Millán, I.S.; Butz, D.; Grocott, M. Muscle Mass and Physical Recovery in ICU: Innovations for Targeting of Nutrition and Exercise. *Curr. Opin. Crit. Care* **2017**, *23*, 269–278. [CrossRef]
113. Taylor, S.; Dumont, N.; Clemente, R.; Allan, K.; Downer, C.; Mitchell, A. Critical care: Meeting protein requirements without overfeeding energy. *Clin. Nutr. ESPEN* **2016**, *11*, e55–e62. [CrossRef]
114. Klein, C.J.; Stanek, G.S.; Wiles, C.E., 3rd. Overfeeding macronutrients to critically ill adults: Metabolic complications. *J. Am. Diet. Assoc.* **1998**, *98*, 795–806. [CrossRef]
115. McClave, S.A.; Snider, H.L. Clinical Use of Gastric Residual Volumes as a Monitor for Patients on Enteral Tube Feeding. *J. Parenter. Enter. Nutr.* **2002**, *26*, S43–S50. [CrossRef]
116. Friedli, N.; Stanga, Z.; Culkin, A.; Crook, M.; Laviano, A.; Sobotka, L.; Kressig, R.W.; Kondrup, J.; Mueller, B.; Schuetz, P. Management and prevention of refeeding syndrome in medical inpatients: An evidence-based and consensus-supported algorithm. *Nutrition* **2018**, *47*, 13–20. [CrossRef]
117. Friedli, N.; Stanga, Z.; Sobotka, L.; Culkin, A.; Kondrup, J.; Laviano, A.; Mueller, B.; Schuetz, P. Revisiting the refeeding syndrome: Results of a systematic review. *Nutrition* **2017**, *35*, 151–160. [CrossRef]
118. Olthof, L.E.; Koekkoek, W.; van Setten, C.; Kars, J.C.N.; van Blokland, D.; van Zanten, A.R.H. Impact of caloric intake in critically ill patients with, and without, refeeding syndrome: A retrospective study. *Clin. Nutr.* **2018**, *37*, 1609–1617. [CrossRef]
119. Doig, G.S.; Simpson, F.; Heighes, P.T.; Bellomo, R.; Chesher, D.; Caterson, I.D.; Reade, M.C.; Harrigan, P.W.; Refeeding Syndrome Trial Investigators Group. Restricted versus continued standard caloric intake during the management of refeeding syndrome in critically ill adults: A randomised, parallel-group, multicentre, single-blind controlled trial. *Lancet Respir. Med.* **2015**, *3*, 943–952. [CrossRef]

120. Mehanna, H.M.; Moledina, J.; Travis, J. Refeeding syndrome: What it is, and how to prevent and treat it. *BMJ* **2008**, *336*, 1495–1498. [CrossRef]
121. Lappas, B.M.; Patel, D.; Kumpf, V.; Adams, D.W.; Seidner, D.L. Parenteral Nutrition: Indications, Access, and Complications. *Gastroenterol. Clin. N. Am.* **2018**, *47*, 39–59. [CrossRef]
122. Davila, J.; Konrad, D. Metabolic Complications of Home Parenteral Nutrition. *Nutr. Clin. Pract.* **2017**, *32*, 753–768. [CrossRef]
123. Pironi, L.; Labate, A.M.; Pertkiewicz, M.; Przedlacki, J.; Tjellesen, L.; Staun, M.; De Francesco, A.; Gallenca, P.; Guglielmi, F.W.; Van Gossum, A.; et al. Prevalence of bone disease in patients on home parenteral nutrition. *Clin. Nutr.* **2002**, *21*, 289–296. [CrossRef]
124. Grau, T.; Bonet, A.; Rubio, M.; Mateo, D.; Farre, M.; Acosta, J.A.; Blesa, A.; Montejo, J.C.; de Lorenzo, A.G.; Mesejo, A.; et al. Liver dysfunction associated with artificial nutrition in critically ill patients. *Crit. Care* **2007**, *11*, R10. [CrossRef]
125. Zhou, X.-D.; Dong, W.-H.; Zhao, C.-H.; Feng, X.-F.; Wen, W.-W.; Tu, W.-Y.; Cai, M.-X.; Xu, T.-C.; Xie, Q.-L. Risk scores for predicting dysphagia in critically ill patients after cardiac surgery. *BMC Anesthesiol.* **2019**, *19*, 7. [CrossRef]
126. Poorjavad, M.; Jalaie, S. Systemic review on highly qualified screening tests for swallowing disorders following stroke: Validity and reliability issues. *J. Res. Med. Sci.* **2014**, *19*, 776–785.
127. Dellinger, R.P.; Levy, M.M.; Rhodes, A.; Annane, D.; Gerlach, H.; Opal, S.M.; Sevransky, J.E.; Sprung, C.L.; Douglas, I.S.; Jaeschke, R.; et al. Surviving Sepsis Campaign: international guidelines for management of severe sepsis and septic shock, 2012. *Intensive Care Med.* **2013**, *39*, 165–228. [CrossRef]
128. Rice, N.; Normand, C. The cost associated with disease-related malnutrition in Ireland. *Public Health Nutr.* **2012**, *15*, 1966–1972. [CrossRef]
129. Turpin, R.S.; Canada, T.; Liu, F.X.; Mercaldi, C.J.; Pontes-Arruda, A.; Wischmeyer, P. Nutrition therapy cost analysis in the US: Pre-mixed multi-chamber bag vs. compounded parenteral nutrition. *Appl. Health Econ. Health Policy* **2011**, *9*, 281–292. [CrossRef]
130. Piquet, M.-A.; Bertrand, P.C.; Roulet, M. Role of a nutrition support team in reducing the inappropriate use of parenteral nutrition. *Clin. Nutr.* **2004**, *23*, 437. [CrossRef]
131. Doig, G.S.; Heighes, P.T.; Simpson, F.; Sweetman, E.A.; Davies, A.R. Early enteral nutrition, provided within 24 h of injury or intensive care unit admission, significantly reduces mortality in critically ill patients: A meta-analysis of randomised controlled trials. *Intensive Care Med.* **2009**, *35*, 2018–2027. [CrossRef]
132. Doig, G.S.; Chevrou-Séverac, H.; Simpson, F. Early enteral nutrition in critical illness: A full economic analysis using US costs. *Clin. Outcomes Res.* **2013**, *5*, 429–436. [CrossRef]
133. Pradelli, L.; Graf, S.; Pichard, C.; Berger, M.M.; Information, P.E.K.F.C. Supplemental parenteral nutrition in intensive care patients: A cost saving strategy. *Clin. Nutr.* **2018**, *37*, 573–579. [CrossRef]
134. Vanderheyden, S.; Casaer, M.P.; Kesteloot, K.; Simoens, S.; De Rijdt, T.; Peers, G.; Wouters, P.J.; Coenegrachts, J.; Grieten, T.; Polders, K.; et al. Early versus late parenteral nutrition in ICU patients: Cost analysis of the EPaNIC trial. *Crit. Care* **2012**, *16*, R96. [CrossRef]
135. Schuetz, P.; Fehr, R.; Baechli, V.; Geiser, M.; Deiss, M.; Gomes, F.; Kutz, A.; Tribolet, P.; Bregenzer, T.; Braun, N.; et al. Individualised nutritional support in medical inpatients at nutritional risk: A randomised clinical trial. *Lancet* **2019**, *393*, 2312–2321. [CrossRef]

# 6

# Nutrition in Cancer Patients

**Paula Ravasco** [1,2,3]

1 University Hospital of Santa Maria, 1649-035 Lisbon, Portugal; p.ravasco@medicina.ulisboa.pt
2 University of Lisbon, 1649-028 Lisbon, Portugal
3 Centre for Interdisciplinary Research in Health (CIIS) of the Portuguese Catholic University, 1649-023 Lisbon, Portugal

**Abstract: Background:** Despite being recognised that nutritional intervention is essential, nutritional support is not widely accessible to all patients. Given the incidence of nutritional risk and nutrition wasting, and because cachexia management remains a challenge in clinical practice, a multidisciplinary approach with targeted nutrition is vital to improve the quality of care in oncology. **Methods:** A literature search in PubMed and Cochrane Library was performed from inception until 26 March. The search consisted of terms on: cancer, nutrition, nutritional therapy, malnutrition, cachexia, sarcopenia, survival, nutrients and guidelines. Key words were linked using "OR" as a Boolean function and the results of the four components were combined by utilizing the "AND" Boolean function. Guidelines, clinical trials and observational studies written in English, were selected. Seminal papers were referenced in this article as appropriate. Relevant articles are discussed in this article. **Results:** Recent literature supports integration of nutrition screening/assessment in cancer care. Body composition assessment is suggested to be determinant for interventions, treatments and outcomes. Nutritional intervention is mandatory as adjuvant to any treatment, as it improves nutrition parameters, body composition, symptoms, quality of life and ultimately survival. Nutrition counselling is the first choice, with/without oral nutritional supplements (ONS). Criteria for escalating nutrition measures include: (1) 50% of intake vs. requirements for more than 1–2 weeks; (2) if it is anticipated that undernourished patients will not eat and/or absorb nutrients for a long period; (3) if the tumour itself impairs oral intake. N-3 fatty acids are promising nutrients, yet clinically they lack trials with homogeneous populations to clarify the identified clinical benefits. Insufficient protein intake is a key feature in cancer; recent guidelines suggest a higher range of protein because of the likely beneficial effects for treatment tolerance and efficacy. Amino acids for counteracting muscle wasting need further research. Vitamins/minerals are recommended in doses close to the recommended dietary allowances and avoid higher doses. Vitamin D deficiency might be relevant in cancer and has been suggested to be needed to optimise protein supplements effectiveness. **Conclusions:** A proactive assessment of the clinical alterations that occur in cancer is essential for selecting the adequate nutritional intervention with the best possible impact on nutritional status, body composition, treatment efficacy and ultimately reducing complications and improving survival and quality of life.

**Keywords:** cancer; nutrition; nutritional therapy; nutritional support; malnutrition; cachexia; sarcopenia; survival

---

## 1. Introduction

Cancer is a complex disease that results from multiple interactions between genes and the environment, and is regarded as one of the current leading causes of mortality worldwide [1,2]. Metabolic and nutritional alterations can influence survival and recovery of cancer patients: malnutrition, sarcopenia and cachexia [3,4]. Malnutrition ensues from an inflammatory state that promotes anorexia and consequently, weight loss. It is highly prevalent in cancer patients [5] as 15 to 40% of patients report weight loss at diagnosis [6]. It is estimated that 40 to 80% of all cancer patients will be malnourished during the course of the disease. Furthermore, malnutrition can influence treatment outcomes, delay wound healing, worsen muscle function and increase the risk of post-operative complications. It can also impair tolerance and response to antineoplastic treatments, which can in turn lead to extended hospital stay, increase the risk for treatment interruptions, and possible reduced survival [7,8]. Sarcopenia is characterised by a decrease in lean body mass with an impact both on strength and physical function that may decrease the quality of life [9]. As cancer-related weight loss in obese patients cannot be identified by a low body mass index (BMI), sarcopenic obesity, defined as low lean body mass in obese patients, is frequently overlooked [10]. In these patients, changes in body composition result in an increased metabolic risk, and it seems to be a significant predictor of treatment related adverse events [11,12]. Cancer cachexia is a complex multifactorial syndrome that results from a combination of metabolic alterations, systemic inflammation and decreased appetite. It is characterised by an involuntary sustained weight loss and loss of skeletal muscle mass, with or without loss of fat mass that are irreversible by conventional nutritional support [13].

In addition to the disease, antineoplastic treatments and/or surgery have a significant impact on patients' nutritional status [14–16]. During chemotherapy (CT), more than 50% of patients experience dysgeusia, nausea, vomiting and mucositis, and radiotherapy (RT) related complications are also common. It is also established that poor nutritional status increases surgical morbidity and post-surgical complications [17]. Nutritional intervention in cancer patients aim to identify, prevent and treat malnutrition through nutritional counselling with or without oral nutritional supplements (ONS) or via artificial nutrition, i.e., enteral or parenteral nutrition [18–20], as well as to address metabolic and nutritional alterations that influence patients' recovery and survival [19,20]. Despite the fact that nutritional intervention is a key component, nutritional support is not widely accessible to all patients at nutritional risk [21–23]. Additionally, given the incidence of nutritional risk in cancer and the fact that the management of cachexia remains a challenge in clinical practice [24], a multidisciplinary approach is vital to define efficient strategies that can improve quality of care in cancer patients. According to the reviewed data and guidelines, nutritional intervention should be central and adjuvant to any treatment and should be included in the multidisciplinary approach mandatory in oncology. This will allow for more adequate and efficient results in these patients. Multidisciplinary follow-up, with early and regular nutritional intervention, is of major importance in oncology, thus being a key factor for successful treatment and recovery. The present article aims to provide insights and an overview of the most recent literature regarding key nutritional aspects in cancer patients.

Based on this framework, a literature search in PubMed and Cochrane Library was performed from inception until 26 March. The search consisted of terms: cancer, nutrition, nutritional therapy, malnutrition, cachexia, sarcopenia, survival, nutrients, guidelines. Key words were linked using "OR" as a Boolean function and the results of the four components were combined by utilizing the "AND" Boolean function. Guidelines, clinical trials and observational studies written in English, were selected. Seminal papers in the area, even if dated outside the search timeline, were referenced in this article as appropriate.

## 2. Results

### *2.1. Nutritional Screening and Assessment*

Screening for nutritional risk as early as possible allows for the identification of patients at risk of becoming malnourished [25]. Screening should be done as early as possible, and recent literature suggests that it should be done at diagnosis or at hospital admission; screening should be repeated in the course of treatment for referral for evaluation if needed [19,21,23,25–27]. Evidence supports the integration of malnutrition screening in cancer patients care. The adequate tool for screening undernutrition should be brief and easy to fill, inexpensive, highly sensitive and have good specificity [25]. MUST (Malnutrition Universal Screening Tool) and NRS-2002 (Nutritional Risk Screening-2002) are considered suitable [28–30]; the MNA (Mini Nutritional Assessment) is a suitable tool for nutritional assessment in the senior population [19,23].

When nutritional risk is present, screening should be followed by comprehensive nutritional assessment to better determine the course of nutritional intervention. It seems there is no consensus on the best method to perform this assessment, but SGA (Subjective Global Assessment) and PG-SGA (Patient Generated-Subjective Global Assessment) have been validated for nutritional assessment of adult oncology patients [25,26,31].

When used isolated, weight loss is ineffective to detect malnutrition, as it has low sensitivity for metabolic changes that occur in cancer patients. Yet, its early and regular assessment, combined with the evaluation of nutritional intake, BMI and inflammatory status is a standard clinical recommendation [19,26]. As for BMI, it has low sensitivity to detect changes in the nutritional status, especially in obese patients, thus it should only be used combined with other assessment tools [26,32].

Body composition provides valuable information in the management of cancer patients, as imaging methods detect loss of muscle mass as well as fatty muscle infiltration [2]. In cancer patients at risk for malnutrition, sarcopenia and cachexia, muscle mass should be assessed [19,21]. Methods available are dual X-ray absorptiometry (DEXA), computed tomography scans at the level of the 3rd vertebra or bioimpedance analysis (BIA). Additionally, it has been recommended that nutritional assessment should be performed for the stages of cancer cachexia, as nutritional intervention is most effective in the stages of precachexia and cachexia [13].

### 2.2. *Nutritional Intervention*

In order to tackle nutritional deterioration, gathering objective data on nutritional status and its evolution throughout the disease course is of prime concern. Different cancer types or locations display different nutritional patterns that require tailored nutritional therapy. Nutritional deterioration is a multifactorial end-result determined by cancer-related and nutrition- and/or metabolic-related factors. Proper nutrition can alleviate symptom burden, improve health across the cancer continuum, support cancer survivorship [33–36] and is a hallmark of successful cancer treatment.

Nutritional interventions will vary according to patients' medical history, type and stage of cancer, as well as to the response to treatment. If the patient can eat and has a functional gastrointestinal tract, nutritional counselling, with or without ONS should be the elected intervention to address altered nutritional demands due to treatment or disease [19,21,26]. ONS may be necessary, as a means to compensate for lower food intake and to try to prevent nutritional deterioration during the course of treatments. Monitoring compliance with the selected nutritional intervention is essential.

#### 2.2.1. Individualised Nutritional Counselling

In clinical practice, oral nutrition is always the priority. Oral nutrition is the preferred route of feeding as it is a significant part of the patient's daily routine and does contribute substantially to the patients' autonomy [19]. It represents a privileged time to spend with family and friends, avoiding the tendency for isolation. The acknowledgement that the prescribed diet is individualized, adapted and adequate to individual needs, empowers the patient with a feeling of control, thus it is also a highly effective approach for psychological modulation. All these factors may potentially contribute to improve the patients' quality of life, and may modulate acute and late treatment morbidity. The referral for a nutrition professional responsible for the individualised dietary counselling should always be based on decision-making plans (Figure 1).

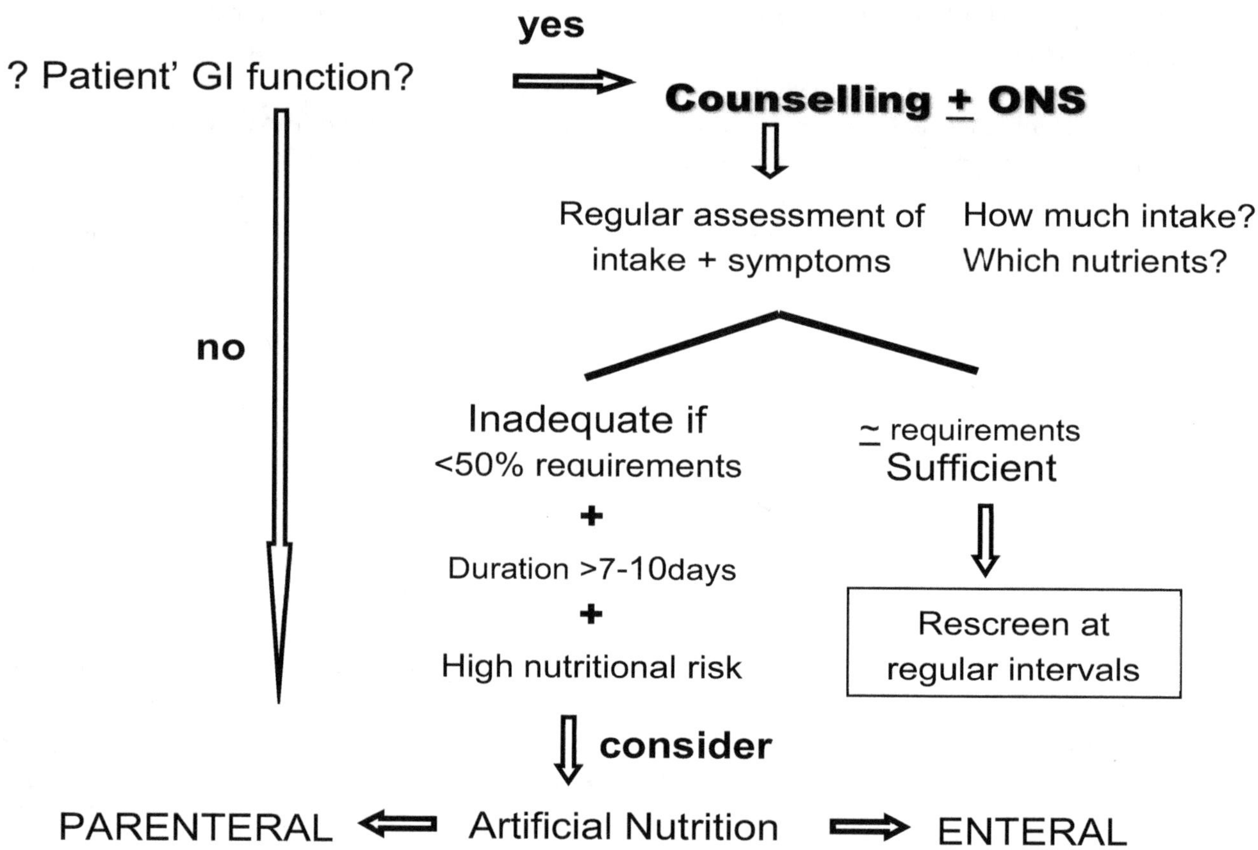


**Figure 1.** Evidence based decision making plan.

As clinicians we have to recognise the dimensions that are determinant for the patients. Indeed, the diet is the only factor that the patient feels he/she can control during the whole course of treatments and interventions. Also, an adequate food intake is recognised by the patient as well as by the family and caregivers, as essential to maintain the daily activity, energy, functional capacity and to overcome treatments more successfully. Notably, nutritional wasting is common regardless of the cancer stage (curative, adjuvant, to palliative) and is an independent predictor of poor physical function, lower quality of life, surgical complications, and reduced survival [3,10,13,37]. Cancer wasting is characterised by muscle mass deterioration that occurs in more than 50% of newly diagnosed cancer patients, in comparison with 15% prevalence in healthy individuals of similar age [38]. Since both muscle mass and adipose tissue play a role in oncological outcomes, strategies to optimize body composition are an important part of successful cancer therapy. Hence, a major goal of nutrition intervention is to favourably influence body composition, with the potential to improve cancer therapy outcomes, morbidities and ultimately, prognosis.

To be effective, individualised counselling has to be based on a thorough assessment of various nutritional and clinical parameters: nutritional status and dietary intake, usual dietary pattern, intolerances or food aversions, patients' psychological status, autonomy, cooperation, need for help or support of others in the act of eating. A thorough symptom assessment is also mandatory (Table 1).

**Table 1.** Common causes for a poor nutrient intake in cancer patients.

- Deterioration in taste, smell and appetite, as a consequence of the tumour and/or therapy
- Altered food preferences/food avoidance/food aversion
- Eating problems (teeth, chewing)
- Dysphagia, odynophagia or partial/total gastrointestinal obstruction
- Early satiety, nausea and vomiting
- Soreness, xerostomia, sticky saliva, painful throat, trismus
- Oral lesions and oesophagitis
- Radiotherapy/chemotherapy induced mucositis
- Acute or chronic radiation enteritis during and after radiotherapy
- Depression, anxiety
- Pain

Individualised nutritional counselling taking into consideration patients' clinical condition and symptoms, was the most effective nutrition intervention, assuring a sustained and adequate diet, which was able to overcome the predictable deterioration subsequent to RT [35,36,39–42]. Positive effects were experienced in the long term with a possible impact of patients' prognosis [43] as recently showed in a randomized trial, the preliminary results of which were presented in the ESPEN Congress in 2018. Another randomised trial of nutritional therapy showed that intervention had an impact in maintaining patients' nutritional status and function [39]. In this study, individualised intensive nutrition counselling was compared with individualised on-demand nutrition counselling by a dietician prior to and during oncologic treatment. On-demand nutrition counselling requested by physician/nurse referral, seemed not inferior to intensive counselling; thus, these results do emphasise the importance of establishing multimodal nutrition teams to effectively and timely screen and orient patients for adequate nutrition [39]. Several guidelines to date do include nutritional counselling as their standard of care for malnourished patients or at risk of malnutrition [19–21,23,26,27] or during anti-neoplastic treatments in head-neck (HNC), oesophageal and colorectal cancers as these patients are in particular risk of malnutrition due to tumour location and irradiated area [14].

If/when oral nutrition is inadequate/insufficient, artificial nutrition should be considered [19–21, 23,26,27]. Criteria for the escalation in nutritional measures are: (1) inadequate food intake (<50% of requirements) is anticipated for more than 10 days due to surgery or chemotherapy (CT)/radiotherapy (RT); (2) if food intake is less than 50% of the requirements for more than one to two weeks; (3) if it is anticipated that undernourished patients will not be able to eat and/or absorb the adequate amount of nutrients for a long period time, due to antineoplastic treatments; (4) if the tumour mass itself impairs oral intake and food progression through the upper GI tract. The decision between enteral nutrition (EN) and parenteral nutrition (PN) must take into account the site of the tumour, its extent, complications, treatment plan and intent, prognosis, patients' overall physical status and the duration of the nutritional support [19–21,23,26,27,44].

### 2.2.2. Artificial Nutrition

If the intestinal functions are preserved, EN should be preferred in order to maintain gut integrity and reduce bacterial translocation [45], as well as to reduce infectious complications [19–21,23,26]. A standard polymeric feeding formula should be preferred. EN is recommended in undernourished or at-risk patients during CT if undernutrition is present or if inadequate food intake is present or anticipated [19,22,23,27,46]. Systematic artificial nutrition during CT treatment is not recommended [19–21,23,26]. In radiation-induced severe mucositis or in obstructive tumours of the head-neck or thorax, either PEG or nasogastric tube are recommended [19,20]. EN is contraindicated in: intestinal obstruction or ileus, severe shock, intestinal ischaemia, high output fistula, severe intestinal haemorrhage, intestinal insufficiency due to radiation enteritis, short bowel syndrome, peritoneal carcinomatosis chylothorax [19,21,23,26]. In these situations, or whenever EN is insufficient, a combination of EN and PN or PN alone should be considered [19,21,23,26].

As for PN, it should be initiated early [19,21,23,26] whenever indicated. PN is the first option of nutritional support in cases of intestinal failure; whenever macro and micronutrient' requirements can only be fulfilled via the parenteral route, long term artificial nutrition as home parenteral nutrition (HPN) is standard recommendation [19,44,47,48].

As for the macronutrients in PN, amino acids (AA) requirement of cancer patients relies on: negative balance between whole body protein synthesis and breakdown, doses of AA closer to 2 g/kg/day may be required to control catabolism and stimulate synthesis vs. 0.8 g/kg/day as recommended for healthy subjects [49], and for older subjects and chronic disease, most recent clinical guidelines recommend >1.0 g/kg/day of protein. Hence, to support protein balance, up to 1.5 g/kg/day or more of protein is the consensual recommendation. In the nutritive PN admixtures, essential AA should be present in approximately 50% of AA and branched chain AA should account for the remainder 50% of total AA [50]. In what concerns fat as an energy substrate, the most consensual regimens have fat accounting for ≈50% of non-protein calories [51,52].

Recently, PN as a supplemental route of nutrient administration (SHPN) emerged as a possible resource to optimise nutrient delivery. Prospective studies [53–57] on SHPN suggest a possible benefit in energy balance, increased body fat, greater maximum exercise capacity and QoL. A recent randomised trial showed that SHPN may prevent loss of MM in patients with incurable gastrointestinal cancer [57]. Hence, there is yet insufficient evidence to recommend SHPN in cancer patients to improve QoL and nutrition parameters. Additionally, practice of HPN differs between countries; most do not consider the use of PN if there is a functional gastrointestinal tract, while others may consider its use if it is according to the will of the patient [58–60].

Refeeding syndrome can occur when severe shifts in fluids and electrolytes happen in severely malnourished patients receiving EN or PN, and it may cause hypophosphatemia, hypokalaemia, hypomagnesaemia, thiamine deficiency, changes in sodium, glucose and fluid balance and also in protein and lipid metabolism [19,21]. Its prevention is recommended when BMI < 16 kg/m$^2$ or in the presence of unintentional weight loss >15% within the last three to six months or whenever there is little or no nutritional intake for more than 10 days or if there are decreased levels of potassium, phosphate or magnesium prior to feeding. If a severe decrease in food intake occurs for at least five days, it is recommended a gradual increase in nutrition over several days, and no more than 50% of the calculated energy requirements should be supplied during the first two days of feeding [19,25]. The identified fluid and electrolytes imbalances should be corrected, and the circulatory volume, fluid balance, heart rate and rhythm, as well as clinical status, should be monitored closely. Attention to the refeeding syndrome risk is currently contemplated in guidelines for cancer management [19–23,26,27].

### 2.2.3. Surgery

In order to minimise the metabolic stress response and catabolism associated with surgery in undernourished patients, the enhanced recovery after surgery program (ERAS) is recommended for all cancer patients undergoing curative or palliative surgery [18,22,61]. Within ERAS protocol the following principles should be followed: Screening for malnutrition and give additional nutritional support if necessary [18,22]; avoid preoperative fasting; preoperative carbohydrate treatment should be considered as well as the reestablishment of oral feeding on the first postoperative day; and early mobilisation [18,22]. To avoid preoperative fasting, patients with no risk of aspiration, are allowed to eat solid food until six hours and drink clear fluids until two hours before anaesthesia [18].

In oncologic surgical patients, with moderate to severe nutritional risk, nutritional support is recommended before and after surgery [18,25]. If severe malnutrition is present, delaying surgery may be necessary [18,25]. When submitted to major surgery, nutritional support should be provided routinely, with particular attention to elderly sarcopenic patients.

Besides the ERAS protocol, an early start of nutritional supplementation can significantly diminish the degree of weight loss and incidence of complications [22,25]. If it is anticipated that after surgery, the patient will be unable to eat for more than seven days, it is advised to start nutrition therapy even in well-nourished patients [18,22,25]. After surgery, oral nutrition should also be preferred to EN and the latter should be preferred to PN. If oral intake is possible, it should start after surgery without interruption, after assessing individual tolerance. If oral nutrition is not possible, EN should be initiated within 24 h, preferring standard polymeric enteral formulae if adequate [25].

#### 2.2.4. Radiotherapy and Chemotherapy

Oral mucositis, dysphagia and diarrhoea are common complications of RT and/or CT treatments [12–22]. During RT, nutritional counselling is also recommended, especially in HNC, thorax and gastrointestinal (GI) tract cancers [12–23]. When deemed necessary, ONS should be provided [62], and when severe mucositis is present, artificial nutrition should be considered [23]. When dietary counselling and ONS are insufficient to reduce weight loss or if in the presence of severe mucositis or obstructive tumours of the head or neck or thorax, artificial nutrition should be considered [19,20,23]. In patients treated with RT or chemoradiotherapy, PN is not recommended [19], and it should only be considered when adequate nutrition cannot be assured with oral or EN [19].

### 2.3. *Specific Nutrients*

Nutritional strategies that potentially allow better management of cancer have been widely investigated, but few have reached conclusive results.

#### 2.3.1. Protein

Many patients with cancer do not meet the recommended intake (1.2–1.5 g/kg/day), and not even the one for healthy individuals (0.8 g/kg/day) [63]. Limited protein intake ensues mainly from nutrition impact symptoms that affect dietary intake [64]. Recent guidelines do suggest a higher range of protein intake (1.2–1.5 g/kg/day), because of the positive results of higher protein intake in protein balancing and in maintaining muscle mass. Of additional interest is a recent study showing an inverse association between red meat consumption and seven-year mortality among 992 individuals with stage III colon cancer [65], suggesting that higher protein intake may actually be beneficial in cancer.

Interventions with amino acids have been tested in cancer, aiming to optimise nutritional status and counteract muscle mass wasting. They include supplementation with branched chain amino acids (leucine, isoleucine and valine) [63], β-hydroxy β-methyl butyrate, carnitine and creatine. Yet further research is needed to clarify potential benefits.

As for glutamine, its supplementation in cases of oral mucositis or to prevent/treat diarrhoea during pelvic RT, is not recommended [19,22,26]. As for its use when PN is required for patients undergoing haematopoietic stem cell transplant, guidelines are not identical: there is a fair graded recommendation for eventual use of 0.2–0.5 g/kg/day [26], and the indication that there is not enough evidence to recommend for or against glutamine to reduce anticancer therapy side effects, especially in high dose protocols [19]. In what concerns its potential to improve muscle mass, there is not enough data to support it.

#### 2.3.2. Eicosapentaenoic Acid and Fish Oil

Eicosapentaenoic acid (EPA) has been identified as a promising nutrient with appointed clinical benefits. Several mechanisms have been proposed to explain the potential benefits of EPA on the body composition: inhibition of catabolic stimuli by modulating the production of pro-inflammatory cytokines and enhancing insulin sensitivity that induces protein synthesis. Intervention studies showed that EPA may attenuate deterioration of nutritional status and may aid in improving calorie and protein intake. Recent systematic reviews found that EPA can reduce inflammation and has a potential to modulate the nutritional status/body composition [66,67]. Furthermore, some studies suggest that n−3 fatty acids inhibit proliferation of cancer cells [68] and might decrease CT toxicity [69]. Given the large number of studies reporting a positive impact of n−3 fatty acids on the muscle mass, it is likely that this would be a practical and effective intervention for preventing loss of muscle without significant side effects [19]. It is noteworthy that the strength of recommendation somewhat differs for the use of n−3 fatty acids supplementation in weight losing cancer patients not responding to standard nutritional therapy. This recommendation has been rated as strong [26] and weak [19]. Nevertheless, both guidelines are inclined to consider supplementation with long chain fatty acids and fish oil to decrease systemic inflammation and improve appetite, food intake and body weight.

Trials with homogeneous patient populations regarding cancer type, stage, anti-neoplastic regimens, supplement dosage and modality of administration are needed to clarify clinical benefits. Indeed, it is noteworthy that in view of the modest survival benefits of CT/RT in some cancers, important issues for physicians are to optimize well-being, quality of life via nutritional status and adequate body composition [70].

#### 2.3.3. Micronutrients

Because of the adverse effects of therapy and restricted diet of many patients, the American Institute for Cancer Research [71], American Cancer Society [72] and the European Society for Clinical Nutrition and Metabolism—ESPEN [19] support the use of a multivitamin-multimineral supplement in doses close to the recommended dietary allowance. High doses of vitamins and minerals are discouraged in the absence of specific deficiencies [19,20]. Vitamin D deficiency might be relevant in cancer [19]; also, an association has been reported between low vitamin D and muscle wasting. As a consequence, vitamin D may be needed to optimise protein supplements effectiveness. In light of the recent literature, vitamin D supplementation with 600–800 international units (RDA) in cancer patients can be beneficial in the context of preventing muscle wasting, but further research is needed.

## 3. Discussion

In cancer, deterioration and muscle wasting result from the combination of reduced nutrient absorption, alterations in appetite, taste and/or dietary intake, hormone-induced metabolic changes and cancer-related immune activation with cytokine release. Regardless of the underlying mechanisms, cancer-related weight loss is a multidimensional manifestation that worsens patients' well-being, tolerance to antineoplastic therapies and prognosis. Clinically speaking, weight loss is frequent in cancer patients, and depending on the location of the tumour, it is present in 15 to 40% of cancer patients at diagnosis. Weight loss is frequently the first sign of the nutritional alterations that occur in the course of the disease and is associated with poor prognosis, reduced quality of life and morbidity [62]. Cancer cachexia can be defined as '*a multi-factorial syndrome defined by an ongoing loss of skeletal muscle mass (with or without loss of fat mass) that cannot be fully reversed by conventional nutritional support. It leads to progressive functional impairment. Its pathophysiology is characterized by a negative protein and energy balance driven by a variable combination of reduced food intake and abnormal metabolism*'. The agreed diagnostic criterion for cachexia was weight loss >5%, or weight loss >2% in individuals already showing depletion of body weight (BMI $< 20$ kg/m$^2$) or of skeletal muscle (sarcopenia). Assessment for classification and clinical management should also include the following domains: 'anorexia/reduced food intake, catabolic drive, muscle mass and strength, functional and psychosocial impairment' [13].

The main nutritional problem in cancer is wasting of muscle mass, acknowledged to be a predictor of lower quality of life, impaired functionality, surgical complications and shortened survival [10,63,73,74]. Of note that sarcopenia occurs independently of loss of weight or of fat mass. Thus, a clinically relevant phenotype that also emerged in cancer is characterised by sarcopenia with excessive fat mass. Additionally, to the previous studies demonstrating the major impact of muscle mass depletion on survival and treatment toxicity [73,74], a recent study in a cohort of head-neck cancer patients, showed that patients with cachexia had a worse disease-free survival compared with non-cachectic patients [12,39].

Bearing this in mind, the clinical efforts and priority given to improve treatment outcomes, will logically have to include nutritional intervention and adequacy of body composition. The search for an effective nutritional intervention that improves body composition (preservation of muscle mass and muscle quality) is of utmost importance for clinicians and patients, given the implications for prognosis. Early detection of malnutrition and cachexia should be part of a multimodal approach to improve both patient-centred and oncology outcomes [47].

## 4. Conclusions

In the present article, the most recent guidelines for the management of cancer patients, as well as original studies in nutrition and cancer, were included. Nutrition is a central factor in oncology, influencing the development of the disease, tumour inherent symptoms, response to, and recovery after anti-neoplastic treatment(s), thus having a strong impact on the quality of life and prognosis of the disease. A main nutritional feature is wasting of muscle mass, strongly associated with decreased functional capacity, higher incidence of chemotherapy toxicity, increased hospitalization and complication rate, as well as mortality. Nutritional risk screening and assessment in cancer patients allows for the early detection of malnourished patients and also for a prompt nutritional intervention aiming to prevent nutritional deterioration and muscle wasting. A proactive assessment of the clinical alterations that occur during treatments and during the disease course, is essential for selecting the adequate nutritional intervention, aiming for the best impact on patients' outcomes. Early tailored intervention has the potential to improve body composition and treatment' efficacy, and as evidence stands, it is an obligatory adjuvant intervention, with the likelihood of improving prognosis of the disease itself.

## References

1. Fearon, K.; Barber, M. Moses A: The cancer cachexia syndrome. *Surg. Oncol. Clin. N. Am.* **2001**, *10*, 109–126. [CrossRef]
2. Mattox, T.W. Cancer Cachexia: Cause, Diagnosis, and Treatment. *Nutr. Clin. Pract.* **2017**, *32*, 599–606. [CrossRef] [PubMed]
3. Brown, J.C.; Caan, B.J.; Meyerhardt, J.A.; Weltzien, E.; Xiao, J.; Feliciano, E.M.C.; Kroenke, C.H.; Castillo, A.; Kwan, M.L.; Prado, C.M. The deterioration of muscle mass and radiodensity is prognostic of poor survival in stage I–III colorectal cancer: A population-based cohort study (C-SCANS). *J. Cachex Sarcopenia Muscle* **2018**, *9*, 664–672. [CrossRef] [PubMed]
4. Demark-Wahnefried, W.; Peterson, B.L.; Winer, E.P.; Marks, L.; Aziz, N.; Marcom, P.K.; Blackwell, K.; Rimer, B.K. Changes in Weight, Body Composition, and Factors Influencing Energy Balance Among Premenopausal Breast Cancer Patients Receiving Adjuvant Chemotherapy. *J. Clin. Oncol.* **2001**, *19*, 2381–2389. [CrossRef] [PubMed]
5. De Wys, W.D.; Begg, C.; Lavin, P.T.; Band, P.R.; Bennett, J.M.; Bertino, J.R.; Cohen, M.H.; Douglass, H.O., Jr.; Engstrom, P.F.; Ezdinli, E.Z.; et al. Prognostic effect of weight loss prior to chemotherapy in cancer patients. *Am. J. Med.* **1980**, *69*, 491–497. [CrossRef]
6. Wigmore, S.J.; Plester, C.E.; Ross, J.A.; Fearon, K.C.H.; Wigmore, S. Contribution of anorexia and hypermetabolism to weight loss in anicteric patients with pancreatic cancer. *BJS* **1997**, *84*, 196–197. [CrossRef]
7. Belghiti, J.; Langonnet, F.; Bourstyn, E.; Fekete, F. Surgical implications of malnutrition and immunodeficiency in patients with carcinoma of the esophagus. *Br. J. Surg.* **1983**, *70*, 339–341. [CrossRef]
8. Mantzorou, M.; Koutelidakis, A.; Theocharis, S.; Giaginis, C. Clinical Value of Nutritional Status in Cancer: What is its Impact and how it Affects Disease Progression and Prognosis? *Nutr. Cancer* **2017**, *69*, 1–26. [CrossRef]
9. Ravasco, P.; Grillo, I.M.; Vidal, P.; Camilo, M. Nutritional Deterioration in Cancer: The Role of Disease and Diet. *Clin. Oncol.* **2003**, *15*, 443–450. [CrossRef]
10. Prado, C.M.; Cushen, S.J.; Orsso, C.E.; Ryan, A.M. Sarcopenia and cachexia in the era of obesity: Clinical and nutritional impact. *Proc. Nutr. Soc.* **2016**, *75*, 188–198. [CrossRef]
11. Bazzan, A.J.; Newberg, A.B.; Cho, W.C.; Monti, D.A. Diet and nutrition in cancersurvivorship and palliative care. *Evid. Based Complement. Alternat. Med.* **2013**, *2013*, 917647. [CrossRef] [PubMed]

12. Orell-Kotikangas, H.; Österlund, P.; Mäkitie, O.; Saarilahti, K.; Ravasco, P.; Schwab, U.; Mäkitie, A.A. Cachexia at diagnosis is associated with poor survival in head and neck cancer patients. *Acta Oto-Laryngol.* **2017**, *137*, 778–785. [CrossRef] [PubMed]
13. Fearon, K.; Strasser, F.; Anker, S.D.; Bosaeus, I.; Bruera, E.; Fainsinger, R.L.; Jatoi, A.; Loprinzi, C.; MacDonald, N.; Mantovani, G.; et al. Definition and classification of cancer cachexia: An international consensus statement. *Lancet Oncol.* **2011**, *12*, 489–495. [CrossRef]
14. Donaldson, S. Nutritional consequences of radiotherapy. *Cancer Res.* **1997**, *37*, 2407–2413.
15. Chao, K.S.C.; Perez, C.A.; Brady, L.W. (Eds.) Fundamentals of patient management. In *Radiation Oncology: Management Decisions*; Lippincot-Raven: Philadelphia, PA, USA, 2014; pp. 1–13.
16. Blauwhoff-Buskermolen, S.; Versteeg, K.S.; De Van Der Schueren, M.A.; Braver, N.R.D.; Berkhof, J.; Langius, J.A.; Verheul, H.M. Loss of Muscle Mass During Chemotherapy Is Predictive for Poor Survival of Patients with Metastatic Colorectal Cancer. *J. Clin. Oncol.* **2016**, *34*, 1339–1344. [CrossRef]
17. Van der Schueren, M.A.; Van Leeuwen, P.A.; Sauerwein, H.P.; Kuik, D.J.; Snow, G.B.; Quak, J.J. Assessment of malnutrition parameters in head and neck cancer patients and their relation to postoperative complications. *Head Neck* **1997**, *19*, 419–425. [CrossRef]
18. Weimann, A.; Braga, M.; Carli, F.; Higashiguchi, T.; Hübner, M.; Klek, S.; Laviano, A.; Ljungqvist, O.; Lobo, D.N.; Martindale, R.; et al. ESPEN guideline: Clinical nutrition in surgery. *Clin. Nutr.* **2017**, *36*, 623–650. [CrossRef]
19. Arends, J.; Bachmann, P.; Baracos, V.; Barthelemy, N.; Bertz, H.; Bozzetti, F.; Fearon, K.; Hütterer, E.; Isenring, E.; Kaasa, S.; et al. ESPEN guidelines on nutrition in cancer patients. *Clin. Nutr.* **2017**, *36*, 11–48. [CrossRef]
20. Arends, J.; Baracos, V.; Bertz, H.; Bozzetti, F.; Calder, P.; Deutz, N.; Erickson, N.; Laviano, A.; Lisanti, M.; Lobo, D.; et al. ESPEN expert group recommendations for action against cancer-related malnutrition. *Clin. Nutr.* **2017**, *36*, 1187–1196. [CrossRef]
21. De Las Peñas, R.; Majem, M.; Perez-Altozano, J.; Virizuela, J.A.; Cancer, E.; Diz, P.; Donnay, O.; Hurtado, A.; Jimenez-Fonseca, P.; Ocon, M.J. SEOM clinical guidelines on nutrition in cancer patients (2018). *Clin. Transl. Oncol.* **2019**, *21*, 87–93. [CrossRef]
22. Raspé, C.; Flöther, L.; Schneider, R.; Bucher, M.; Piso, P. Best practice for perioperative management of patients with cytoreductive surgery and HIPEC. *Eur. J. Surg. Oncol.* **2017**, *43*, 1013–1027. [CrossRef]
23. French Speaking Society of Clinical Nutrition and Metabolism (SFNEP). Clinical nutrition guidelines of the French Speaking Society of Clinical Nutrition and Metabolism (SFNEP): Summary of recommendations for adults undergoing non-surgical anticancer treatment. *Dig. Liver Dis.* **2014**, *46*, 667–674. [CrossRef]
24. Prado, C.M.; Sawyer, M.B.; Ghosh, S.; Lieffers, J.R.; Esfandiari, N.; Antoun, S.; Baracos, V. Central tenet of cancer cachexia therapy: Do patients with advanced cancer have exploitable anabolic potential? *Am. J. Clin. Nutr.* **2013**, *98*, 1012–1019. [CrossRef]
25. Benoist, S.; Brouquet, A. Nutritional assessment and screening for malnutrition. *J. Visc. Surg.* **2015**, *152* (Suppl. 1), S3–S7. [CrossRef]
26. Thompson, K.L.; Elliott, L.; Fuchs-Tarlovsky, V.; Levin, R.M.; Voss, A.C.; Piemonte, T. Rd Oncology Evidence-Based Nutrition Practice Guideline for Adults. *J. Acad. Nutr. Diet.* **2017**, *117*, 297–310. [CrossRef]
27. Talwar, B.; Donnelly, R.; Skelly, R.; Donaldson, M. Nutritional management in head and neck cancer: United Kingdom National Multidisciplinary Guidelines. *J. Laryngol. Otol.* **2016**, *130*, S32–S40. [CrossRef]
28. Orell-Kotikangas, H.; Österlund, P.; Saarilahti, K.; Ravasco, P.; Schwab, U.; Mäkitie, A.A. NRS-2002 for pre-treatment nutritional risk screening and nutritional status assessment in head and neck cancer patients. *J. Support. Care Cancer* **2015**, *23*, 1495–1502. [CrossRef]
29. Boléo-Tomé, C.; Monteiro Grillo, I.; Camilo, M.E.; Ravasco, P. Validation of the Malnutrition Universal Screening Tool (MUST) in cancer. *Br. J. Nutr.* **2012**, *108*, 343–348. [CrossRef]
30. Boléo-Tomé, C.; Chaves, M.; Monteiro-Grillo, I.; Camilo, M.; Ravasco, P. Teaching Nutrition Integration: MUST Screening in Cancer. *Oncologist* **2011**, *16*, 239–245. [CrossRef]
31. Ottery, F. Definition of standardised nutritional assessment and interventional pathways in oncology. *Nutrition* **1996**, *12*, s15–s19. [CrossRef]
32. Ortiz, C. Analysis of clinical guidelines in oncology. *Nutr. Hosp.* **2016**, *33* (Suppl. 1), 40–49.
33. Ravasco, P.; Monteiro-Grillo, I.; Camilo, M.E. Does nutrition influence quality of life in cancer patients undergoing radiotherapy? *Radiother. Oncol.* **2003**, *67*, 213–220. [CrossRef]

34. Monteiro-Grillo, I.; Vidal, P.M.; Camilo, M.E.; Ravasco, P. Cancer: Disease and nutrition are key determinants of patients' quality of life. *Support. Care Cancer* **2004**, *12*, 246–252. [CrossRef]
35. Ravasco, P.; Monteiro Grillo, I.; Marques Vidal, P.; Camilo, M.E. Dietary conseling improves patient outcomes: A prospective, randomized, controlled trial in colorectal cancer patients undergoing radiotherapy. *J. Clin. Oncol.* **2005**, *23*, 1431–1438. [CrossRef]
36. Ravasco, P.; Vidal, P.M.; Camilo, M.E.; Monteiro-Grillo, I.; Monteiro-Grillo, I. Impact of nutrition on outcome: A prospective randomized controlled trial in patients with head and neck cancer undergoing radiotherapy. *Head Neck* **2005**, *27*, 659–668. [CrossRef]
37. Martin, L.; Senesse, P.; Gioulbasanis, I.; Antoun, S.; Bozzetti, F.; Deans, C.; Strasser, F.; Thoresen, L.; Jagoe, R.T.; Chasen, M.; et al. Diagnostic criteria for the classification of cancer-associated weight loss. *J. Clin. Oncol.* **2015**, *33*, 90–99. [CrossRef]
38. Von Haehling, S.; Morley, J.E.; Anker, S.D. An overview of sarcopenia: Facts and numbers on prevalence and clinical impact. *J. Cachexia Sarcopenia Muscle* **2010**, *1*, 129–133. [CrossRef]
39. Orell-Kotikangas, H.; Österlund, P.; Saarilahti, K.; Ravasco, P.; Schwab, U.; Mäkitie, A.A. Nutritional Counseling for Head and Neck Cancer Patients Undergoing (Chemo) Radiotherapy-A Prospective Randomized Trial. *Front. Nutr.* **2019**, *18*, 22. [CrossRef]
40. Van Bokhorst-de van der Schueren, M.A. Nutritional support strategies for malnourished cancer patients. *Eur. J. Oncol. Nurs.* **2005**, *9* (Suppl. 2), S74–S83. [CrossRef]
41. Bauer, J.; Isenring, E.; Ferguson, M. Dietary counseling: Evidence in chemotherapy patients. *Support. Oncol.* **2008**, *6*, 354–355.
42. Isenring, E.A.; Bauer, J.D.; Capra, S. Nutrition Support Using the American Dietetic Association Medical Nutrition Therapy Protocol for Radiation Oncology Patients Improves Dietary Intake Compared with Standard Practice. *J. Am. Diet. Assoc.* **2007**, *107*, 404–412. [CrossRef]
43. Ravasco, P.; Monteiro Grillo, I.; Camilo, M. Dietary individualized counseling benefits in colorectal cancer: The long term follow-up of a randomized controlled trial of nutritional therapy. *Am. J. Clin. Nutr.* **2012**, *96*, 1346–1353. [CrossRef]
44. Staun, M.; Pironi, L.; Bozzetti, F.; Baxter, J.; Forbes, A.; Joly, F.; Jeppesena, P.; Morenog, J.; Hebuterne, X.; Pertkiewicz, M.; et al. ESPEN Guidelines on Parenteral Nutrition: Home Parenteral Nutrition (HPN) in Adult Patients. Available online: http://espen.info/documents/0909/HomeParenteralNutritioninadults.pdf (accessed on 17 July 2019).
45. Souza, N.C.S.; Simões, B.P.; Júnior, A.A.J.; Chiarello, P.G. Changes in Intestinal Permeability and Nutritional Status after Cytotoxic Therapy in Patients with Cancer. *Nutr. Cancer* **2014**, *66*, 576–582. [CrossRef]
46. O'Reilly, D.; Fou, L.; Hasler, E.; Hawkins, J.; O'Connell, S.; Pelone, F.; Callaway, M.; Campbell, F.; Capel, M.; Charnley, R.; et al. Diagnosis and management of pancreatic cancer in adults: A summary of guidelines from the UK National Institute for Health and Care Excellence. *Pancreatology* **2018**, *18*, 962–970. [CrossRef]
47. Lis, C.G.; Gupta, D.; Lammersfeld, C.A.; Markman, M.; Vashi, P.G. Role of nutritional status in predicting quality of life outcomes in cancer—A systematic review of the epidemiological literature. *Nutr. J.* **2012**, *11*, 27. [CrossRef]
48. Nightingale, J.; Young, A.; Hawthorne, B.; McKee, R.; McKinlay, A.; Rafferty, G.; Protheroe, S.; Culkin, A.; Eastwood, J.; Farrer, K.; et al. Position Statement from BIFA Committee. Available online: https://www.bapen.org.uk/nutrition-support/parenteral-nutrition/position-statement-from bifa-committee (accessed on 17 July 2019).
49. Bozzetti, F.; Bozzetti, V. Is the intravenous supplementation of amino acid to cancer patients adequate? A critical appraisal of literature. *Clin. Nutr.* **2013**, *32*, 142–146. [CrossRef]
50. Wolfe, R.R. The 2017 Sir David P Cuthbertson lecture. Amino acids and muscle protein metabolism in critical care. *Clin. Nutr.* **2018**, *37*, 1093–1100. [CrossRef]
51. Körber, J.; Pricelius, S.; Heidrich, M.; Muller, M.J. Increased lipid utilization in weight losing and weight stable cancer patients with normal body weight. *Eur. J. Clin. Nutr.* **1999**, *53*, 740–745. [CrossRef]
52. Cao, D.-X.; Wu, G.-H.; Zhang, B.; Quan, Y.-J.; Wei, J.; Jin, H.; Jiang, Y.; Yang, Z.-A. Resting energy expenditure and body composition in patients with newly detected cancer. *Clin. Nutr.* **2010**, *29*, 72–77. [CrossRef]
53. Finocchiaro, C.; Gervasio, S.; Agnello, E.; Appiano, S.; Bertetto, O.; Ciuffreda, L.; Montrucchio, G.; Luisa, A.M.; D'andrea, F.; Domeniconi, D.; et al. Multicentric study on home parenteral nutrition in advanced cancer patients. *Riv. Ital. Nutr. Parenter. Enter.* **2002**, *20*, 98–107.

54. Seys, P.; Tadmouri, A.; Senesse, P.; Radji, A.; Rotarski, M.; Balian, A.; Culine, S.; Dufour, P.; Chambrier, C. Home parenteral nutrition in elderly patients with cancer: An observational prospective study. *Bull. Cancer* **2014**, *101*, 243–249. [CrossRef]
55. Culine, S.; Chambrier, C.; Tadmouri, A.; Senesse, P.; Seys, P.; Radji, A.; Rotarski, M.; Balian, A.; Dufour, P. Home parenteral nutrition improves quality of life and nutritional status in patients with cancer: A French observational multicentre study. *Support. Care Cancer* **2014**, *22*, 1867–1874. [CrossRef]
56. Vashi, P.G.; Dahlk, S.; Popiel, B.; Lammersfeld, C.A.; Ireton-Jones, C.; Gupta, D. A longitudinal study investigating quality of life and nutritional outcomes in advanced cancer patients receiving home parenteral nutrition. *BMC Cancer* **2014**, *14*, 593. [CrossRef]
57. Girke, J.; Seipt, C.; Markowski, A.; Luettig, B.; Schettler, A.; Momma, M.; Schneider, A.S. Quality of Life and Nutrition Condition of Patients Improve Under Home Parenteral Nutrition: An Exploratory Study. *Nutr. Clin. Pract.* **2016**, *31*, 659–665. [CrossRef]
58. Keane, N.; Fragkos, K.C.; Patel, P.S.; Bertsch, F.; Mehta, S.J.; Di Caro, S.; Rahman, F. Performance status, prognostic scoring, and parenteral nutrition requirements predict survival in patients with advanced cancer receiving home parenteral nutrition. *Nutr. Cancer* **2018**, *70*, 73–82. [CrossRef]
59. Bozzetti, F.; Arends, J.; Lundholm, K.; Micklewright, A.; Zürcher, G.; Muscaritoli, M. ESPEN Guidelines on Parenteral Nutrition: Non-surgical oncology. *Clin. Nutr.* **2009**, *28*, 445–454. [CrossRef]
60. Scolapio, J.; Picco, M.; Tarrosa, V. Enteral versus parenteral nutrition: The patient's preference. *J. Parenter. Enter. Nutr.* **2002**, *26*, 248–250. [CrossRef]
61. Obermair, A.; Simunovic, M.; Isenring, L.; Janda, M. Nutrition interventions in patients with gynecological cancers requiring surgery. *Gynecol. Oncol.* **2017**, *145*, 192–199. [CrossRef]
62. Baldwin, C.; Weekes, C.E. Dietary counselling with or without oral nutritional supplements in the management of malnourished patients: A systematic review and meta-analysis of randomised controlled trials. *J. Hum. Nutr. Diet.* **2012**, *25*, 411–426. [CrossRef]
63. Deutz, N.E.; Safar, A.; Schutzler, S.; Memelink, R.; Ferrando, A.; Spencer, H.; Van Helvoort, A.; Wolfe, R.R. Muscle protein synthesis in cancer patients can be stimulated with a specially formulated medical food. *Clin. Nutr.* **2011**, *30*, 759–768. [CrossRef]
64. Omlin, A.; Blum, D.; Wierecky, J.; Haile, S.R.; Ottery, F.D.; Strasser, F. Nutrition impact symptoms in advanced cancer patients: Frequency and specific interventions, a case–control study. *J. Cachex Sarcopenia Muscle* **2013**, *4*, 55–61. [CrossRef]
65. Van Blarigan, E.L.; Fuchs, C.S.; Niedzwiecki, D.; Zhang, S.; Saltz, L.B.; Mayer, R.J.; Mowat, R.B.; Whittom, R.; Hantel, A.; Benson, A.; et al. Association of Survival with Adherence to the American Cancer Society Nutrition and Physical Activity Guidelines for Cancer Survivors After Colon Cancer Diagnosis: The CALGB 89803/Alliance Trial. *JAMA Oncol.* **2018**, *4*, 783–790. [CrossRef]
66. Papallardo, G.; Almeida, A.; Ravasco, P. Eicosapentaenoic acid in cancer: Does it improve body composition and modulate metabolism? *Nutrition* **2015**, *31*, 549–555. [CrossRef]
67. Ravasco, P.; Lavriv, D.; Neves, P. Should omega-3 be used in cancer cachexia? *Clin. Nutr. ESPEN* **2018**, *25*, 18–25.
68. Hering, J.; Garrean, S.; Dekoj, T.R.; Razzak, A.; Saied, A.; Trevino, J.; Babcock, T.A.; Espat, N.J. Inhibition of Proliferation by Omega-3 Fatty Acids in Chemoresistant Pancreatic Cancer Cells. *Ann. Surg. Oncol.* **2007**, *14*, 3620–3628. [CrossRef]
69. Murphy, R.A.; Mourtzakis, M.; Mazurak, V.C. n-3 polyunsaturated fatty acids: The potential role for supplementation in cancer. *Curr. Opin. Clin. Nutr. Metab. Care* **2012**, *15*, 246–251. [CrossRef]
70. Geisler, C.; Prado, C.; Müller, M. Inadequacy of Body Weight-Based Recommendations for Individual Protein Intake—Lessons from Body Composition Analysis. *Nutrients* **2017**, *9*, 23. [CrossRef]
71. Norman, H.A.; Butrum, R.R.; Feldman, E.; Picciano, M.F.; Rivlin, R.; Simopoulos, A.; Wargovich, M.J.; Weisburger, E.K.; Zeisel, S.H.; Heber, D.; et al. The Role of Dietary Supplements during Cancer Therapy. *J. Nutr.* **2003**, *133*, 3794S–3799S. [CrossRef]
72. Rock, C.L.; Doyle, C.; Demark-Wahnefried, W.; Meyerhardt, J.; Courneya, K.S.; Schwartz, A.L.; Bandera, E.V.; Hamilton, K.K.; Grant, B.; McCullough, M.; et al. Nutrition and physical activity guidelines for cancer survivors. *CA Cancer J. Clin.* **2012**, *62*, 242–274. [CrossRef]

73. Stene, G.B.; Helbostad, J.L.; Amundsen, T.; Sørhaug, S.; Hjelde, H.; Kaasa, S.; Grønberg, B.H. Changes in skeletal muscle mass during palliative chemotherapy in patients with advanced lung cancer. *Acta Oncol.* **2015**, *54*, 340–348. [CrossRef]
74. Lieffers, J.R.; Bathe, O.F.; Fassbender, K.; Winget, M.; Baracos, V.E. Sarcopenia is associated with postoperative infection and delayed recovery from colorectal cancer resection surgery. *Br. J. Cancer* **2012**, *107*, 931–936. [CrossRef]

# 7

# Nutritional Risk Screening and Assessment

**Emilie Reber [1,*,†], Filomena Gomes [2,†], Maria F. Vasiloglou [3], Philipp Schuetz [4,5] and Zeno Stanga [1]**

[1] Department of Diabetes, Endocrinology, Nutritional Medicine and Metabolism, Bern University Hospital, and University of Bern, Freiburgstrasse 15, 3010 Bern, Switzerland
[2] The New York Academy of Sciences, 250 Greenwich Sweet, 40th floor, New York, NY 10007, USA
[3] Diabetes Technology Research Group, ARTORG Center for Biomedical Engineering Research, University of Bern, Murtenstrasse 50, 3008 Bern, Switzerland
[4] Medical University Department, Division of General Internal and Emergency Medicine, Kantonsspital Aarau, Tellstrasse 25, 5000 Aarau, Switzerland
[5] Department for Clinical Research, Medical Faculty, University of Basel, 4001 Basel, Switzerland
* Correspondence: emilie.reber@insel.ch
† Contributed equally to this manuscript.

**Abstract:** Malnutrition is an independent risk factor that negatively influences patients' clinical outcomes, quality of life, body function, and autonomy. Early identification of patients at risk of malnutrition or who are malnourished is crucial in order to start a timely and adequate nutritional support. Nutritional risk screening, a simple and rapid first-line tool to detect patients at risk of malnutrition, should be performed systematically in patients at hospital admission. Patients with nutritional risk should subsequently undergo a more detailed nutritional assessment to identify and quantify specific nutritional problems. Such an assessment includes subjective and objective parameters such as medical history, current and past dietary intake (including energy and protein balance), physical examination and anthropometric measurements, functional and mental assessment, quality of life, medications, and laboratory values. Nutritional care plans should be developed in a multidisciplinary approach, and implemented to maintain and improve patients' nutritional condition. Standardized nutritional management including systematic risk screening and assessment may also contribute to reduced healthcare costs. Adequate and timely implementation of nutritional support has been linked with favorable outcomes such as a decrease in length of hospital stay, reduced mortality, and reductions in the rate of severe complications, as well as improvements in quality of life and functional status. The aim of this review article is to provide a comprehensive overview of nutritional screening and assessment methods that can contribute to an effective and well-structured nutritional management (process cascade) of hospitalized patients.

**Keywords:** nutritional risk screening; nutritional assessment; malnutrition

---

## 1. Introduction

Nutrition is a basic need of life and thus plays an important role in health promotion and disease prevention. Nutritional intake and its controlling mechanisms (e.g., appetite, satiety) are highly complex physiological processes. These processes have a strong influence on nutritional status, which in turn depends on nutritional intake, its balanced supply of macro and micronutrients, and fluid intake. For various reasons, ill people may struggle to meet their nutritional and hydration requirements, and as a consequence, 20–50% of patients are malnourished or at high risk of malnutrition upon hospital admission [1]. One in five patients does not consume enough food to cover their energy or protein needs [2]. The underlying disease may directly impair nutritional intake and may induce metabolic and/or psychological disorders, which increase the nutritional needs or decrease food intake [3–5].

Frequent problems such as chewing and swallowing issues, immobility, and side effects of drugs and polypharmacy should not be underestimated in this regard [6,7]. A protracted decline in nutritional status results in a catabolic metabolism and chronic low-grade inflammation, potentially leading to several harmful consequences, such as loss of fat-free mass, immune dysfunction, higher complications and mortality rates, reduced quality of life, and prolonged hospital stays [8,9]. Malnutrition also influences the efficacy or tolerance of several treatments, such as antibiotic therapy, chemotherapy, radiotherapy, and surgery. The increased metabolism due to the stress of eventual surgical procedures further aggravates the nutritional metabolic risk, and is characterized by activation of the sympathetic nervous system, endocrine responses, and immunological and hematological changes—all leading to a hypermetabolic state, which may further increase patients' nutritional needs. In addition, the fasting periods before many examinations and interventions, as well as inappropriate meal services, inadequate quality and flexibility of hospital catering, and insufficient assistance provided by the health care staff to the most vulnerable patients, lead to further inadequate food intake and deterioration of patients' nutritional status.

Malnutrition should be considered and treated as an additional disease, as it has been shown to worsen clinical outcomes and to increase morbidity, mortality, and complication rates, thus causing additional costs [3,4,7,10–14]. However, malnutrition is preventable and mostly reversible with early adequate nutritional therapy. It often remains undetected due to lack of awareness, knowledge, and clinical protocols to identify and treat this problem within hospitals. The identification of malnutrition has typically been based on anthropometric, biochemical, and physical parameters, among others. However, there is currently no universally accepted gold standard (best method) for the assessment of nutritional status [15,16].

A systematic and standardized approach to identifying this condition is needed, and that is where nutritional screening tools play an important role [17]. When malnutrition is diagnosed, an individual nutritional care plan should be established by a nutrition specialist (e.g., dietitian, expert clinician) in consultation with a multidisciplinary team, and monitored regularly throughout the hospital stay. To improve the overall outcomes from nutritional treatment it is necessary to select patients with overt malnutrition, and those at most risk of developing nutritional deficiencies during their hospitalization. A systematic approach to addressing malnutrition in hospitals should start with the screening of all patients on admission, proceeding to a detailed assessment of nutritional status in those found to be at increased risk. In patients who are identified as malnourished or at nutritional risk, an appropriate nutritional intervention tailored to the individual patient's needs should follow. Unfortunately, although the need for this process is well-recognized and forms part of several national and international guidelines, it is not carried out everywhere. In the well-known cross-sectional "NutriDay" survey conducted in 2007–2008, 21,007 patients from 325 hospitals in 25 European countries were included. Results showed that a screening routine existed in only half (53%) of the hospitals in the different regions, mostly performed with locally developed methods. While the routine screening of patients for malnutrition on hospital admission existed for 93% of units in the United Kingdom, less than 33% of units had this practice in Austria, Germany, and the South Eastern region. In addition, more than a quarter of all patients (27%) were considered to be at risk of malnutrition, and energy goals were not met in almost half (43%) of the surveyed population [18]. It remains necessary to raise awareness of malnutrition and to improve the outcomes of patients' nutritional treatments.

We aimed to provide an extensive and critical overview of the nutritional screening and nutritional assessment methods of hospitalized patients, complemented by the description of the most novel technological approaches developed to improve the accuracy of dietary assessment. We hope that this review will be helpful to update clinicians involved in the nutritional care of this patient population.

## 2. Screening

Nutritional risk screening tools are very helpful in the daily routine to detect potential or manifest malnutrition in a timely manner. Such tools should be easy to use, quick, economical, standardized, and validated. Screening tools should be both sensitive and specific, and if possible, predictors of the success of the nutritional therapy. Nutritional screening should be part of a defined clinical protocol that results in a plan of action if the screening result is positive.

Diverse scores and screening systems were established in past decades for use in various clinical settings and patient populations (inpatients, community, geriatrics, etc.). Screening should be performed within the first 24–48 h after hospital admission and at regular intervals thereafter (e.g., weekly), in order to rapidly and accurately identify individuals who should be referred to the nutrition specialist (e.g., dietitian, expert clinician) for further assessment. Nutritional screening should include dynamic parameters rather than static ones—for example, recent weight loss, current body mass index (BMI), recent food intake, and disease severity. According to the systematic review conducted by van Bokhorst-de van der Schueren et al., at least 33 different nutritional risk screening tools exist [19]. The present work will use three as examples. The present work will use three examples thereof, which the European Society for Clinical Nutrition and Metabolism (ESPEN) recommends: the Nutritional Risk Screening 2002 (NRS-2002) for the inpatient setting, the Malnutrition Universal Screening Tool (MUST) for the ambulatory setting and the Mini Nutritional Assessment (MNA) for institutionalized geriatric patients [20].

One of the nutritional risk screening tools used most often in hospitals worldwide is the NRS-2002 (Table 1). The NRS-2002 was developed by Kondrup et al., and is meant to be a generic tool in the hospital setting—that is, useful in detecting most of the patients who would benefit from nutritional therapy [21]. This was recently shown in a large multicenter randomized controlled study in a medical inpatient population, which demonstrated a reduction of important clinical outcomes, including mortality, in patients at risk of malnutrition as determined by the NRS-2002 [22]. The NRS-2002 is a simple and well-validated tool which incorporates pre-screening with four questions. If one of these is answered positively, a screening follows which includes surrogate measures of nutritional status, with static and dynamic parameters and data on the severity of the disease (stress metabolism). For each parameter, a score from 0 to 3 can result. Age over 70 years is considered as a risk factor, and is included in the screening tool as well, giving 1 point. A total score of ≥3 points means that the patient is at risk of malnutrition or already malnourished and therefore a nutritional therapy is indicated. The NRS-2002 has been assessed and validated in hundreds of studies, including randomized controlled trials, and has been shown to be very reliable if administered by trained staff.

The MUST (Table 2) was developed to identify malnourished individuals in all care settings (hospitals, nursing homes, home care, etc.) [23]. It was the basis for the NRS-2002 [21]. Recent food intake is not included, and calculations of the weight loss percentage may be a barrier for the busy healthcare staff on the wards.

The MNA is the screening tool most frequently used in institutionalized geriatric patients (Table 3). It combines screening and assessment features. Unlike the NRS-2002, the MNA includes diverse components (loss of appetite, altered sense of taste and smell, loss of thirst, frailty, depression) often relevant for the nutritional status of older people. It also includes anthropometric measurements, nutritional habits, general condition, and self-evaluation. Both the MNA (complete form) as well as a short-form MNA (MNA-SF) are available. The complete MNA includes eighteen items in four domains (Appendix A). The MNA-SF includes only six items, but is quicker and as effective as the long version. If the total score is 11 points or less, the patient is considered at risk of malnutrition or malnourished and the full version (assessment) should be performed.

It is important for clinicians to understand how the tools were validated and for which population and care setting they were developed in order to determine if the tool is appropriate for use in their institution [24]. For example, a study that aimed to identify the most appropriate nutritional screening tool for predicting unfavorable clinical outcomes in 705 patients admitted to a Brazilian hospital compared the performance of NRS-2002, MNA-SF, and MUST. The authors observed that the NRS-2002 and MNA-SF had similar performance in predicting complications, very long length of hospital stay, and mortality, but the NRS-2002 had the best yield, and therefore recommended the use of this tool in the Brazilian inpatient population [25].

**Table 1.** Nutritional Risk Screening 2002. APACHE: acute physiology and chronic health evaluation; BMI: body mass index; COPD: chronic obstructive pulmonary disease; ONS: oral nutritional supplement.

| **Pre-Screening** | | | |
|---|---|---|---|
| Is the BMI of the patient < 20.5 kg/m$^2$ | | | Yes |
| Did the patient lose weight in the past 3 months? | | | Yes |
| Was the patient's food intake reduced in the past week? | | | Yes |
| Is the patient critically ill? | | | Yes |
| If yes to one of those questions, proceed to screening.<br>If no for all answers, the patient should be re-screened weekly. | | | |
| **Screening** | | | |
| Nutritional status | score | Stress metabolism (severity of the disease) | score |
| None | 0 | None | 0 |
| Mild<br>Weight loss >5% in 3 months<br>OR<br>50–75% of the normal food intake in the last week | 1 | Mild stress metabolism<br>Patient is mobile<br>Increased protein requirement can be covered with oral nutrition<br>*Hip fracture, chronic disease especially with complications e.g., liver cirrhosis, COPD, diabetes, cancer, chronic hemodialysis* | 1 |
| Moderate<br>Weight loss >5% in 2 months<br>OR<br>BMI 18.5–20.5 kg/m$^2$ AND reduced general condition<br>OR<br>25–50% of the normal food intake in the last week | 2 | Moderate stress metabolism<br>Patient is bedridden due to illness<br>Highly increased protein requirement, may be covered with ONS<br>*Stroke, hematologic cancer, severe pneumonia, extended abdominal surgery* | 2 |
| Severe<br>Weight loss >5% in 1 month<br>OR<br>BMI <18.5 kg/m$^2$ AND reduced general condition<br>OR<br>0–25% of the normal food intake in the last week | 3 | Severe stress metabolism<br>Patient is critically ill (intensive care unit)<br>Very strongly increased protein requirement can only be achieved with (par)enteral nutrition<br>*APACHE-II >10, bone marrow transplantation, head traumas* | 3 |
| Total (A) | | Total (B) | |
| **Age** | | | |
| <70 years: 0 pt<br>≥70 years: 1 pt | | | |
| **TOTAL = (A) + (B) + Age** | | | |
| ≥3 points: patient is at nutritional risk. Nutritional care plan should be set up<br><3 points: repeat screening weekly | | | |

**Table 2.** The Malnutrition Universal Screening Tool.

| **Malnutrition Universal Screening Tool (MUST)** | | | | |
|---|---|---|---|---|
| BMI (kg/m²) | | Unintentional weight loss in the past 3–6 months | | Acute illness with reduced food intake (estimated) for ≥5 days |
| ≥20 | 0 | ≤5% | 0 | No = 0 |
| 18.5–20.0 | 1 | 5–10% | 1 | Yes = 2 |
| ≤18.5 | 2 | ≥10% | 2 | |
| **Overall Risk for Malnutrition** | | | | |
| Total | Risk | Procedure | Implementation | |
| 0 | Low | Routine clinical care | Clinic: weekly<br>Nursing home: monthly<br>Outpatient: yearly in at-risk patient groups, e.g., age >75 years | |
| 1 | Medium | Observe | Clinic, nursing home, and outpatient:<br>Document dietary intake for 3 days.<br>If adequate: little concern and repeat screening (hospital weekly, care home at least monthly, community at least every 2–3 months).<br>If inadequate: clinical concern. Follow local policy, set goals, improve and increase overall nutritional intake, monitor and review care plan regularly. | |
| ≥2 | High | Treat | Clinic, nursing home, and outpatient:<br>Refer to dietitian, Nutritional Support Team, or implement local policy. Set goals, improve and increase overall nutritional intake. Monitor and review care plan (hospital weekly, care home monthly, community monthly). | |

**Table 3.** The Mini Nutritional Assessment Short-Form.

| **Screening** | | |
|---|---|---|
| A | Has food intake declined over the past 3 months due to loss of appetite, digestive problems, or chewing or swallowing difficulties? | 0 = severe decrease in food intake<br>1 = moderate decrease in food intake<br>2 = no decrease in food intake |
| B | Weight loss during the last 3 months | 0 = weight loss greater than 3 kg<br>1 = does not know<br>2 = weight loss between 1 and 3 kg<br>3 = no weight loss |
| C | Mobility | 0 = bedridden or chair bound<br>1 = able to get out of bed/chair but does not go out<br>2 = goes out |
| D | Has the patient suffered psychological stress or acute disease in the past 3 months? | 0 = yes<br>2 = no |
| E | Neuropsychological problems | 0 = severe dementia or depression<br>1 = mild dementia<br>2 = no psychological problems |
| F1 | Body mass index (BMI) | 0 = BMI less than 19<br>1 = BMI 19 to less than 21<br>2 = BMI 21 to less than 23<br>3 = BMI 23 or greater |
| *If BMI is not available, replace question F1 with F2. Do not answer F2 if F1 is already completed.* | | |
| F2 | Calf circumference (CC) in cm | 0 = CC less than 31<br>3 = CC 31 or greater |
| **Screening Score** | | |
| 12–14 points | Normal nutritional status | |
| 8–11 points | At risk of malnutrition | |
| 0–7 points | Malnourished | |

## 3. Assessment

Nutritional assessment should be performed in patients identified as at nutritional risk according to the first step (i.e., screening for risk of malnutrition). Assessment allows the clinician to gather more information and conduct a nutrition-focused physical examination in order to determine if there is truly a nutrition problem, to name the problem, and to determine the severity of the problem [26]. The data collected in a nutritional assessment are often similar to data collected in the screening process, but in more depth. Screening assesses risk whereas assessment actually determines nutritional status [26]. The observation and documentation of oral nutritional intake, including qualitative and quantitative aspects, and measurement of energy, protein, and micronutrient intake, is an important part of nutritional assessment.

There is a limited number of tools used for the assessment of nutritional status. The most-used tool is the Subjective Global Assessment (SGA), which includes information on a medical history (weight loss; dietary intake change; gastrointestinal and functional impairment) and physical examination (loss of subcutaneous fat; muscle wasting; ankle edema, sacral edema, and ascites). Each patient is classified as either well nourished (SGA A), moderately or suspected of being malnourished (SGA B), or severely malnourished (SGA C). A limitation of using SGA is that it only classifies subjects into three general groups, and it does not reflect subtle changes in nutritional status. Furthermore, it is subjective, does not account for biochemical values (e.g., visceral protein levels), and its sensitivity, precision, and reproducibility over time have not been extensively studied in some patient populations. Thus, here we describe the several components that should be part of the nutritional assessment process and interpreted by specialized clinical staff (e.g., dietitians) [27–29].

Most of these components have limited sensitivity and specificity when used individually; therefore, methods for identifying malnourished patients require the use of several parameters and the clinical judgment of experienced and specialized clinical staff. Detailed evaluation leads to an understanding of the nature and cause of the nutrition-related problem, and will inform the design of a personalized nutritional care plan [30].

### 3.1. *Anthropometric Measurements*

#### 3.1.1. Body Weight and Body Mass Index

Body weight, height, and the resulting BMI are important parameters which are relatively easy to obtain from patients with acute as well as chronic diseases. If height cannot be assessed (e.g., in bedridden patients or patients that are unable to stand), knee height or demi-span (also recommended by the MNA) may be used to estimate height by means of standard formulas [31,32]. The body weight measurement should be standardized (e.g., measured at the same time of day and with the same amount of light clothing) to obtain a reliable weight trend. The BMI is an indicator of chronic malnutrition. Europeans are considered underweight when BMI is <18.5 kg/m$^2$. BMI values under this cutoff are associated with poor outcome and higher mortality rates, as are BMI values greater than 30 kg/m$^2$ (typically classified as obesity). In older adults the cut-off for the definition of underweight is higher, that is, <22 kg/m$^2$, as carrying some extra weight seems to be protective in this population. However, the BMI has some limitations. For example, it may be biased by fluid overload and edemas, and does not describe body composition (for example, a high BMI can be seen in fat individuals and also in very muscular athletes). Thus, the BMI does not reflect potentially pathological weight loss nor the patient's actual food intake. Unintentional weight loss is paramount for the assessment of nutritional status, as it points to a catabolic metabolic situation and is associated with higher morbidity and mortality rates.

#### 3.1.2. Skinfold Measurements

One of the easiest and lowest-priced non-invasive methods is the measurement of the circumference of a limb (e.g., mid-arm, calf) and of skinfold thickness (SFT). The subcutaneous fat tissues normally account for half of the entire body fat mass, and the measurement of SFT gives information on the energy stores of the body, mainly fat stores (i.e., triglycerides). To estimate the total amount of body fat, four skinfolds need to be measured [33]:

- Biceps skinfold (front side of the middle upper arm);
- Triceps skinfold (back side of the middle upper arm);
- Subscapular skinfold (under the lowest point of the shoulder blade); and
- Suprailiac skinfold (above the upper bone of the hip).

The measurement of SFT requires trained staff and defined conditions. The high interindividual variability is a clear disadvantage of this method, as age, gender, and ethnicity influence the fat mass. The mid-upper-arm muscle circumference (MAMC) reflects the muscle mass, while the mid-arm muscle area (MAMA) gives information about the muscle protein stores, as half of the body's proteins are stored in the skeletal muscles. The MAMA is calculated from the MAMC and the triceps SFT (MAMA = MAMC − (0.314 × SFT)). The decrease in MAMA shows the loss of muscle mass, as a mobilization of the endogenous proteins. This method is not reliable in patients with fluid overload, however, nor does it represent short-term modifications of the nutritional status. The reliability of both the SFT and the MAMA strongly depend on the reference values. For these reasons, triceps skin fold and MAMA are mostly used for research purposes and not in daily clinical routine, as they give validated data—especially when measurements are performed by the same investigator and repeated in a given time period.

### 3.1.3. Body Composition

Body weight—including weight loss, calculation of the BMI, and measurement of the length, circumference, or thickness of various body parts—is useful for the assessment of nutritional status. Body composition describes the body compartments, such as fat mass, fat-free mass, muscle mass, and bone mineral mass, depending on the body composition model used (Figure 1). Body composition measurements may serve as an early diagnostic tool, as quantification, or as a follow-up method that helps to assess nutritional status [34]. Such measurements contribute to the diagnosis of sarcopenia and sarcopenic adiposity, and may establish reference values (energy expenditure/kg fat-free mass (FFM) or power/g muscle). Body composition may change due to disease, age, physical activity, and starvation. There are several methods available to determinate body composition, more or less invasively, as described in the following section (Table 4).

### 3.1.4. Bioelectrical Impedance Analysis (BIA)

Bioelectrical impedance analysis (BIA) is a simple, inexpensive, non-invasive method of estimating body composition. It is suitable for bedside measurements which depend on the body's proportions of fat, muscle, and water. BIA relies on the conduction of an alternating electrical current by the human body. The current passes easily through tissues containing a lot of water and electrolytes like blood and muscles, whereas fat tissues, air, and bone are harder to pass through. Therefore, the larger the fat-free mass, the greater the capacity of the body to conduct the current. BIA gives good information about total body water, body cell mass, and fat mass when correcting for age, sex, and ethnicity. However, BIA is not recommended in patients with fluid overload, in patients at extremes of BMI (<16 or >34 kg/m$^2$), in intensive care unit patients, or in the elderly [35,36]. The newly developed bioelectrical impedance vector analysis (BIVA) provides information about hydration status, body cell mass, and cell integrity through the vector length and position. Both malnutrition and obesity are clearly reflected by BIVA, making it attractive to assess and monitor patients' nutritional status.

### 3.1.5. Creatinine Height Index (CHI)

Creatine is metabolized to creatinine at a more or less stable rate, and reflects the amount of muscle mass [37]. Creatinine excretion correlates with lean body mass and body weight. The creatinine height index (CHI) [38] is a measure of lean body mass and is calculated as follows: CHI (%) = measured 24 h urinary creatinine × 100/normal 24 h urinary creatinine. Urinary creatinine excretion may be influenced by several factors, such as renal insufficiency, meat consumption, physical activity, fever, infections, and trauma. Additionally, the collection of 24-h urine is challenging in daily practice and further limits the use of this method.

### 3.1.6. Dual Energy X-ray Absorptiometry (DXA)

DXA is currently considered the gold standard of body composition measurement. It is increasingly used in clinical practice and in research, despite some exposure to radiation. DXA depends on radiological density analysis (usually in the hip and spine) and is a useful, indirect method of measuring fat mass, fat-free mass, and bone mineral mass.

### 3.1.7. Magnetic Resonance Tomography (MRT) and Computed Tomography (CT)

Magnetic resonance tomography (MRT) and computed tomography (CT) allow the quantification of fat mass and fat-free mass, giving information about the fat distribution and enabling an estimation of skeletal muscle mass. Unlike CT, MRT does not require ionizing radiation. These two methods are mainly used in research due to their restricted availability, their cost, and the time expended [39]. However, it is often possible to obtain nutritional information from scans taken for general diagnostic purposes.

### 3.1.8. Further Methods Used to Measure Body Composition

Several other methods are available, mainly for research purposes due to their complexity. These demanding and expensive methods include air displacement plethysmography (ADP), dilution methods, the measurement of total body potassium, and in vivo neutron activation analysis [40].

Air displacement plethysmography (ADP) is a method to determine the body density (body weight/body volume). It is based on the determination of the body volume by means of air displacement having regard to the residual air volume in the lungs and the gastrointestinal tract. Since the density of fat differs from the density of fat free mass, they can both be determined using a two-compartment model. ADP may also be used in ill patients, unlike other densitometry measurement using hydrodensitometry.

The dilution methods aim to determinate the total body water by means of dilution of non-radioactive isotopes (e.g., deuterium). Such tracers are given orally or parenterally, and their concentrations in urine and blood are measured after a defined time. Extracellular water can then be determined using bromide or sulfate, allowing the definition of intracellular water.

Since potassium is mostly found intracellularly and the natural isotope $^{40}K$ is present in constant fraction, the measurement of the potassium allows the calculation of the body cell mass and thus enables the very accurate determination of the body cell mass.

With the in vivo neutron activation, the body is irradiated with neutron radiation, inducing the emission of a characteristic spectrum of gamma-radiations. This expensive method allows the quantification of single elements such as nitrogen, calcium, sodium, etc.

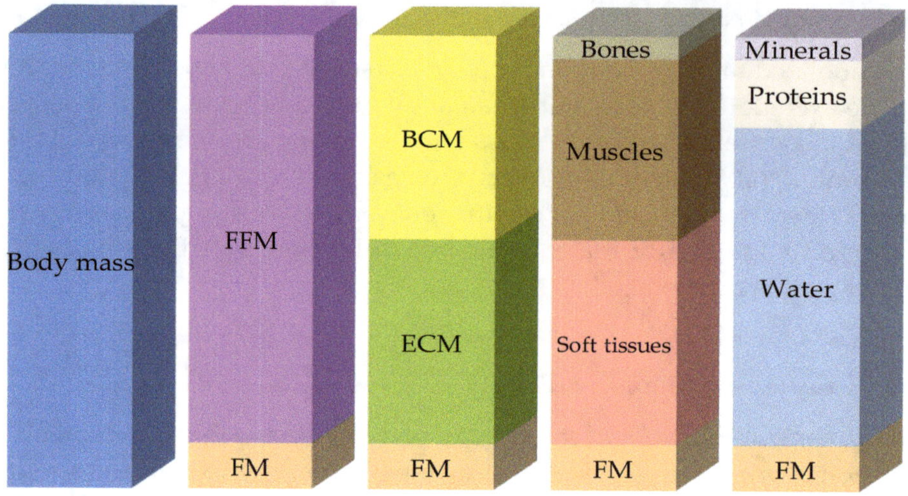


**Figure 1.** Compartment models of body composition. FFM: fat-free mass, FM: fat mass, BCM: body cell mass, ECM: extracellular cell mass. Modified after [40].

**Table 4.** Advantages and disadvantages of methods used to assess body composition.

| Method | Target | Precision | Expenditure (Time/Apparatus) | Costs |
|---|---|---|---|---|
| Anthropometrics | FM, fat distribution, MM | ↓ | ↓ | ↓↓ |
| Bioelectrical impedance analysis | TBW, FM, FFM, BCM phase angle | ↑ | ↓ | ↓ |
| Creatinine height index | MM | ↓ | - | ↓ |
| Dual energy X-ray absorptiometry | FM, bone mineral content, soft tissues, bone density | ↑ | ↑ | ↑ |
| Magnetic resonance tomography | MM, FM, fat distribution | ↑ | ↑ | ↑↑ |
| Computed tomography | FM, fat distribution, MM | ↑ | ↑ | ↑ |
| Dilution method | TBW, FM, FFM (deuterium) ECW, ICW (bromide) | ↑ | ↑ | - |
| Potassium count | BCM, FFM, FM | ↑ | ↑ | ↑↑ |
| Neutron activation | Ca, Na, Cl, $PO_4$, N, H, O, C | ↑ | ↑ | ↑↑ |

FM: fat mass; FFM: fat-free mass; MM: muscle mass; TBW: total body water; BCM: body cell mass; ECW: extracellular water; ICW: intracellular water; Ca: calcium; Na: sodium; Cl: chloride; $PO_4$: phosphate; N: nitrogen; H: hydrogen; O: oxygen; C: carbon.

### *3.2. Biochemical Analysis*

There is no single parameter that can thoroughly assess nutritional status or monitor nutritional therapy. However, a set of laboratory parameters in the clinical routine (e.g., complete blood count, lipid profile, electrolytes, liver parameters) may provide valuable information about a patient's nutritional status (e.g., proof of nutrient deficiency, information about the etiology of malnutrition, follow-up nutritional therapy), about the severity and activity of the disease, and about changes in body composition (Table 5) [41]. Laboratory values—particularly in chronically malnourished patients—may help to detect deficiencies in vitamins (C, D, E, K, thiamine, B6, B12, and folic acid) and trace elements (zinc, selenium, and iron) and help to monitor current substitution therapies. In the early phase of refeeding, potassium, phosphate, and magnesium deficiencies may occur, potentially leading to severe complications (e.g., refeeding syndrome); hence, there is a need for close monitoring of these electrolytes.

**Table 5.** Laboratory values to detect malnutrition and monitor nutritional status [41].

| Laboratory Value | Nutrition Independent Factors | Half-Life | Appropriateness to Detect Malnutrition | Appropriateness to Monitor Nutritional Therapy |
|---|---|---|---|---|
| Albumin | ↑ dehydration<br>↓ inflammation, infections, trauma, heart failure, edema, liver dysfunction, nephrotic syndrome | 20 d | +/++<br>Not appropriate in case of anorexia and acute illness | Not appropriate due to high suggestibility and long half-life |
| Transferrin | ↑ renal failure, iron status, acute hepatitis, hypoxia<br>↓ inflammation, chronic infections hemochromatosis, nephrotic syndrome, liver dysfunction | 10 d | +<br>Low sensitivity and specificity | +<br>Concentration is independent of the energy and protein intake |
| Prealbumin/Transthyretin (TTR) | ↑ renal dysfunction, dehydration, corticosteroid therapy<br>↓ inflammation, hyperthyreosis, liver disease, overhydration | 2 d | ++<br>Not appropriate to detect anorexia Subnormal values within one week in case of fasting | ++/+++<br>One of the most appropriate proteins |
| Retinol binding protein (RBP) | ↑ kidney failure, alcohol abuse<br>↓ hyperthyreosis, chronic liver diseases, vitamin A deficiency, selenium deficiency | 12 h | Idem prealbumin | Idem prealbumin |
| Insulin-like growth factor 1 (IGF-1) | ↑ kidney failure<br>↓ liver diseases, severe catabolic status, age | 24 h | ++<br>Rapid decrease in fasting periods | +++<br>More specific than retinol-binding protein and prealbumin/transthyretin |
| Urinary creatinine | ↑ collection time >24h, infection, trauma<br>↓ insufficient collection time, acute kidney failure | - | 1 mmol of creatinine is derived from 1.9 kg of skeletal muscle mass | Not appropriate, very slow |
| Lymphocytes | ↑ healing phase after infection, hematologic diseases<br>↓ sepsis, hematologic disease, immune suppressants, steroids | - | +<br>Very unspecific | Not appropriate, very slow |

Laboratory values are mostly delayed and costly, and largely dependent on the analytic method and the analyzing laboratory. Additionally, numerous non-nutrition-related factors may influence the laboratory parameters (e.g., inflammatory markers such as CRP), leading to distorted values. Thus, laboratory values must always be interpreted within the clinical context.

## 3.3. *Clinical Evaluation*

### 3.3.1. Patient Clinical History

The patient's clinical history is a subjective and retrospective description of the patient's condition. It is the starting point of the nutritional assessment. Factors leading to malnutrition such as pain, gastrointestinal symptoms (e.g., diarrhea, vomiting, constipation), weight loss, loss of appetite, inability to chew or swallow, and poor dentition/oral health are discussed with the patient. The patient's clinical history should include previous medical condition (chronic or acute disease, symptoms of psychiatric illness, presence of conditions that may lead to metabolic stress (e.g., infection), as well as the actual functional capacity and physiological changes possibly influencing nutritional requirements or body composition (e.g., loss of muscle mass).

### 3.3.2. Physical Examination

Physical examination is an objective method of detecting clinical signs and symptoms of nutritional deficiencies of vitamins and minerals (e.g., poor muscle control, night vision impairment, vertical lip cracks, depression), and allows the assessment of tolerance to nutritional support (e.g., abdominal distention, vomiting, diarrhea) [42]. Some clinical signs are specific to a specific disease or nutrient deficiency. Others are non-specific and need further tests to elucidate their etiology (Table 6). Physical examination includes the control of vital parameters, the inspection and palpation for water retention (edema and ascites), and a rough assessment of muscle mass and subcutaneous fat stores.

**Table 6.** Clinical signs and symptoms of micronutrient deficiencies [40,42].

| Body Region | Signs | Possible Deficiencies |
|---|---|---|
| Skin | Petechiae | Vitamins A, C |
| | Purpura | Vitamins C, K |
| | Pigmentation | Niacin |
| | Edema | Protein, vitamin B1 |
| | Pallor | Folic acid, iron, biotin, vitamins B12, B6 |
| | Decubitus | Protein, energy |
| | Seborrheic dermatitis | Vitamin B6, biotin, zinc, essential fatty acids |
| | Unhealed wounds | Vitamin C, protein, zinc |
| Nails | Pallor or white coloring<br>Clubbing, spoon-shape, or transverse ridging/banding; excessive dryness, darkness in nails, curved nail ends | Iron, protein, vitamin B12 |
| Head/Hair | Dull/lackluster; banding/sparse; alopecia; depigmentation of hair; scaly/flaky scalp | Protein and energy, biotin, copper, essential fatty acid |
| Eyes | Pallor conjunctiva | Vitamin B12, folic acid, iron |
| | Night vision impairment | Vitamin A |
| | Photophobia | Zinc |
| Oral cavity | Glossitis | Vitamins B2, B6, B12, niacin, iron, folic acid |
| | Gingivitis | Vitamin C |
| | Fissures, stomatitis | Vitamin B2, iron, protein |
| | Cheilosis | Niacin, vitamins B2, B6, protein |
| | Pale tongue | Iron, vitamin B12 |
| | Atrophied papillae | Vitamin B2, niacin, iron |
| Nervous system | Mental confusion | Vitamins B1, B2, B12, water |
| | Depression, lethargy | Biotin, folic acid, vitamin C |
| | Weakness, leg paralysis | Vitamins B1, B6, B12, pantothenic acid |
| | Peripheral neuropathy | Vitamins B2, B6, B12 |
| | Ataxia | Vitamin B12 |
| | Hyporeflexia | Vitamin B1 |
| | Muscle cramps | Vitamin B6, calcium, magnesium |
| | Fatigue | Energy, biotin, magnesium, iron |

### 3.3.3. Physical Function

Functional measurements are increasingly important in nutritional assessment. Indeed, muscle strength and cognitive functions all influence quality of life. Energy deficiency diminishes muscle strength and power, as well as overall physical condition. It is therefore very relevant to have information about muscle function and strength in the clinical setting. Muscle function tests are very sensitive to nutritional deficiencies, and therefore also to nutritional interventions. Changes can therefore be noticed much earlier than through body composition tests, for example. Hand dynamometry has been validated as a nutritional marker, correlates very well with the nutritional status, and is simultaneously a good predictor of surgical outcome, increased hospital length of stay, higher re-hospitalization rates, and decreased physical status. It is additionally a good predictor for short- and long-term mortality [43]. This test is easy, quick, and low-priced, but largely depends on the patient's cooperation. Other possible measurements are knee extension, hip flexion strength, or peak expiratory flow. Measurement of the distance walked in a given time (e.g., at a 4-m gait speed) may also provide good information on the global condition [44].

#### 3.3.4. Medication

A patient's prescribed medications (including vitamin/mineral/botanical supplements) should be examined regarding potential drug–nutrient interactions and nutrition-related side effects (interactions with appetite, gastrointestinal function or symptoms).

### *3.4. Dietary History, Current Dietary Intake, and Innovative Dietary Assessment Methods*

The dietary history includes the patient's dietary habits and preferences, including cultural and religious habits, special diets, as well as food allergies or intolerances. Fluid and alcohol intake should also be recorded.

The energy and protein balance and the comparison between food intake and energy expenditure reflect the current nutritional status—whether the patient's dietary intake is sufficient or not.

The quantification of food intake is one of the key approaches to assessing nutritional risk in individual patients. The assessment of macronutrients (fat, carbohydrates, and proteins) is as important as the assessment of micronutrients (vitamins, trace elements). There are numerous standardized methods of measuring food intake, such as 24 h food recall, food frequency questionnaires, and direct observation (food records are frequently used by nurses for institutionalized patients). These provide (semi-) quantitative information. The accurate assessment of food intake is difficult and error-prone. There is a growing need for more accurate dietary assessment methods. High-quality data are essential for research on the association between diet and health, for an understanding of dietary patterns, and for the identification of nutrition-related health problems [45].

Innovative technologies that improve dietary assessment have been proposed recently, and can be classified into four principal groups according to the technological features that each of them incorporate [46–50]:

- *Manual dietary assessment*—The user inserts all required data (e.g., portion size estimation, type of food) on a web page, smartphone app, etc. [50]. This method replaces the paper-based methods of dietary assessment into an electronic form by the use of pictures, video, text, or voice without the inclusion of automatic features.
- *Dietitian-supported assessment*—The user takes photos of the food and sends them to the dietitian. These data are then analyzed by nutrition experts who use standardized methods (e.g., nutritional software) to estimate the corresponding amount of nutrients [51]. No automation features are usually incorporated.
- *Wearable devices monitoring food intake*—Devices that directly measure eating behavior [52], such as detection systems which identify eating gestures (ear-based chewing and swallowing) in order to complement self-reporting of nutrient intake.
- *Computer-aided assessment—this includes*:

  (i) Systems that incorporate some degree of automation. These either use bar-code readers in order to automatically recognize packaged food labels [50], or utilize smartphone applications that integrate the automatic recognition of food items. In this case, the user takes photos of the food and the system recognizes the type of food. Typically, in this situation the user needs to manually insert or select the volume/portion of the food items in order for the system to be able to translate the information into macronutrients and energy [53].

  (ii) Systems that are completely based on artificial intelligence. In a typical scenario, the user takes photo(s) of the food and then the system automatically and in real-time identifies the different food items (identification), recognizes the type of each of them (labeling), and creates a 3D model of each of them (3D reconstruction) [54–58]. Supported by food composition databases, food images are translated into nutrient values such as grams of macronutrients or calories [54,56].

These new technologies have several advantages. They do not (fully) rely on a respondent's memory; they are based on a number of automatic data-processing steps, thus minimizing user-related variability [45]; there is minimal participant burden; and there are reduced research and administrative costs [50]. Additionally, these technologies offer portability and greater social acceptability than paper-based methods [59]. Some additional advantages of computer-aided methods include decreased workload and costs (excluding costs for software development) [48], minimization of researchers' transcription errors [60], reduced paper waste and postage costs, and the optimization of space, security, and organization required for paper file storage [61].

However, there are also some limitations for each group. The manual dietary assessment methods provide all the disadvantages of paper-based methods except for expenditures related to paper usage. Body sensor monitoring provides no input about the type or quality of the food that is captured [50]. What is more, dietician-supported assessment is labor-intense and expensive to analyze [50]. Moreover, with the AI-based systems, it is not possible to capture all the basic nutrient information (including cooking methods) with one single image [45], and the majority of the existing apps are manual or semi-automatic in terms of food logging, and non-automatic in portion size estimation. Individuals tend to estimate portion size inaccurately [62]; almost half of the errors found in food records are attributed to such faulty estimations [63]. Other possible disadvantages are under-reporting due to either poor image quality or user negligence in taking an adequate number of pictures before and after food and drink consumption [64]. In addition, some food types such as mixed foods or liquids are difficult to analyze with automated image analysis [58]. Tools that include only some AI components are usually non-validated; they include a limited number of food categories, and questions relating to the used nutrient databases arise [50]. The most important limitation of the majority of these technologies is the need for a tech-savvy user [45].

Several studies have compared dietary assessment by traditional methods versus innovative technologies. Some of them conclude that electronic records would be a useful tool, both for large-scale epidemiological studies and in the clinical context [61]. Others conclude that apps could replace the traditional 24-h recall and serve as feasible tools for dieticians investigating dietary intake at a population level [65]. The longer the app recording periods are, the better the correlation between the traditional and the innovative methods seems to be [66]. However, novel technologies for dietary assessment appear valid at the population level rather than for individualized support [67–69]. Even though there are an increasing number of studies in the domain of innovative technologies, sample sizes are relatively low, and duration is usually short. Therefore, there is a need for well-designed long-term studies to explore and analyze the combination of traditional methods and state-of-the-art technological tools which characterizes the new era of nutritional assessment.

Energy requirements are calculated from the basal energy requirement multiplied by an activity factor. They can be calculated with formulae (e.g., the Harris–Benedict formula [70]) or through a simplified general rule based on energy values between 25–35 kcal per kg of body weight per day, with adjustment for underweight and overweight patients (30 × body weight, +20% if BMI $<20$ kg/m$^2$ or −20% if BMI $>30$ kg/m$^2$) [71]. These formulae cannot be used in special situations (e.g., in ICU patients). The protein requirement may be estimated by using 1.2–1.5 g/kg body weight per day (0.8 g/kg/d in case of chronic kidney failure) [22]. The specific macronutrient requirements are described in Table 7. Indirect calorimetry remains the gold standard for the assessment of energy requirements, but in many clinical settings this option is not available, as indirect calorimeters may not be easy to operate and may not be portable or affordable.

**Table 7.** Macronutrient requirements for adults.

| Macronutrient | Energy Content/g | Recommended Amount/kg Body Weight/d |
|---|---|---|
| Proteins | 4 kcal | 1.0–1.5 g |
| Carbohydrates | 4 kcal | max. 3–5 g |
| Fats | 9 kcal | 0.8–1.5 g |

Several conditions may impair food intake and should be taken into account as well. Among these are chewing and/or swallowing problems and functional limitations impairing independent eating. Additionally, cognitive changes affecting appetite and ability to feed oneself, and physiological changes that affect the desire to eat, may negatively impact the dietary intake.

### 3.5. Quality of Life

The assessment of quality of life is a more subjective parameter that is being increasingly included in nutritional assessment. It reflects the current health status, and may be used as an outcome parameter to monitor nutritional therapy. It is based on the perception of wellbeing in different domains—for example, symptoms (pain), physical (mobility, strength), psychological (anxiety, depression), and social (isolation), all potentially having an effect on eating. There are many questionnaires available, but there is no established consensus on which should optimally be used.

## 4. Conclusions and Outlook

Malnutrition is a frequent threat in hospitals, and is associated with negative outcomes. However, it remains a mostly treatable condition when there is adequate nutritional management. It is crucial to identify patients who are at nutritional risk or malnourished as early as possible, allowing the start of timely and effective nutritional support. Identifying patients at risk of malnutrition is the first step in the nutritional care process within a multimodal care system. Nutritional risk screening with simple and rapid tools should be performed systematically in each patient at hospital admission to detect patients who are nutritionally at risk or malnourished. Comprehensive detailed nutritional assessment should be performed thereafter in those patients identified as at risk of malnutrition or who are malnourished. This screening should be performed by a specialist (e.g., a dietician) using subjective and objective parameters such as clinical history, physical examination, body composition measurements, functional assessment, and laboratory values. New assessment methods may be very helpful, as they are accurate and quick. A nutritional care plan should be drawn up using an interdisciplinary approach and implemented to improve the patient's condition. Systematic nutritional risk screening and standardized nutritional management may also contribute to reduced healthcare costs.

**Author Contributions:** Conceptualization, E.R. and Z.S.; writing—original draft preparation E.R. and F.G.; writing—review and editing, M.V., P.S., and Z.S.; supervision, Z.S.

## Appendix A

**Table A1.** MNA full screening tool.

| Screening | | |
|---|---|---|
| A | Has food intake declined over the past 3 months due to loss of appetite, digestive problems, chewing or swallowing difficulties? | 0 = severe decrease in food intake<br>1 = moderate decrease in food intake<br>2 = no decrease in food intake |
| B | Weight loss during the past 3 months | 0 = weight loss greater than 3 kg<br>1 = does not know<br>2 = weight loss between 1 and 3 kg<br>3 = no weight loss |

**Table A1.** *Cont.*

| | | |
|---|---|---|
| C | Mobility | 0 = bedridden or chair bound<br>1 = able to get out of bed/chair but does not go out<br>2 = goes out |
| D | Has suffered psychological stress or acute disease in the past 3 months? | 0 = yes<br>2 = no |
| E | Neuropsychological problems | 0 = severe dementia or depression<br>1 = mild dementia<br>2 = no psychological problems |
| F1 | Body mass index (BMI) | 0 = BMI less than 19<br>1 = BMI 19 to less than 21<br>2 = BMI 21 to less than 23<br>3 = BMI 23 or greater |
| **Screening Score (subtotal max. 14 points)** | | |
| 12–14 points | Normal nutritional status | |
| 8–11 points | At risk of malnutrition | |
| 0–7 points | Malnourished | |
| For a more in-depth assessment, continue with questions G-R | | |
| **Assessment** | | |
| G | Lives independently (not in nursing home or hospital) | 0 = yes<br>1 = no |
| H | Takes more than 3 prescription drugs per day | 0 = yes<br>1 = no |
| I | Pressure sores or skin ulcers | 0 = yes<br>1 = no |
| J | How many full meals does the patient eat daily? | 0 = 1 meal<br>1 = 2 meals<br>2 = 3 meals |
| K | Selected consumption markers for protein intake | 0.0 = if 0 or 1 yes<br>0.5 = if 2 yes<br>1.0 = if 3 yes |
| | • Meat, fish or poultry every day | Yes/No |
| | • ≥1 serving of dairy products (milk, cheese, yoghurt) per day | Yes/No |
| | • ≥2 servings of legumes or eggs per week | Yes/No |
| L | Consumes ≥2 servings of fruit or vegetables per day? | 0 = yes<br>1 = no |
| M | How much fluid (water, juice, coffee, tea, milk...) is consumed per day? | 0.0 = less than 3 cups<br>0.5 = 3 to 5 cups<br>1.0 = more than 5 cups |
| N | Mode of feeding | 0 = unable to eat without assistance<br>1 = self-fed with some difficulty<br>2 = self-fed without any problem |
| O | Self view of nutritional status | 0 = views self as being malnourished<br>1 = is uncertain of nutritional status<br>2 = views self as having no nutritional problem |
| P | In comparison with other people of the same age, how does the patient consider his/her health status? | 0.0 = not as good<br>0.5 = does not know<br>1.0 = as good<br>2.0 = better |
| Q | Mid-arm circumference (MAC) in cm | 0.0 = MAC less than 21<br>0.5 = MAC 21 to 22<br>1.0 = MAC greater than 22 |
| R | Calf circumference (CC) in cm | 0 = CC less than 31<br>1 = CC 31 or greater |
| **Malnutrition Indicator Score** | | |
| 24–30 points | Normal nutritional status | |
| 17–23.5 points | At risk of malnutrition | |
| <17 points | Malnourished | |

## References


1. Sorensen, J.; Kondrup, J.; Prokopowicz, J.; Schiesser, M.; Krahenbuhl, L.; Meier, R.; Liberda, M.; EuroOOPS Study Group. EuroOOPS: An international, multicentre study to implement nutritional risk screening and evaluate clinical outcome. *Clin. Nutr.* **2008**, *27*, 340–349. [CrossRef]
2. Dupertuis, Y.M.; Kossovsky, M.P.; Kyle, U.G.; Raguso, C.A.; Genton, L.; Pichard, C. Food intake in 1707 hospitalised patients: A prospective comprehensive hospital survey. *Clin. Nutr.* **2003**, *22*, 115–123. [CrossRef]
3. Schwegler, I.; von Holzen, A.; Gutzwiller, J.P.; Schlumpf, R.; Muhlebach, S.; Stanga, Z. Nutritional risk is a clinical predictor of postoperative mortality and morbidity in surgery for colorectal cancer. *Br. J. Surg.* **2010**, *97*, 92–97. [CrossRef]
4. Sun, Z.; Kong, X.J.; Jing, X.; Deng, R.J.; Tian, Z.B. Nutritional Risk Screening 2002 as a predictor of postoperative outcomes in patients undergoing abdominal surgery: A systematic review and meta-analysis of prospective cohort studies. *PLoS ONE* **2015**, *10*, e0132857. [CrossRef]
5. Imoberdorf, R.; Meier, R.; Krebs, P.; Hangartner, P.J.; Hess, B.; Staubli, M.; Wegmann, D.; Rühlin, M.; Ballmer, P.E. Prevalence of undernutrition on admission to Swiss hospitals. *Clin. Nutr.* **2010**, *29*, 38–41. [CrossRef]
6. Studley, H.O. Percentage of weight loss: A basic indicator of surgical risk in patients with chronic peptic ulcer. 1936. *Nutr Hosp.* **2001**, *16*, 141–143.
7. Meguid, M.M.; Debonis, D.; Meguid, V.; Hill, L.R.; Terz, J.J. Complications of abdominal operations for malignant disease. *Am. J. Surg.* **1988**, *156*, 341–345. [CrossRef]
8. Pikul, J.; Sharpe, M.D.; Lowndes, R.; Ghent, C.N. Degree of preoperative malnutrition is predictive of postoperative morbidity and mortality in liver transplant recipients. *Transplantation* **1994**, *57*, 469–472. [CrossRef]
9. Soeters, P.B.; Schols, A.M. Advances in understanding and assessing malnutrition. *Curr. Opin. Clin. Nutr. Metab. Care* **2009**, *12*, 487–494. [CrossRef]
10. Guo, W.; Ou, G.; Li, X.; Huang, J.; Liu, J.; Wei, H. Screening of the nutritional risk of patients with gastric carcinoma before operation by NRS 2002 and its relationship with postoperative results. *J. Gastroenterol. Hepatol.* **2010**, *25*, 800–803. [CrossRef]
11. Lieffers, J.R.; Bathe, O.F.; Fassbender, K.; Winget, M.; Baracos, V.E. Sarcopenia is associated with postoperative infection and delayed recovery from colorectal cancer resection surgery. *Br. J. Cancer* **2012**, *107*, 931–936. [CrossRef]
12. Schiesser, M.; Kirchhoff, P.; Muller, M.K.; Schafer, M.; Clavien, P.A. The correlation of nutrition risk index, nutrition risk score, and bioimpedance analysis with postoperative complications in patients undergoing gastrointestinal surgery. *Surgery* **2009**, *145*, 519–526. [CrossRef]
13. Schiesser, M.; Muller, S.; Kirchhoff, P.; Breitenstein, S.; Schafer, M.; Clavien, P.A. Assessment of a novel screening score for nutritional risk in predicting complications in gastro-intestinal surgery. *Clin. Nutr.* **2008**, *27*, 565–570. [CrossRef]
14. Sungurtekin, H.; Sungurtekin, U.; Balci, C.; Zencir, M.; Erdem, E. The influence of nutritional status on complications after major intraabdominal surgery. *J. Am. Coll. Nutr.* **2004**, *23*, 227–232. [CrossRef]
15. Donini, L.M.; Savina, C.; Rosano, A.; Cannella, C. Systematic review of nutritional status evaluation and screening tools in the elderly. *J. Nutr. Health. Aging* **2007**, *11*, 421–432.
16. Foley, N.C.; Salter, K.L.; Robertson, J.; Teasell, R.W.; Woodbury, M.G. Which reported estimate of the prevalence of malnutrition after stroke is valid? *Stroke* **2009**, *40*, E66–E74. [CrossRef]
17. Bauer, J.M.; Kaiser, M.J.; Sieber, C.C. Evaluation of nutritional status in older persons: Nutritional screening and assessment. *Curr. Opin. Clin. Nutr. Metab. Care* **2010**, *13*, 8–13. [CrossRef]
18. Schindler, K.; Pernicka, E.; Laviano, A.; Howard, P.; Schutz, T.; Bauer, P.; Grecu, I.; Jonkers, C.; Kondrup, J.; Ljungqvist, O.; et al. How nutritional risk is assessed and managed in European hospitals: A survey of 21,007 patients findings from the 2007–2008 cross-sectional nutritionDay survey. *Clin. Nutr.* **2010**, *29*, 552–559. [CrossRef]
19. Van Bokhorst-de van der Schueren, M.A.E.; Guaitoli, P.R.; Jansma, E.P.; de Vet, H.C.W. Nutrition screening tools: Does one size fit all? A systematic review of screening tools for the hospital setting. *Clin. Nutr.* **2014**, *33*, 39–58. [CrossRef]

20. Kondrup, J.; Allison, S.P.; Elia, M.; Vellas, B.; Plauth, M. ESPEN guidelines for nutrition screening 2002. *Clin. Nutr.* **2003**, *22*, 415–421. [CrossRef]
21. Kondrup, J.; Rasmussen, H.H.; Hamberg, O.; Stanga, Z. Nutritional risk screening (NRS 2002): A new method based on an analysis of controlled clinical trials. *Clin. Nutr.* **2003**, *22*, 321–336. [CrossRef]
22. Schuetz, P.; Fehr, R.; Baechli, V.; Geiser, M.; Gomes, F.; Kutz, A.; Tribolet, P.; Bregenzer, T.; Braun, N.; Hoess, C.; et al. Individualized nutritional support in medical inpatients at nutritional risk: A randomized clinical trial. *Lancet* **2019**, *393*, 2312–2321. [CrossRef]
23. Weekes, C.E.; Elia, M.; Emery, P.W. The development, validation and reliability of a nutrition screening tool based on the recommendations of the British, Association for Parenteral and Enteral Nutrition (BAPEN). *Clin. Nutr.* **2004**, *23*, 1104–1112.
24. Anthony, P.S. Nutrition screening tools for hospitalized patients. *Nutr. Clin. Pract.* **2008**, *23*, 373–382. [CrossRef]
25. Raslan, M.; Gonzalez, M.C.; Dias, M.C.; Nascimento, M.; Castro, M.; Marques, P.; Segatto, S.; Torrinhas, R.S.; Cecconello, I.; Waitzberg, D.L.; et al. Comparison of nutritional risk screening tools for predicting clinical outcomes in hospitalized patients. *Nutrition* **2010**, *26*, 721–726. [CrossRef]
26. Charney, P. Nutrition screening vs. nutrition assessment: How do they differ? *Nutr. Clin. Pract.* **2008**, *23*, 366–372. [CrossRef]
27. Detsky, A.S.; McLaughlin, J.R.; Baker, J.P.; Johnston, N.; Whittaker, S.; Mendelson, R.A.; Jeejeebhoy, K.N. What is subjective global assessment of nutritional status? 1987. *Classical article. Nutr. Hosp.* **2008**, *23*, 400–407.
28. Koom, W.S.; Ahn, S.D.; Song, S.Y.; Lee, C.G.; Moon, S.H.; Chie, E.K.; et al. Nutritional status of patients treated with radiotherapy as determined by subjective global assessment. *Radiat. Oncol. J.* **2012**, *30*, 132–139. [CrossRef]
29. National Kidney Foundation. KDOQI Clinical Practice Guidelines for Nutrition in Chronic Renal Failure 2000. Available online: https://kidneyfoundation.cachefly.net/professionals/KDOQI/guidelines_nutrition/nut_a09.html (accessed on 24 June 2019).
30. British Dietetic Association. *Parenteral and Enteral Nutrition Group. A Pocket Guide to Clinical Nutrition*, 4th ed.; Parenteral and Enteral Nutrition Group of the British Dietetic Association: Birmingham, UK, 2011.
31. Han, T.S.; Lean, M.E. Lower leg length as an index of stature in adults. *Int. J. Obes. Relat. Metab. Disord.* **1996**, *20*, 21–27.
32. Reeves, S.L.; Varakamin, C.; Henry, C.J. The relationship between arm-span measurement and height with special reference to gender and ethnicity. *Eur. J. Clin. Nutr.* **1996**, *50*, 398–400.
33. Maastricht UMC+. Nutritional Assessment Body Composition Skinfold Measurements 2019. Available online: https://nutritionalassessment.mumc.nl/en/skinfold-measurements (accessed on 12 July 2019).
34. Bosy-Westphal, A.; Kromeyer-Hausschild, K.; Pirlich, M.; Schlattmann, A.; Scholz, G. Body composition analysis—What can be measured with practical value? *Aktuel Ernahrungsmed.* **2004**, *1*, 189–195.
35. Kyle, U.; Bosaeus, I.; De Lorenzo, A.; Deurenberg, P.; Elia, M.; Gomez, J.; Heitmann, B.L.; Kent-Smith, L.; Melchior, J.C.; Pirlich, M.; et al. Bioelectrical impedance analysis—Part I: Review of principles and methods. *Clin. Nutr.* **2004**, *23*, 1226–1243. [CrossRef]
36. Kyle, U.; Bosaeus, I.; De Lorenzo, A.; Deurenberg, P.; Elia, M.; Manuel Gomez, J.; Lilienthal Heitmann, B.; Kent-Smith, L.; Melchior, J.C.; Pirlich, M.; et al. Bioelectrical impedance analysis—Part II: Utilization in clinical practice. *Clin. Nutr.* **2004**, *23*, 1430–1453. [CrossRef]
37. Forbes, G.B.; Bruining, G.J. Urinary creatinine excretion and lean body mass. *Am. J. Clin. Nutr.* **1976**, *29*, 1359–1366. [CrossRef]
38. Stratton, R.J.; Green, C.J.; Elia, M. *Disease-Related Malnutrition: An Evidence-Based Approach to Treatment*; CABI Publishing: Wallingford, UK, 2003.
39. MacDonald, A.J.; Greig, C.A.; Baracos, V. The advantages and limitations of cross-sectional body composition analysis. *Curr. Opin. Support Palliat. Care.* **2011**, *5*, 342–349. [CrossRef]
40. Pirlich, M.; Norman, K. *Bestimmung des Ernährungszustands (inkl. Bestimmung der Körperzusammensetzung und ernährungsmedizinisches Screening) in Biesalski, rnährungsmedizin*; Georg Thieme Verlag KG: Stuttgart, Germany, 2018.
41. Leuenberger, M.S.; Joray, M.L.; Kurmann, S.; Stanga, Z. How to assess the nutritional status of my patient. *Praxis (Bern 1994)* **2012**, *101*, 307–315. [CrossRef]

42. Esper, D.H. Utilization of nutrition-focused physical assessment in identifying micronutrient deficiencies. *Nutr. Clin. Pract.* **2015**, *30*, 194–202. [CrossRef]
43. Norman, K.; Stobaus, N.; Gonzalez, M.C.; Schulzke, J.D.; Pirlich, M. Hand grip strength: Outcome predictor and marker of nutritional status. *Clin. Nutr.* **2011**, *30*, 135–142. [CrossRef]
44. Studenski, S.; Perera, S.; Wallace, D.; Chandler, J.M.; Duncan, P.W.; Rooney, E.; Fox, M.; Guralnik, J.M. Physical performance measures in the clinical setting. *J. Am. Geriatr. Soc.* **2003**, *51*, 314–322. [CrossRef]
45. Food and Agriculture Organization of the United Nations. *Dietary Assessment: A Resource Guide to Method Selection and Application in Low Resource Settings*; Food and Agriculture Organization of the United Nations: Rome, Italy, 2018.
46. Forster, H.; Walsh, M.C.; Gibney, M.J.; Brennan, L.; Gibney, E.R. Personalised nutrition: The role of new dietary assessment methods. *Proc. Nutr. Soc.* **2016**, *75*, 96–105. [CrossRef]
47. Gemming, L.; Utter, J.; Ni Mhurchu, C. Image-assisted dietary assessment: A systematic review of the evidence. *J. Acad. Nutr. Diet.* **2015**, *115*, 64–77. [CrossRef]
48. Illner, A.K.; Freisling, H.; Boeing, H.; Huybrechts, I.; Crispim, S.P.; Slimani, N. Review and evaluation of innovative technologies for measuring diet in nutritional epidemiology. *Int. J. Epidemiol.* **2012**, *41*, 1187–1203. [CrossRef]
49. Stumbo, P.J. New technology in dietary assessment: A review of digital methods in improving food record accuracy. *Proc. Nutr. Soc.* **2013**, *72*, 70–76. [CrossRef]
50. Archundia Herrera, M.C.; Chan, C.B. Narrative Review of New Methods for Assessing Food and Energy Intake. *Nutrients* **2018**, *10*, 1064. [CrossRef]
51. Martin, C.K.; Correa, J.B.; Han, H.; Allen, H.R.; Rood, J.C.; Champagne, C.M.; Gunturk, B.K.; Bray, G.A. Validity of the Remote Food Photography Method (RFPM) for estimating energy and nutrient intake in near real-time. *Obesity (Silver Spring)* **2012**, *20*, 891–899. [CrossRef]
52. Dong, Y.; Hoover, A.; Scisco, J.; Muth, E. A new method for measuring meal intake in humans via automated wrist motion tracking. *Appl Psychophysiol. Biofeedback* **2012**, *37*, 205–215. [CrossRef]
53. Kawano, Y.; Yanai, K. FoodCam: A real-time food recognition system on a smartphone. *Multimed. Tool. Appl.* **2015**, *74*, 5263–5287. [CrossRef]
54. Anthimopoulos, M.; Dehais, J.; Shevchik, S.; Ransford, B.H.; Duke, D.; Diem, P.; Mougiakakou, S. Computer vision-based carbohydrate estimation for type 1 patients with diabetes using smartphones. *J. Diabetes Sci. Technol.* **2015**, *9*, 507–515. [CrossRef]
55. Bally, L.; Dehais, J.; Nakas, C.T.; Anthimopoulos, M.; Laimer, M.; Rhyner, D.; Rosenberg, G.; Zueger, T.; Diem, P.; Mougiakakou, S.; et al. Carbohydrate Estimation Supported by the GoCARB System in Individuals With Type 1 Diabetes: A Randomized Prospective Pilot Study. *Diabetes Care* **2017**, *40*, e6–e7. [CrossRef]
56. Dehais, J.; Anthimopoulos, M.; Shevchik, S.; Mougiakakou, S. Two-view 3D reconstruction for food volume estimation. *IEEE Trans. Multimed.* **2017**, *19*, 1090–1099. [CrossRef]
57. Rhyner, D.; Loher, H.; Dehais, J.; Anthimopoulos, M.; Shevchik, S.; Botwey, R.H.; Duke, D.; Stettler, C.; Diem, P.; Mougiakakou, S.; et al. Carbohydrate Estimation by a Mobile Phone-Based System Versus Self-Estimations of Individuals With Type 1 Diabetes Mellitus: A Comparative Study. *J. Med. Int. Res.* **2016**, *18*, e101. [CrossRef]
58. Vasiloglou, M.F.; Mougiakakou, S.; Aubry, E.; Bokelmann, A.; Fricker, R.; Gomes, F.; Guntermann, C.; Meyer, A.; Studerus, D.; Stanga, Z. A Comparative Study on Carbohydrate Estimation: GoCARB vs. Dietitians. *Nutrients* **2018**, *10*, 741. [CrossRef]
59. Ambrosini, G.L.; Hurworth, M.; Giglia, R.; Trapp, G.; Strauss, P. Feasibility of a commercial smartphone application for dietary assessment in epidemiological research and comparison with 24-h dietary recalls. *Nutr. J.* **2018**, *17*, 5. [CrossRef]
60. Bucher Della Torre, S.; Carrard, I.; Farina, E.; Danuser, B.; Kruseman, M. Development and Evaluation of e-CA, an Electronic Mobile-Based Food Record. *Nutrients* **2017**, *9*, 76.
61. Bejar, L.M.; Sharp, B.N.; Garcia-Perea, M.D. The e-EPIDEMIOLOGY Mobile Phone App for Dietary Intake Assessment: Comparison with a Food Frequency Questionnaire. *JMIR Res. Protoc.* **2016**, *5*, e208. [CrossRef]
62. Poslusna, K.; Ruprich, J.; de Vries, J.H.; Jakubikova, M.; van't Veer, P. Misreporting of energy and micronutrient intake estimated by food records and 24 hour recalls, control and adjustment methods in practice. *Br. J. Nutr.* **2009**, *101*, S73–85. [CrossRef]

63. Beasley, J.; Riley, W.T.; Jean-Mary, J. Accuracy of a PDA-based dietary assessment program. *Nutrition* **2005**, *21*, 672–677. [CrossRef]
64. Casperson, S.L.; Sieling, J.; Moon, J.; Johnson, L.; Roemmich, J.N.; Whigham, L. A mobile phone food record app to digitally capture dietary intake for adolescents in a free-living environment: Usability study. *JMIR Mhealth Uhealth* **2015**, *3*, e30. [CrossRef]
65. Ashman, A.M.; Collins, C.E.; Brown, L.J.; Rae, K.M.; Rollo, M.E. Validation of a Smartphone Image-Based Dietary Assessment Method for Pregnant Women. *Nutrients* **2017**, *9*, 73. [CrossRef]
66. Recio-Rodriguez, J.I.; Rodriguez-Martin, C.; Gonzalez-Sanchez, J.; Rodriguez-Sanchez, E.; Martin-Borras, C.; Martinez-Vizcaino, V.; Arietaleanizbeaskoa, M.S.; Magdalena-Gonzalez, O.; Fernandez-Alonso, C.; Maderuelo-Fernandez, J.A.; et al. EVIDENT Smartphone App, a New Method for the Dietary Record: Comparison With a Food Frequency Questionnaire. *JMIR Mhealth Uhealth* **2019**, *7*, e11463. [CrossRef]
67. Carter, M.C.; Burley, V.J.; Nykjaer, C.; Cade, J.E. 'My Meal Mate' (MMM): Validation of the diet measures captured on a smartphone application to facilitate weight loss. *Br. J. Nutr.* **2013**, *109*, 539–546. [CrossRef]
68. Conrad, J.; Nothlings, U. Innovative approaches to estimate individual usual dietary intake in large-scale epidemiological studies. *Proc. Nutr. Soc.* **2017**, *76*, 213–219. [CrossRef]
69. Lemacks, J.L.; Adams, K.; Lovetere, A. Dietary Intake Reporting Accuracy of the Bridge2U Mobile Application Food Log Compared to Control Meal and Dietary Recall Methods. *Nutrients* **2019**, *11*, 199. [CrossRef]
70. Harris, J.A.; Benedict, F.G. A Biometric Study of Human Basal Metabolism. *Proc. Natl. Acad. Sci. USA* **1918**, *4*, 370–373. [CrossRef]
71. Druml, W.; Jadrna, K. *Recommendations for Enteral and Parenteral Nutrition in Adults*; English Edition/Pocket Version; Austrian Society of Clinical Nutrition (AKE): Vienna, Austria, 2008.

# 8

# Nutritional Management of Medical Inpatients

**Emilie Reber [1,*,†], Filomena Gomes [2,†], Lia Bally [1], Philipp Schuetz [3,4] and Zeno Stanga [1]**

1 Department of Diabetes, Endocrinology, Nutritional Medicine and Metabolism, Bern University Hospital, and University of Bern, 3010 Bern, Switzerland
2 The New York Academy of Sciences, New York, NY 10007, USA
3 Department of Medical University, Division of General Internal and Emergency Medicine, Kantonsspital Aarau, 5000 Aarau, Switzerland
4 Department for Clinical Research, Medical Faculty, University of Basel, 4001 Basel, Switzerland
* Correspondence: emilie.reber@insel.ch
† These authors contributed equally to the manuscript.

**Abstract:** Malnutrition is a common condition in hospitalized patients that is often underdiagnosed and undertreated. Hospital malnutrition has multifactorial causes and is associated with negative clinical and economic outcomes. There is now growing evidence from clinical trials for the efficiency and efficacy of nutritional support in the medical inpatient population. Since many medical inpatients at nutritional risk or malnourished are polymorbid (i.e., suffer from multiple comorbidities), this makes the provision of adequate nutritional support a challenging task, given that most of the clinical nutrition guidelines are dedicated to single diseases. This review summarizes the current level of evidence for nutritional support in not critically ill polymorbid medical inpatients.

**Keywords:** malnutrition; nutritional management; nutritional therapy

---

## 1. Introduction

Hippocrates of Kos, one of the most outstanding figures in the history of medicine in the fourth to fifth century BCE stated that "The patient ought likewise to be consider'd, whether he is able to hold out with the prescribed diet, even in the height of the disease; for if the diet is not sufficient, the patient will grow too faint, and be overcome by the disease." [1]. He considered nutritional interventions to cure diseases as reflected in his well-known statement "Let food be thy medicine and medicine be thy food".

Around 80 years ago, Studley described weight loss of >20% of body weight as a factor increasing mortality (+33%) in chronic peptic ulcer patients undergoing non-emergency surgery, "regardless of the appearance of the individual" [2]. Some years later, more than 30 years ago, concerns regarding prevalence and adverse effects of disease-related malnutrition (malnutrition triggered by illness or disease) and in hospitalized patients were first reported [3–5]. Nowadays, the link between malnutrition and clinical negative outcomes, e.g., muscle wasting, higher infection rates, longer length of hospital stay, morbidity and mortality rates, is clearly established [6–10]. In high-income countries, where access to food should not be limited, every third patient is at risk for malnutrition or already malnourished at hospital admission [11]. Most patients further lose weight during their hospital stay, and, as consequence, their nutritional status deteriorates. A study of Barton et al. showed that 40% of the hospital food served to patients is left on the plates and returned, thus resulting in patients eating less than 80% of their individual energy and protein requirements [12]. There are several factors leading to progressive unintentional weight loss, such as gastrointestinal symptoms, inactivity, depression or low mood, advanced age, effects of illness on protein and energy homeostasis, protein catabolism, inflammation, hormonal function and loss of appetite [13]. Loss of appetite may develop during hospital stays either as a consequence of an underlying disease or treatment or preexist as a primary condition. This loss of appetite arises as a physiological response to acute illness and predisposes inpatients to serious caloric and protein deficits [14]. In combination with immobilization and a pronounced inflammatory and endocrine stress response, these nutritional deficits contribute to muscle wasting and progressive deterioration of metabolic and functional status, particularly in medical inpatients with multiple morbidities [9,15]. An initial loss of appetite does, however, not confer a risk to fail achievement of nutritional targets since this improves quite rapidly after the initiation of nutritional support [16].

There is some evidence from high-quality trials in critical care settings reporting harmful effects of hypercaloric replacement nutrition strategies [14]. These negative effects might be explained by suppression of autophagy with inadequate clearance of acute cell damage associated with illness [17]. Autophagy is a body mechanism to get rid of damaged cells organelles and toxic products. Loss of appetite may therefore be a protective mechanism in an acute disease with the goals to accelerate recovery from disease by improving autophagy. Importantly, in patients suffering from chronic diseases, this protective physiological response may have been exaggerated thereby causing malnutrition. Thus, in patients with multiple chronic diseases, who have milder disease severities, lost weight and muscle mass over time, use of an adequate eucaloric nutritional support has a potentially positive effect. They might have better metabolism and nutrients use due to decreased insulin resistance and decreased risk that nutrition would interfere with autophagy [7,18]. Thus, since critically ill patients have different nutritional needs from the patients on the medical wards, this review focuses on the nutritional support of non-critically ill medical inpatients; as such, the critically ill population is the focus of another publication in this special issue ("Kopp-Lugli et al. Nutrition therapy in critically ill patients treated on intensive and intermediate care units: a literature review").

Understanding the optimal use of nutritional support is highly complex because timing, route of delivery, and the amount and type of nutrients may all have important roles and potentially affect patient's outcomes. Furthermore, it has been questioned whether nutritional support in polymorbid medical inpatients differs from the ones suffering from a single disease. Polymorbidity (or multimorbidity) is mostly defined as the co-occurrence of at least two chronic medical conditions in one patient. Polymorbidity is frequent in hospitals and, despite being common in older people, is not necessarily associated with higher age. Nevertheless, older adult patients require special attention, as they tend to be more polymorbid than younger patients are. In addition to the disease burden, older patients often experience malnutrition by multifactor, such as anorexia of aging, presbyphagia and dysphagia due to sarcopenia [19–21]. While there are plenty of clinical nutrition guidelines available focusing on individual diseases, [22–26] Gomes et al. recently published new guidelines for the nutritional support in polymorbid medical inpatients [13].

## 2. Today's Clinical Evidence Level

Recent meta-analyses, which investigated the effects of nutritional support on clinical outcomes concluded that nutritional support leads to an increase in energy and protein intake, an increase in body weight but there were no significant effects on clinical outcomes such as mortality and morbidity, and only little effect on non-elective hospital readmissions [27,28]. The results showed no benefit in critical ill patients, possibly due to a suppression of autophagy and increased risk of refeeding syndrome [28]. In fact, these systematic reviews found (from the included heterogeneous trials and with high risk for bias) an important lack of evidence in this area, as high quality randomized, interventional trials, needed to establish causal relationships, were missing. Thus, the lack of significant results regarding mortality and morbidity may be rather due to methodological issues and low statistical power, and not lack of effectiveness per se.

In fact, other recent studies showed results that are more promising. The multicenter randomized placebo controlled double-blind "NOURISH-trial", conducted by Deutz and his colleagues, evaluated the effect of specialized, energy-dense ONS on postdischarge outcomes including nonelective readmission and mortality in initially hospitalized, malnourished, older adults. Patients were randomly allocated to receive during hospitalization and after discharge either a specialized, energy-dense ONS or a carbohydrate-only ONS. Results showed that energy-dense, specialized ONS extending beyond discharge improved body weight but could not reduce readmission rate. A significant reduction in 90-day mortality in the intervention group compared to the placebo group (4.8% vs. 9.7%) resulting in a number needed to treat (NNT) of 20 [29]. However, it remains unclear whether this beneficial effect is attributable to the specific formula (containing a leucine metabolite) used in this study or the high protein and energy amount provided by the oral nutritional supplement, given that control patients received a low protein and calorie placebo product. The very recently published open-label, non-blinded, multicenter, randomized-controlled trial, the "EFFORT trial", conducted by Schuetz and colleagues, assessed the effect of a protocol-guided individualized nutritional support to reach nutritional needs (determined either with the Harris-Benedict formula or with indirect calorimetry) of medical inpatients. Protocol-guided nutritional support reduced the primary outcome (all-cause mortality, admission to intensive care, non-elective hospital readmission, major complications, and decline in functional status) by 4% (22.9% vs. 26.9%) by 30 days when compared to usual care, translating into a NNT of 25 to prevent one severe complication [30]. Additionally, mortality rate was significantly lower in the intervention group compared to the control group (7.2% vs. 9.9%, NNT of 37) and notable improvements in functional outcomes and in quality of life measures were observed. Notably, in the nutrition support group, 91% received oral nutrition, and, perhaps most importantly, an individualized nutritional care plan from a specialist dietitian. Conversely, enteral or parenteral nutrition was used in eight and 12 participants respectively [30]. The effect of nutritional support on the risk for the primary endpoint was consistent across predefined subgroups. Thus, these results provide strong evidence for the concept of systematically screening medical inpatients on hospital admission in terms of nutritional risk, independent of the medical condition, followed by a nutritional assessment and initiation of individualized nutritional support in at-risk patients. The results also contradict the hypothesis that provision of nutritional support during the acute phase of illness would have harmful effects—at least in the non-critically ill setting [30]. Unlike the NOURISH trial that investigated the effect of a specific formula of an oral nutritional supplement, within EFFORT a variety of nutritional support strategies were used by trained dieticians to reach the individual nutritional goals of each patient. Thus, EFFORT does not provide evidence regarding single nutritional components or types of foods, but rather proves that the overall strategy of providing tailored nutritional support to reach the nutritional requirements during the acute phase of illness is beneficial for medical inpatients [30].

## 3. Nutritional Therapy

Since there is growing evidence for the positive effect of nutritional therapy (Figure 1), proper definition and thus diagnosis are lacking. The Global Leadership Initiative on Malnutrition (GLIM) working group recently published an umbrella approach to diagnose malnutrition in various clinical settings [31]. This aims to early identify nutritional risk in polymorbid patients to individually treat them and improve their clinical outcome [31]. The GLIM working group supports a two-step process with screening and assessment, targeting a standardization of nutritional support [31].

There are differences of prognosis of nutritional status and nutritional strategy among the etiology of malnutrition; malnutrition with severe inflammation (e.g., severe infection, multiple trauma), with persistent inflammation due to chronic disease (e.g., cancer, congestive heart failure), malnutrition with minimum or no inflammation in chronic disease patients (e.g., short bowel syndrome, dysphagia after stroke and anorexia nervosa) and malnutrition due to simple starvation (e.g., poverty, dementia, lack of appropriate nutrition care in the hospital/facilities). Patients with severe inflammation are often difficult to recover their nutritional status by only nutritional support, so the goal of nutrition support is to minimize deterioration of nutritional status. On the other hand, nutritional status of the patients with no or minimum inflammation, or those after simple starvation, can be improved if appropriate nutrition support provided by the nutrition specialists.

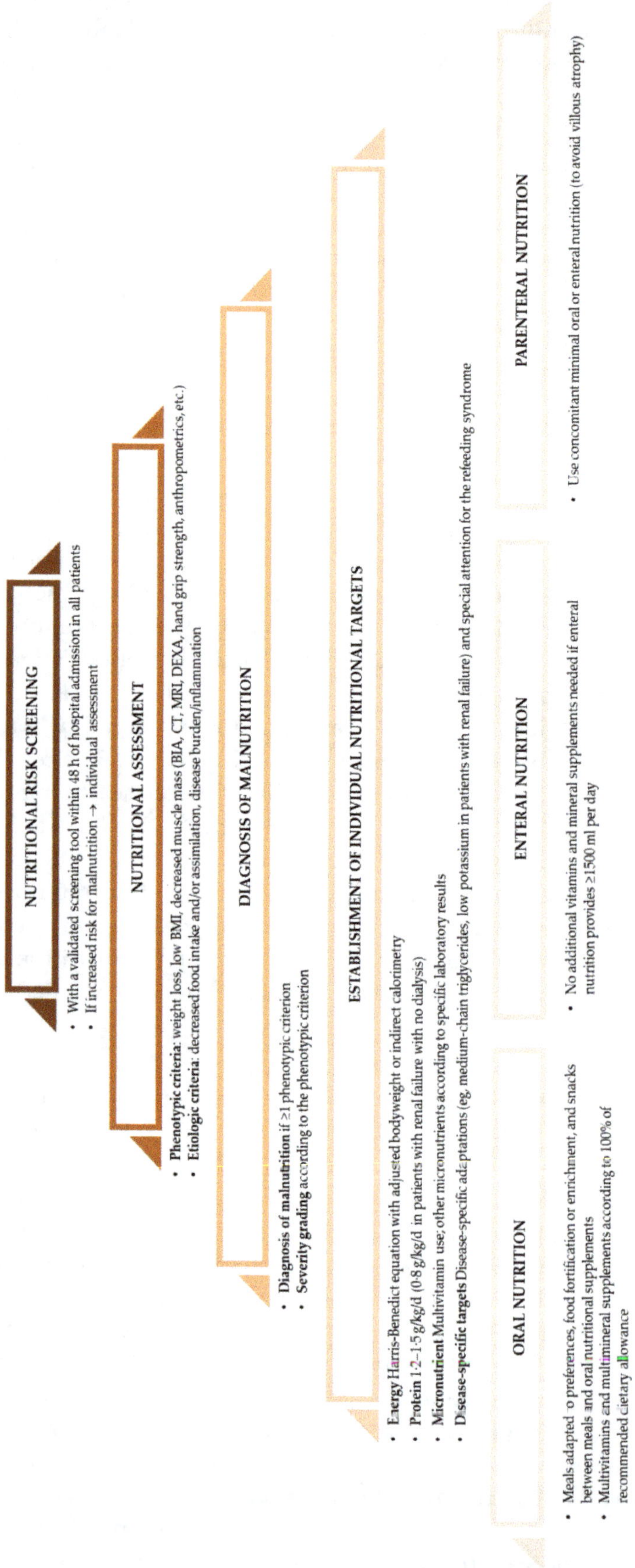


**Figure 1.** Nutritional algorithm, after [30].

### 3.1. Organization of Nutritional Support

Nutritional support in hospitals ideally relies on two main structures: A hospital nutrition steering committee and multidisciplinary nutritional support teams. The nutrition steering committee is working within the clinical governance framework (sets nutritional standards, protocols and guidelines) and has a direct access to hospital management. Members of the nutrition steering committee should be drawn from the management, and include senior representation from medical staff, catering, nursing, dietetics, pharmacy and other healthcare professionals [32,33]. A nutritional support team has an executive function within the hospital, implementing standards, protocols and guidelines in daily clinical practice. Such a team consisting of physicians, dieticians, nurses, and pharmacists, ensures and improves nutritional treatments quality and safety, and is continuously checking and optimizing procedures of nutritional management (see dedicated manuscript in this special issue). Interdisciplinary cooperation and good communication between healthcare professionals is important and mandatory to provide an individualized nutritional support to all patients who need it.

### 3.2. Screening and Assessment

The identification of malnutrition has been typically based on anthropometric, biochemical and physical parameters, among others. There is no universally accepted gold standard (best method) for the assessment of nutritional status [34,35]. Commonly used criteria include unintentional weight loss (percentage of body weight) in the past 3–6 months, low BMI, reduced muscle mass, reduced dietary intake in the past week, reduced absorptive capacity, and disease burden/inflammation [31].

Standardized procedures are needed in order to initiate a timely and adequate nutritional therapy [36]. Systematic screening for nutritional risk, followed by a comprehensive nutritional assessment should be implemented and lead to the development of a personalized nutritional care plan (see dedicated manuscript in this special issue: Reber et al., Nutritional screening and assessment) [13,33,37]. Nutrition screening is the first step in determining nutritional problems. Screening should rapidly and accurately identify individuals who should be referred to the nutrition specialist (e.g., dietitian, expert clinician) for a further assessment, where it would be possible to gather more information and determine if there truly is a nutrition problem, to understand the cause of the problem and to determine its severity. Nutritional screening should be done with validated screening tools, such as malnutrition universal screening (MUST), mini nutritional assessment short form (MNA-SF) and nutritional risk screening 2002 (NRS-2002), each of them having strength and limitations and may not be sufficiently validated in specific populations like polymorbid patients (see dedicated manuscript in this special issue: Reber et al., Nutritional screening and assessment) [38,39]. In general, nutritional assessment continues the data gathering process initiated in the screen. The types of data collected in nutritional assessment are often similar to data collected in the screening process but in more depth [40]. In summary, nutritional support should be initiated with a detailed nutritional care plan (appropriate monitoring procedures and clear guidelines for action e.g., food record charts or dietetic referral) in people who are at risk of malnutrition or manifestly malnourished according to the result of the nutritional risk screening and assessment results [41].

### 3.3. Nutritional Targets

Meeting the nutritional requirement is important to maintain or gain weight, muscle mass and function, to improve clinical outcomes, and reduce complications and rehospitalization rates.

Dietitians and medical staff trained in nutrition support should ensure that the patients' dietary intake meets the individual energy, protein, fluid, electrolyte, mineral, micronutrients and fiber needs [33]. The activity levels and the underlying clinical condition (e.g., catabolism, pyrexia, gastrointestinal tolerance, potential metabolic instability), as well as the likely duration of nutrition support, should also be taken into account.

3.3.1. Energy

Determining the patients' energy requirements is a central point of nutritional assessment. The total energy expenditure consists of the resting energy expenditure, diet-induced thermogenesis and the energy expended during physical activity [13]. The gold standard to measure energy requirements is the indirect calorimetry, but when not possible, these may be calculated with published prediction equations adjusted for age sex, and weight (e.g., Harris-Benedict formula) in addition to activity and stress factors, or roughly estimated weight-based formulae (it has been suggested 27 kcal/kg/day for polymorbid older patients) [13]. In individuals with very low BMI, the higher value of 30 kcal/kg/d should slowly be targeted [13]. Reaching the energy targets too quickly and/or feeding at too high rates potentially lead to complications such as the refeeding syndrome or overfeeding [42].

3.3.2. Proteins

The general protein requirement is 1 g/kg/d for the polymorbid medical inpatient population. In case of acute or chronic kidney failure, protein requirements may have to be reduced to 0.8–1 g/kg/d unless dialysis, but there are no specific recommendations for polymorbid patients suffering from kidney failure [13]. In case of dialysis, the protein requirements are the same as normal and there is a need for 20 g of proteins after the dialysis (dialytic loss). For older patients suffering acute or chronic disease, recommendations are 1.2–15. g/kg/d [43,44]. An individual target has to be defined for each patient, since other factors such as hypermetabolism can change protein requirements (e.g., major trauma and burns). Patients undergoing paracentesis need 10 g proteins per liter ascites.

3.3.3. Micronutrients

In malnourished polymorbid inpatients, micronutrients requirements may be higher due to reduced food intake or due to higher needs (disease-depending). Micronutrients should be supplemented according to the recommended daily intake, and/or substituted if deficiencies are occurring [13]. The daily micronutrients requirements are considered to be covered in case of the amount of enteral nutrition is ≥1500 mL per day. Vitamins and trace elements should be provided to patients receiving parenteral nutrition since there are none in the nutritional solutions.

*3.4. Nutritional Route*

Oral nutrition should be the first-line choice of nutritional support, including meals adapted to the individual patient preferences, additional energy dense snacks (e.g., "homemade" milkshakes), food fortification with powdered carbohydrate and protein supplements, and the commercial oral nutritional supplements [13]. The use of the convenient commercial oral nutritional supplements have been shown to maintain the muscle mass, to lower the complication rate and hospital readmission rate after six months [13,45–48], but a combination of oral nutritional support strategies (using both traditional and commercially available products) also results in the improvement of important clinical outcomes [30].

If oral nutrition is not possible, safe or sufficient, enteral and eventually parenteral nutrition should be considered, whereas the enteral nutrition should be the preferred route due to lower risk of infectious and non-infectious complications [13]. The energy and protein intake should be assessed every 24–48 h and escalated after 5 days if the patient does not meet at least 75% of his/her requirements [49].

*3.5. Nutrition for Specific Medical Conditions*

Patients with renal failure need restrictions in potassium and phosphate. Patients with congestive heart failure may benefit from sodium and water restrictions in given cases.

There is weak evidence to support the use of specialized oral nutritional supplements or enteral nutrition formulas in polymorbid medical inpatients. Arginine, glutamine, and beta-hydroxy-beta-metylbuturate (HMB) may be used in patients suffering from pressure ulcers [13,50].

Arginine (semi-essential amino acid) is required for promotion of nitrogen balance, cell proliferation, T lymphocyte function and collagen accumulation. It also changes into nitric oxide, which is known for its vasodilatory and angiogenic properties. Glutamine (conditionally essential amino acid) plays a key role in the immune system, and its deficiency may significantly slow the healing process. HMB (metabolite of leucine, an essential amino acid) supplementation was associated with increased muscle mass accretion by inhibiting muscle proteolysis and modulating protein turnover. A mixture of soluble and insoluble fibers can be used in older polymorbid patients receiving enteral nutrition and suffering from diarrhea or constipation, which are frequent complications of enteral nutrition [13]. Special attention should then be paid to the hydration state as it may cause obstipation [51].

### 3.6. Timing

An early start of nutritional support (within 48 h after hospital admission) is recommended to maintain or improve patient's nutritional and functional status, and prevent sarcopenia [13]. Even though the optimal length of the nutritional support is still unclear, it is usually recommended to treat beyond hospital discharge, as this continued nutritional intervention is known to increase patients' quality of life and nutritional and functional status, and in the older (>65 years) polymorbid patients it results in lower mortality rates [13,52,53].

### 3.7. Monitoring

Experienced clinical teams with the relevant skills and training in nutritional monitoring should review the indications, route, risks, benefits and goals of nutrition support at regular intervals. This interval depends on the patient and the parameter that is being monitored (e.g., nutritional, anthropometric, biochemical, clinical condition), and may increase when the patient's condition is stable under nutritional treatment. For example, nutrient intake from oral, enteral or parenteral nutrition (including any change in conditions that are affecting food intake) is recommended to be monitored daily initially, reducing to twice weekly when stable [33]. Similarly, laboratory parameters (e.g., sodium, potassium, urea, creatinine) should be monitored more frequently initially, i.e., at baseline and daily until stable, and then reduced to 1 or 2 times a week. In addition to the nutritional parameters used to monitor responses to nutritional support, functional indices (e.g., handgrip strength) should be used regularly to asses other clinical outcomes (i.e., survival, quality of life) in polymorbid medical inpatients.

## 4. Barriers to the Adequate Provision of Nutritional Support

The awareness about malnutrition must be raised primarily among hospital medical staff, where nutritional support is not seen as being part of the medical treatment. Malnutrition is often unrecognized as a diagnosis and is, subsequently, being under-reported and not being treated. Clearly defined protocols and responsibilities are needed to address this hidden problem, starting with a systematic nutritional risk screening and nutritional assessment for all patients on admission to hospital. Malnutrition should become a topic in the education and training of medical staff. At the same time, because the causes of malnutrition are often multifactorial (from depression and lack of appetite to inability to self-feed), communication and collaboration should be improved between the different members of the multidisciplinary team and between the team and the patient, in order to efficiently address those causes [16]. A recently published study showed that 78% of the hospitals and 22% of the nursing homes in Switzerland have a nutritional steering committee, and 92% and 14%, respectively, have dieticians available. Around 80% of the hospitals and nursing homes did not implement a systematic nutritional risk screening procedure, resulting in around 60% of the patients being screened at least at one time point (in hospitals and nursing homes); 25% of the hospital do screen the patients as they feel a problem [54]. Further, 56% of the institutions monitor the food intake of their patients and 50% monitor and document the nutritional status [54]. The nutritionDay survey 2018, a survey on nutritional care conducted worldwide (https://www.nutritionday.org/en/network/imprint/index.html;

Table 1) showed that 76.4% of the participating centers had NST available on site, and that 61.6% of the participating centers use a specific screening tool to screen the patients at hospital admission.

**Table 1.** National reports from the nutritionDay 2018, available from https://www.nutritionday.org/en/about-nday/national-reports/index.html.

| Country | Number of Participating Centers | Percentage of Hospitals with NST Present on Site | Percentage of Screening at Hospital Admission |
|---|---|---|---|
| Australia | 1 | 100 | 100 |
| Austria | 4 | 100 | 45.5 |
| Belgium | 52 | 88 | 77.3 |
| Brazil | 12 | 100 | 80.0 |
| Bulgaria | 1 | 66.7 | 0 |
| China | 9 | 100 | 56.5 |
| Colombia | 35 | 69.1 | 56.6 |
| Croatia | 3 | 55.6 | 20.0 |
| Germany | 36 | 60.9 | 49.5 |
| Greece | 3 | 100 | 0 |
| India | 13 | 7.7 | 50.1 |
| Japan | 9 | 100 | 50 |
| Netherlands | 1 | 100 | 0 |
| Poland | 4 | 0 | 60 |
| Portugal | 4 | 100 | 66.7 |
| Singapore | 1 | 0 | 82.6 |
| Spain | 5 | 100 | 50.0 |
| Sweden | 2 | 100 | 100 |
| Switzerland | 1 | 66.7 | 16.7 |
| Thailand | 1 | 100 | 66.7 |
| United States of America | 16 | 62.5 | 96.0 |

Individual factors such as patients' symptoms, disease severity (e.g., causing dysphagia and loss of appetite), mood and orientation, impaired functional and cognitive status, social environment (e.g., isolation, loneliness, lack of family support) may all significantly reduce the food (and nutrient) intake of hospitalized patients and contribute for the deterioration of their nutritional status. Polypharmacy, especially in polymorbid patients, may further influence their nutritional status, causing drug–drug and drug–nutrients interactions as well as gastrointestinal symptoms. This calls for the need of frequent monitoring of the nutritional status of the hospitalized patient (e.g., weekly monitoring of the body weight). For those patients receiving nutritional support, regular visits by the dietitian allow the patient to receive the encouragement to comply with the nutritional care plan, and the adaptation of this plan to the changing needs of the patient [55].

## 5. Conclusions and Outlook

Nutritional support has been shown to be a highly effective treatment option to prevent and/or treat malnutrition, decreasing morbidity and mortality rates. Nutritional interventions deserve as much attention as any other therapeutic interventions, and clinicians should aim to maximize their efficacy and minimize side effects. Further studies should also investigate the cost-effectiveness of nutritional interventions in medically ill patients. It will be equally important to determine which medical inpatients have the most benefit from nutritional support interventions through metabolomics and microbiome research, walking towards an evidence-based personalized nutrition approach.

**Author Contributions:** Conceptualization, E.R. and Z.S.; writing—original draft preparation, E.R.; writing—review and editing, F.G. and L.B. and P.S. and Z.S.; supervision, Z.S.

## References


1. Sprengell, C. *Hippocrates: The Aphorisms of Hippocrates, and The Sentences of Celsus; with Explanations and References to the Most Considerable Writers*, 2nd ed.; Wilkin, F., Bonwick, F., Eds.; Gale Ecco: London, UK, 1735.
2. Studley, H.O. Percentage of weight loss: A basic indicator of surgical risk in patients with chronic peptic ulcer. *J. Am. Med. Assoc.* **1936**, *106*, 458–460. [CrossRef]
3. McWhirter, J.P.; Pennington, C.P. Incidence and recognition of malnutrition in hospital. *Br. Med. J.* **1994**, *308*, 945–948. [CrossRef] [PubMed]
4. Hill, G.L.; Pickford, I.; Young, G.A.; Schorah, C.J.; Blackett, R.L.; Burkinshaw, L.; Warren, J.V.; Morgan, D.B. Malnutrition in surgical patients: An unrecognised problem. *Lancet* **1977**, *309*, 689–692. [CrossRef]
5. Bistrian, B.R.; Blackburn, G.L.; Vitale, J.; Cochran, D.; Naylor, J. Prevalence of malnutrition in general medical patients. *JAMA* **1976**, *235*, 1567–1570. [CrossRef] [PubMed]
6. Kubrak, C.; Jensen, L. Malnutrition in acute care patients: A narrative review. *Int. J. Nurs. Stud.* **2007**, *44*, 1036–1054. [CrossRef]
7. Schutz, P.; Bally, M.; Stanga, Z.; Keller, U. Loss of appetite in acutely ill medical inpatients: Physiological response or therapeutic target? *Swiss Med. Wkly.* **2014**, *144*, w13957. [CrossRef]
8. Casaer, M.P.; Hermans, G.; Wilmer, A.; Van den Berghe, G. Impact of early parenteral nutrition completing enteral nutrition in adult critically ill patients (EPaNIC trial): A study protocol and statistical analysis plan for a randomized controlled trial. *Trials* **2011**, *12*, 21. [CrossRef]
9. Felder, S.; Lechtenboehmer, C.; Bally, M.; Fehr, R.; Deiss, M.; Faessler, L.; Kutz, A.; Steiner, D.; Rast, A.C.; Laukemann, S.; et al. Association of nutritional risk and adverse medical outcomes across different medical inpatient populations. *Nutrition* **2015**, *31*, 1385–1393. [CrossRef]
10. Villet, S.; Chiolero, R.L.; Bollmann, M.D.; Revelly, J.P.; Cayeux, M.C.; Delarue, J.; Berger, M.M. Negative impact of hypocaloric feeding and energy balance on clinical outcome in ICU patients. *Clin. Nutr.* **2005**, *24*, 502–509. [CrossRef]
11. Sorensen, J.; Kondrup, J.; Prokopowicz, J.; Schiesser, M.; Krahenbuhl, L.; Meier, R.; Liberda, M. EuroOOPS: An international, multicentre study to implement nutritional risk screening and evaluate clinical outcome. *Clin. Nutr.* **2008**, *27*, 340–349. [CrossRef]
12. Barton, A.D.; Beigg, C.L.; Macdonald, I.A.; Allison, S.P. High food wastage and low nutritional intakes in hospital patients. *Clin. Nutr.* **2000**, *19*, 445–449. [CrossRef] [PubMed]
13. Gomes, F.; Schuetz, P.; Bounoure, L.; Austin, P.; Ballesteros-Pomar, M.; Cederholm, T.; Fletcher, J.; Laviano, A.; Norman, K.; Poulia, K.A.; et al. ESPEN guidelines on nutritional support for polymorbid internal medicine patients. *Clin. Nutr.* **2018**, *37*, 336–353. [CrossRef] [PubMed]
14. Casaer, M.P.; Van den Berghe, G. Nutrition in the acute phase of critical illness. *N. Engl. J. Med.* **2014**, *370*, 1227–1236. [CrossRef] [PubMed]
15. Felder, S.; Braun, N.; Stanga, Z.; Kulkarni, P.; Faessler, L.; Kutz, A.; Steiner, D.; Laukemann, S.; Haubitz, S.; Huber, A.; et al. Unraveling the Link between Malnutrition and Adverse Clinical Outcomes: Association of Acute and Chronic Malnutrition Measures with Blood Biomarkers from Different Pathophysiological States. *Ann. Nutr. Metab.* **2016**, *68*, 164–172. [CrossRef] [PubMed]
16. Tribolet, P.; Fehr, R.; Bächli, V.; Geiser, M.; Toplak, H.; Stanga, Z.; Schuetz, P. What are Barriers of Nutritional Therapy in Malnourished Medical Inpatients? An Observational Study. *Aktuel Ernahr.* **2017**, *42*, 167–179.
17. Schetz, M.; Casaer, M.P.; Van den Berghe, G. Does artificial nutrition improve outcome of critical illness? *Crit. Care* **2013**, *17*, 302. [CrossRef]
18. Russell, R.C.; Yuan, H.X.; Guan, K.L. Autophagy regulation by nutrient signaling. *Cell Res.* **2014**, *24*, 42–57. [CrossRef] [PubMed]
19. Fujishima, I.; Fujiu-Kurachi, M.; Arai, H.; Hyodo, M.; Kagaya, H.; Maeda, K.; Mori, T.; Nishioka, S.; Oshima, F.; Ogawa, S.; et al. Sarcopenia and dysphagia: Position paper by four professional organizations. *Geriatr. Gerontol. Int.* **2019**, *19*, 91–97. [CrossRef]
20. Morley, J.E. Defining Undernutrition (Malnutrition) in Older Persons. *J. Nutr. Health Aging* **2018**, *22*, 308–310. [CrossRef]
21. Ortega, O.; Martin, A.; Clave, P. Diagnosis and Management of Oropharyngeal Dysphagia Among Older Persons, State of the Art. *J. Am. Med. Direct. Assoc.* **2017**, *18*, 576–582. [CrossRef]

22. Arends, J.; Bachmann, P.; Baracos, V.; Barthelemy, N.; Bertz, H.; Bozzetti, F.; Fearon, K.; Hutterer, E.; Isenring, E.; Kaasa, S.; et al. ESPEN guidelines on nutrition in cancer patients. *Clin. Nutr.* **2017**, *36*, 11–48. [CrossRef] [PubMed]
23. Forbes, A.; Escher, J.; Hebuterne, X.; Klek, S.; Krznaric, Z.; Schneider, S.; Shamir, R.; Stardelova, K.; Wierdsma, N.; Wiskin, A.E.; et al. ESPEN guideline: Clinical nutrition in inflammatory bowel disease. *Clin. Nutr.* **2017**, *36*, 321–347. [CrossRef] [PubMed]
24. Meier, R.; Beglinger, C.; Layer, P.; Gullo, L.; Keim, V.; Laugier, R.; Friess, H.; Schweitzer, M.; Macfie, J. ESPEN guidelines on nutrition in acute pancreatitis. European Society of Parenteral and Enteral Nutrition. *Clin. Nutr.* **2002**, *21*, 173–183. [CrossRef] [PubMed]
25. Plauth, M.; Bernal, W.; Dasarathy, S.; Merli, M.; Plank, L.D.; Schutz, T.; Bischoff, S.C. ESPEN guideline on clinical nutrition in liver disease. *Clin. Nutr.* **2019**, *38*, 485–521. [CrossRef] [PubMed]
26. Turck, D.; Braegger, C.P.; Colombo, C.; Declercq, D.; Morton, A.; Pancheva, R.; Robberecht, E.; Stern, M.; Strandvik, B.; Wolfe, S.; et al. ESPEN-ESPGHAN-ECFS guidelines on nutrition care for infants, children, and adults with cystic fibrosis. *Clin. Nutr.* **2016**, *35*, 557–577. [CrossRef] [PubMed]
27. Bally, M.R.; Blaser Yildirim, P.Z.; Bounoure, L.; Gloy, V.L.; Mueller, B.; Briel, M.; Schuetz, P. Nutritional Support and Outcomes in Malnourished Medical Inpatients: A Systematic Review and Meta-analysis. *JAMA Intern. Med.* **2016**, *176*, 43–53. [CrossRef] [PubMed]
28. Feinberg, J.; Nielsen, E.E.; Korang, S.K.; Halberg Engell, K.; Nielsen, M.S.; Zhang, K.; Didriksen, M.; Lund, L.; Lindahl, N.; Hallum, S.; et al. Nutrition support in hospitalised adults at nutritional risk. *Cochrane Database Syst. Rev.* **2017**, *5*, Cd011598. [CrossRef]
29. Deutz, N.E.; Matheson, E.M.; Matarese, L.E.; Luo, M.; Baggs, G.E.; Nelson, J.L.; Hegazi, R.A.; Tappenden, K.A.; Ziegler, T.R. Readmission and mortality in malnourished, older, hospitalized adults treated with a specialized oral nutritional supplement: A randomized clinical trial. *Clin. Nutr.* **2016**, *35*, 18–26. [CrossRef]
30. Schuetz, P.; Fehr, R.; Baechli, V.; Geiser, M.; Gomes, F.; Kutz, A.; Tribolet, P.; Bregenzer, T.; Hoess, C.; Pavlicek, V.; et al. Individualized nutritional support in medical inpatients at nutritional risk: A randomized clinical trial. *Lancet* **2019**, *393*, 2312–2321. [CrossRef]
31. Cederholm, T.; Jensen, G.L.; Correia, M.; Gonzalez, M.C.; Fukushima, R.; Higashiguchi, T.; Baptista, G.; Barazzoni, R.; Blaauw, R.; Coats, A.J.S.; et al. GLIM criteria for the diagnosis of malnutrition—A consensus report from the global clinical nutrition community. *J. Cachexia Sarcopenia Muscle* **2019**, *10*, 207–217. [CrossRef]
32. Ten Dam, S.; Droop, A.; Arjaans, W.; de Groot, S.; van Bokhorst-de van der Schueren, M. Module 11.1 Organisation of a Nutritional Support Team. In *ESPEN LLL, Organisation of Nutritional Care Ethical and Legal Aspects: ESPEN*; 2012; Available online: https://lllnutrition.com/mod/page/view.php?id=3422, (accessed on 29 July 2019).
33. National Institute for Health and Clinical Excellence. *Nutrition Support for Adults: Oral Nutrition Support, Enteral Tube Feeding and Parenteral Nutrition (Clinical Guidance 32) London: National Collaborating Centre for Acute Care (UK)*; National Institute for Health and Clinical Excellence: London, UK, 2006.
34. Donini, L.M.; Savina, C.; Rosano, A.; Cannella, C. Systematic review of nutritional status evaluation and screening tools in the elderly. *J. Nutr. Health Aging* **2007**, *11*, 421–432. [PubMed]
35. Foley, N.C.; Salter, K.L.; Robertson, J.; Teasell, R.W.; Woodbury, M.C. Which Reported Estimate of the Prevalence of Malnutrition After Stroke Is Valid? *Stroke* **2009**, *40*, E66–E74. [CrossRef] [PubMed]
36. Bauer, J.M.; Kaiser, M.J.; Sieber, C.C. Evaluation of nutritional status in older persons: Nutritional screening and assessment. *Curr. Opin. Clin. Nutr. Metab. Care* **2010**, *13*, 8–13. [CrossRef] [PubMed]
37. Weekes, C.E.; Elia, M.; Emery, P.W. The development, validation and reliability of a nutrition screening tool based on the recommendations of the British Association for Parenteral and Enteral Nutrition (BAPEN). *Clin. Nutr.* **2004**, *23*, 1104–1112. [PubMed]
38. Power, L.; Mullally, D.; Gibney, E.R.; Clarke, M.; Visser, M.; Volkert, D.; Bardon, L.; de van der Schueren, M.A.E.; Corish, C.A. A review of the validity of malnutrition screening tools used in older adults in community and healthcare settings—A MaNuEL study. *Clin. Nutr. ESPEN* **2018**, *24*, 1–13. [CrossRef] [PubMed]
39. Van Bokhorst-de van der Schueren, M.A.; Guaitoli, P.R.; Jansma, E.P.; de Vet, H.C. Nutrition screening tools: Does one size fit all? A systematic review of screening tools for the hospital setting. *Clin. Nutr.* **2014**, *33*, 39–58. [CrossRef] [PubMed]
40. Charney, P. Nutrition screening vs. nutrition assessment: How do they differ? *Nutr. Clin. Pract.* **2008**, *23*, 366–372. [CrossRef] [PubMed]

41. Elia, M. *Guidelines for Detection and Management of Malnutrition*; British Association for Parenteral and Enteral Nutrition: Redditch, UK, 2000.
42. Friedli, N.; Stanga, Z.; Culkin, A.; Crook, M.; Laviano, A.; Sobotka, L.; Kressig, R.W.; Kondrup, J.; Mueller, B.; Schuetz, P. Management and prevention of refeeding syndrome in medical inpatients: An evidence-based and consensus-supported algorithm. *Nutrition* **2018**, *47*, 13–20. [CrossRef] [PubMed]
43. Deutz, N.E.; Bauer, J.M.; Barazzoni, R.; Biolo, G.; Boirie, Y.; Bosy-Westphal, A.; Cederholm, T.; Cruz-Jentoft, A.; Krznaric, Z.; Nair, K.S.; et al. Protein intake and exercise for optimal muscle function with aging: Recommendations from the ESPEN Expert Group. *Clin. Nutr.* **2014**, *33*, 929–936. [CrossRef] [PubMed]
44. Volkert, D.; Beck, A.M.; Cederholm, T.; Cruz-Jentoft, A.; Goisser, S.; Hooper, L.; Kiesswetter, E.; Maggio, M.; Raynaud-Simon, A.; Sieber, C.C.; et al. ESPEN guideline on clinical nutrition and hydration in geriatrics. *Clin. Nutr.* **2019**, *38*, 10–47. [CrossRef] [PubMed]
45. Gariballa, S.; Forster, S.; Walters, S.; Powers, H. A randomized, double-blind, placebo-controlled trial of nutritional supplementation during acute illness. *Am. J. Med.* **2006**, *119*, 693–699. [CrossRef] [PubMed]
46. Hegerova, P.; Dedkova, Z.; Sobotka, L. Early nutritional support and physiotherapy improved long-term self-sufficiency in acutely ill older patients. *Nutrition* **2015**, *31*, 166–170. [CrossRef] [PubMed]
47. Starke, J.; Schneider, H.; Alteheld, B.; Stehle, P.; Meier, R. Short-term individual nutritional care as part of routine clinical setting improves outcome and quality of life in malnourished medical patients. *Clin. Nutr.* **2011**, *30*, 194–201. [CrossRef] [PubMed]
48. Volkert, D.; Hubsch, S.; Oster, P.; Schlierf, G. Nutritional support and functional status in undernourished geriatric patients during hospitalization and 6-month follow-up. *Aging Clin. Exp. Res.* **1996**, *8*, 386–395. [CrossRef]
49. Bounoure, L.; Gomes, F.; Stanga, Z.; Keller, U.; Meier, R.; Ballmer, P.; Fehr, R.; Mueller, B.; Genton, L.; Bertrand, P.C.; et al. Detection and treatment of medical inpatients with or at-risk of malnutrition: Suggested procedures based on validated guidelines. *Nutrition* **2016**, *32*, 790–798. [CrossRef] [PubMed]
50. Wong, A.; Chew, A.; Wang, C.M.; Ong, L.; Zhang, S.H.; Young, S. The use of a specialised amino acid mixture for pressure ulcers: A placebo-controlled trial. *J. Wound Care* **2014**, *23*, 259–260. [CrossRef] [PubMed]
51. Vandewoude, M.F.; Paridaens, K.M.; Suy, R.A.; Boone, M.A.; Strobbe, H. Fibre-supplemented tube feeding in the hospitalised elderly. *Age Ageing* **2005**, *34*, 120–124. [CrossRef] [PubMed]
52. Beck, A.M.; Holst, M.; Rasmussen, H.H. Oral nutritional support of older (65 years+) medical and surgical patients after discharge from hospital: Systematic review and meta-analysis of randomized controlled trials. *Clin. Rehabil.* **2013**, *27*, 19–27. [CrossRef] [PubMed]
53. Munk, T.; Tolstrup, U.; Beck, A.M.; Holst, M.; Rasmussen, H.H.; Hovhannisyan, K.; Thomsen, T. Individualised dietary counselling for nutritionally at-risk older patients following discharge from acute hospital to home: A systematic review and meta-analysis. *J. Hum. Nutr. Diet.* **2016**, *29*, 196–208. [CrossRef] [PubMed]
54. Aubry, E.; Mareschal, J.; Gschweitl, M.; Zvingelis, M.; Schuetz, P.; Stanga, Z. Facts zum Management der Klinischen Ernährung—Eine Online-Befragung. *Aktuel Ernahr.* **2018**, *42*, 452–460. [CrossRef]
55. Lobo, D.N. Improving outcomes with a little EFFORT. *Lancet* **2019**, *393*, 2278–2280. [CrossRef]

# 9

# Clinical Value of Muscle Mass Assessment in Clinical Conditions Associated with Malnutrition

**Julie Mareschal [1,*], Najate Achamrah [2], Kristina Norman [3,4] and Laurence Genton [5,*]**

1 Clinical Nutrition, Geneva University Hospitals, 1205 Geneva, Switzerland
2 Department of Clinical Nutrition, Rouen University Hospital, Normandie University, 76000 Rouen, France
3 Research Group on Geriatrics, Charité Universitätsmedizin Berlin, Corporate Member of Freie Universität Berlin, Humboldt-Universität zu Berlin, and Berlin Institute of Health, 13347 Berlin, Germany
4 Department of Nutrition and Gerontology, German Institute for Human Nutrition Potsdam-Rehbrücke, 14558 Nuthetal, Germany
5 Clinical Nutrition, Geneva University Hospital, 1205 Geneva, Switzerland
* Correspondence: julie.mareschal@hcuge.ch (J.M.); laurence.genton@hcuge.ch (L.G.)

**Abstract:** Malnutrition results from a reduction of food intake or an alteration of nutrient assimilation and leads to decreased lean mass. Strong evidence shows that malnutrition associated with loss of muscle mass negatively impacts clinical outcomes. The preservation or improvement of muscle mass represents a challenge. This review aims to (1) describe current methods to assess muscle mass in clinical practice, (2) describe the associations between muscle mass and clinical outcomes, and (3) describe the impact of interventions aiming at increasing muscle mass on clinical outcomes. It highlights the importance of assessing muscle mass as part of the screening and the follow-up of malnutrition in clinical practice.

**Keywords:** mid-arm muscle circumference; bioelectrical impedance analysis; dual-energy X-ray absorptiometry; computed tomography; fat-free mass; appendicular skeletal muscle mass; lean soft tissue; skeletal muscle index; chronic disease; old

---

## 1. Introduction

Malnutrition results from a reduction of food intake or alteration of nutrient assimilation and leads to decreased lean mass, either combined or not with the loss of fat mass. Potential causes include diseases, starvation, or aging. This condition may be associated with other homeostasis disorders such as inflammation [1]. Malnutrition negatively impacts clinical outcomes, mortality, length of stay, and costs [2]. In hospitalized patients, the prevalence ranges from 20 to 50% [3].

To standardize the definition of malnutrition and its diagnostic criteria, the Global Leadership Initiative on Malnutrition (GLIM) has recently convened experts of major worldwide clinical nutrition societies. They suggested defining malnutrition with one phenotypic criterion (bodyweight loss, low body mass index (BMI), or reduced muscle mass) associated to one etiologic criterion (reduced food intake/assimilation or inflammation/disease burden) [4]. Thus, the experts promote the use of body composition measurement as part of a nutritional assessment to evaluate muscle mass.

This narrative review aims to (1) describe current methods to assess muscle mass in clinical practice, (2) describe the associations between muscle mass and clinical outcomes, and (3) describe the impact of interventions aiming at increasing muscle mass on clinical outcomes.

## 2. Methods to Assess Muscle Mass in Clinical Practice

In clinical practice, several tools and techniques are available to assess body composition. BMI is often used due to its simplicity. Indeed, the U-shaped association between BMI and all-cause mortality has been well described, as subjects with the highest and lowest BMIs have the highest mortality rates [5]. However, BMI does not allow the measurement of body composition compartments and tends to underestimate fat-free mass (FFM) depletion [6–8]. Other anthropometric measurements such as skinfold thickness and waist-hip ratio can also be used. Even though these tools are convenient, quick, and inexpensive, they do not provide direct information on muscle mass [9,10]. Therefore, other methods are required to assess muscle mass in clinical practice. In this section, we focused on portable techniques which can be used at patient bedsides, such as mid-arm muscle circumference and bioelectrical impedance analysis. We concentrated also on dual-energy X-ray absorptiometry and computed tomography, non-portable techniques used for other clinical diagnostic purposes, but allows for the simultaneous assessment of body composition. The characteristics of each method are compared in Table 1. Other methods to assess muscle mass were not introduced because they are rarely used in clinical practice.

**Table 1.** Principal characteristics of main clinical methods to assess muscle mass.

| | MAMC | BIA | DXA | CT |
|---|---|---|---|---|
| Accuracy | - | + | ++ | +++ |
| Interobserver variability | +++ | + | - | - |
| Simplicity | ++ | ++ | + | - |
| Radiation | - | - | + | +++ |
| Cost | | | | |
| *If device already available* | - | - | - [1] | + [2] |
| *If device not available* | - | + | ++ | +++ |
| Time to measurement | 5 min | 5 min | 5–10 min [3] | 10–15 min [3] |

"-": weak/low; "+": high; [1] Body composition software usually included in the device; [2] Related to the purchase of the software; [3] To obtain body composition analysis in addition to a routine exam; MAMC: mid-arm muscle circumference; BIA: bioelectrical impedance analysis; DXA: dual-energy X-ray absorptiometry; CT: computed tomography; Adapted from Guglielmi and al. [11].

### 2.1. *Mid-Arm Muscle Circumference*

Mid-arm muscle circumference (MAMC) is obtained by using the formula: MAMC (mm) = mid-arm circumference (mm) − (3.14 × triceps skinfold(mm)) [12]. Measurements are usually performed in standing position, on the dominant arm, at the mid-point between the acromion and the olecranon. Mid-arm circumference is measured using a plastic metric tape and triceps skinfold using a skinfold caliper. For both parameters, the average of three consecutive measurements is recorded [12]. MAMC provides an estimation of upper extremity skeletal muscle mass, which strongly correlates to dual-energy X-ray absorptiometry results [13,14].

This method is quick, portable, inexpensive, and easy to perform. It requires simple equipment, minimal training, and is useful in patients with ascites and edema. The main disadvantages are interobserver variations [15]. For instance, in obese people, accuracy is low due to the difficulty of the required triceps skinfold measurement [16].

### 2.2. *Bioelectrical Impedance Analysis*

Several bioelectrical impedance analysis (BIA) methods are available (single frequency, multi-frequency, segmental, or vector BIA). We focused on single-frequency 50 kHz tetrapolar BIA, as this is the most used method in clinical practice, and on BIA devices with hand-to-foot surface electrodes, as these BIA devices provide raw electrical data. BIA allows to obtain whole FFM, which refers to all body compartments except fat mass, and appendicular skeletal muscle mass (ASMM) defined as the sum of the lean soft tissue of the four limbs.

Principles and methods of BIA have been previously detailed in the guidelines of the European Society for Clinical Nutrition and Metabolism [17]. BIA is based on the concept that adipose tissue is more resistant to the conduction of the current compared to other tissues and fluids. Briefly, the patient, lying on the back, is exposed to a low-intensity alternating current between surface electrodes. The BIA device measures resistance and reactance, or impedance and phase angle. To estimate FFM and ASMM, several population-specific equations using these electrical parameters in addition to age, sex, weight, and height have been developed and validated against dual-energy X-ray absorptiometry (DXA) [18–21]. FFM and ASMM can be divided by height squared to be converted into FFM index (FFMI) and ASMM index (ASMMI), in order to compare people of different heights.

As a portable non-invasive bedside method, BIA is convenient in clinical practice. It is safe, cheap and not technically demanding. The small interobserver variability, 0.02 kg for FFM, is an advantage compared to anthropometry methods [22,23]. This device also allows the calculation of phase angle, supposed to be an indicator of cellular integrity, associated with clinical prognosis [24]. FFM assessment using BIA does, however, bear some limitations. BIA is not accurate in patients with altered hydration (e.g., ascites, edema, fluid loss) and with extreme BMI ($<16$ kg/m$^2$ and $>34$ kg/m$^2$) [25]. BIA formulas are population-specific. Finally, multiple devices of BIA are commercially available, but integrated algorithms are not always released by the manufacturer, thus questioning the reliability of the results measured by these devices [26,27].

### 2.3. *Dual-Energy X-ray Absorptiometry*

Dual-energy X-ray absorptiometry (DXA) allows the measurement of bone, lean soft tissue, and fat mass. Compared to FFM, lean soft tissue contains essential and non-essential lipids, but not bone mass. DXA device uses X-rays of low- and high-photon energy. As they cross the body, they are attenuated according to the composition and thickness of the encountered body tissues. A detector on the opposite side of the body analyzes the transmitted photon intensity. Complex algorithms allow then to differentiate bone, fat mass, and lean soft tissue, as detailed previously [28]. This method, initially used for bone density measurement, is often considered as the reference method to assess body composition in clinical research [29].

In clinical practice, DXA allows accurate, fast, and non-invasive lean soft tissue assessment. This device is often available in developed countries. Measurement is achieved in supine position. Irradiation is acceptable (2–5 μSv), which is low compared to the daily background radiation of 5–7 μSv [28]. Besides whole-body composition, DXA also allows for the measurement of ASMM. As DXA calculations are based on a constant hydration of lean soft tissue, hydration level variations may impact the results. However, this effect seems to be negligible [30]. Finally, measurements may be influenced by the thickness of the tissue with potential underestimation of fat mass and overestimation of muscle mass in obese patients [31].

### 2.4. *Computed Tomography*

Computed tomography (CT) to assess muscle mass is becoming more common [32]. As cutoff values have been defined at the third lumbar vertebrae (L3) level, an area reflective of whole-body tissue distribution, we focused only on muscle assessment at this anatomic landmark [33,34]. L3 muscle mass area is usually normalized to the patients' height squared to determine skeletal muscle index (SMI).

CT is a medical imaging technique, performed in supine position, which measures tissue absorption of X-rays emitted through a rotating beam. Computer processing then reconstructs cross-sectional images of anatomical structures by 2D and 3D maps of pixels. According to the attenuation of the different tissues, each pixel is associated with a numerical value (Hounsfield Unit). Tissues are identified in the cross-sectional images by their specific absorption Hounsfield Unit ranges [35,36]. Muscle mass area is obtained by cross-sectional analysis using standard radiology software [37].

CT provides high-quality images and precise assessment of muscle mass [38,39]. Its advantages compared to other methods are to evaluate muscle mass quality by measuring fat infiltration in muscle. CT images are frequently available in cancer and other chronic disease patients, as part of the routine diagnosis or follow-up of these diseases [26]. Major drawbacks are high radiation exposure (10 mSv), cost, non-portability, and need for qualified technicians and specific software. Moreover, a recent systematic review highlighted the lack of consensus and high variability of CT-based methods of muscle mass assessment [32].

## 3. Impact of Muscle Mass on Clinical Outcomes

The impact of muscle mass on clinical outcomes is well described in different populations. In this section, we focused on chronic diseases such as chronic obstructive pulmonary disease (COPD), chronic heart failure (CHF), cancer, and on older adults. This choice was related to the fact that the prevalence of malnutrition is particularly high in these populations [40–42]. We made an update of the latest observational studies and subjectively considered articles from the last three years.

### 3.1. *Chronic Diseases*

The prevalence of malnutrition is significant in patients with chronic diseases, such as for instance, COPD, CHF or solid tumors cancer. It ranges respectively from 20–35%, 60–69% and 14–66% according to the tumor site [43–45].

#### 3.1.1. Chronic Obstructive Pulmonary Disease

In patients with COPD, the influence of muscle mass on the severity of the disease and the prognosis has been described by Munhoz et al. [46]. In this study, disease severity was evaluated with the Global Initiative for Obstructive Lung Disease (GOLD) index based on airflow limitation, exacerbation history, symptom burden, and prognosis with the body mass index/airflow obstruction/dyspnea/exercise capacity score (BODE), known to predict disease severity and mortality. Interestingly, ASMMI assessed by DXA decreased significantly according to the worsening of GOLD and BODE indexes. In another study, Matkovic et al. have been interested in the association between body composition and physical performance [47]. In 111 moderate to very severe COPD patients, FFMI, assessed by DXA, were significantly associated with a low capacity exercise and physical activity defined, respectively, by a 6-minute walk distance ≤350 m and a daily step count ≤7128 steps/day (=median). Finally, emphysema severity in COPD patients, characterized by a loss of lung tissue, seems to be related to muscle mass and prognosis [48]. Patients in the higher quartiles of emphysema severity had lower FFMI, evaluated by BIA, and a worse BODE index. Thus, in patients with COPD, muscle mass is associated with disease severity, prognosis, and physical performance.

#### 3.1.2. Chronic Heart Failure

As for patients with COPD, muscle mass also appears to be a good predictor of exercise capacity in patients with chronic heart failure [49]. In 117 patients with heart failure and preserved left ventricular ejection fraction, ASMM measured by DXA was significantly associated with a 6-minute walk test <400 m. Tsuchida et al. have studied the association between muscle mass obtained by DXA and severity of acute decompensated heart failure characterized by brain natriuretic peptide (BNP) > 500 pg/mL [50]. Low ASMMI was defined as two standard deviations below the mean reference values of healthy Japanese subjects [51]. After adjustment for anemia and atrial fibrillation, a low ASMMI was related to a higher BNP level, indicative of poor prognosis in CHF patients [52]. In patients with heart failure, muscle mass is associated with physical performance, severity of the disease, and prognosis.

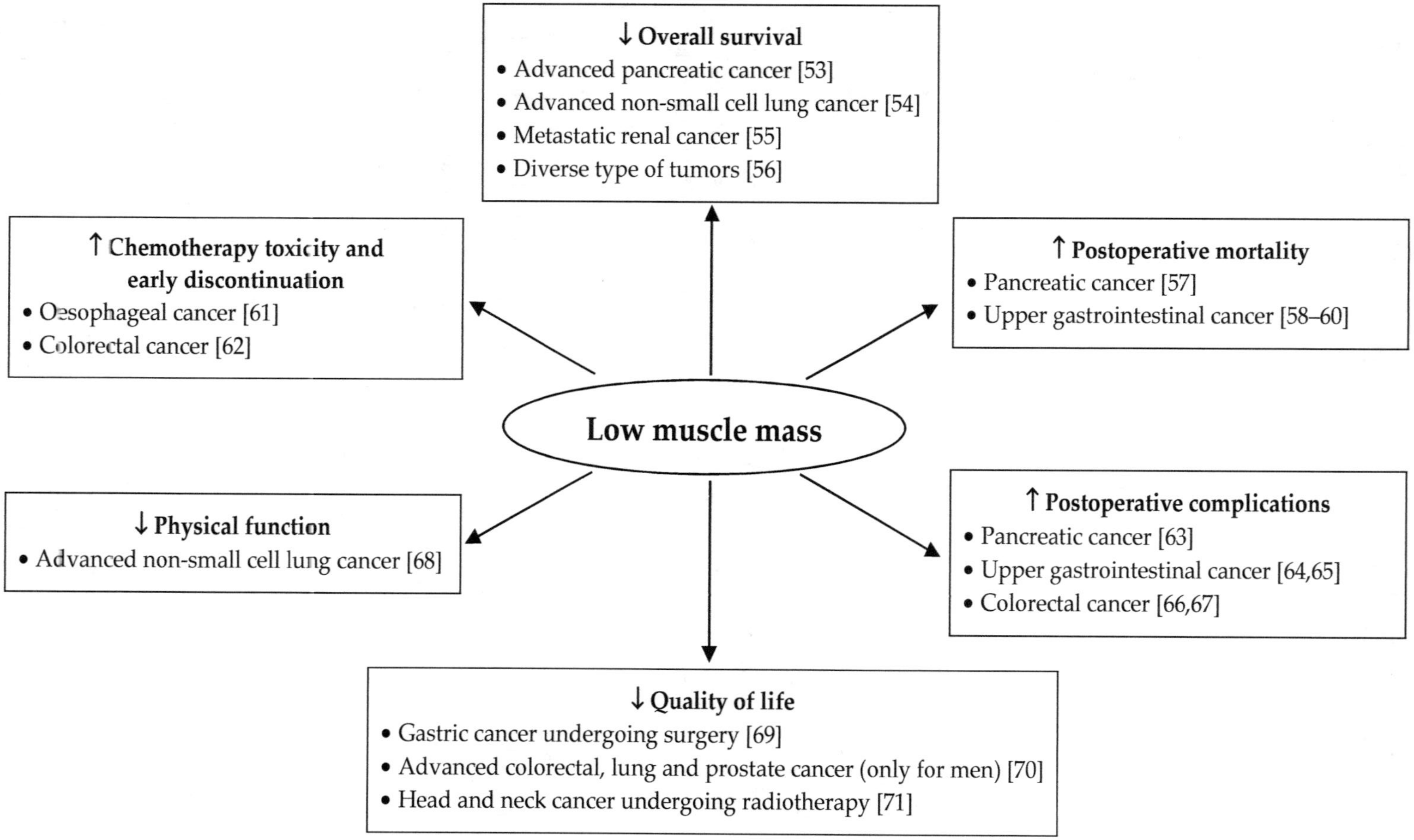


**Figure 1.** Association between low muscle mass and clinical outcomes in solid tumor cancer patients [53–71]. Muscle mass was quantified by computed tomography at the L3 level except for references [56] and [71] for which bioelectrical impedance analysis and mid-arm muscle circumference were respectively used.

#### 3.1.3. Cancer

Figure 1 highlights the association between muscle mass and clinical outcomes in patients with cancer. In diverse solid tumor types, muscle mass is related with mortality, surgical complications, and quality of life. For advanced cell lung cancer, an association between muscle mass and physical function has been reported. Interestingly, early chemotherapy discontinuation and delayed chemotherapy also appear to be related to the amount of muscle mass. In summary, maintaining muscle mass is essential in cancer patients to improve overall survival, quality of life, physical exercise capacity, tolerance to cancer treatments, and to decrease postoperative mortality as well as complications.

### *3.2. Older Adults*

Due to aging, the risk of muscle mass depletion is high in older adults. In this population, malnutrition ranges from 29% to 61% according to the diagnostic criteria [40]. Recently, muscle mass has been included in the definition of sarcopenia published by the European Working Group on Sarcopenia in Older People [72]. Over the last three years, we found over 80 studies dealing with muscle mass in older adults. Due to the large amount of publications, Figure 2 considers studies including more than 100 participants and illustrates the effect of low muscle mass according to the clinical setting. Studies including fewer participants showed a similar impact.

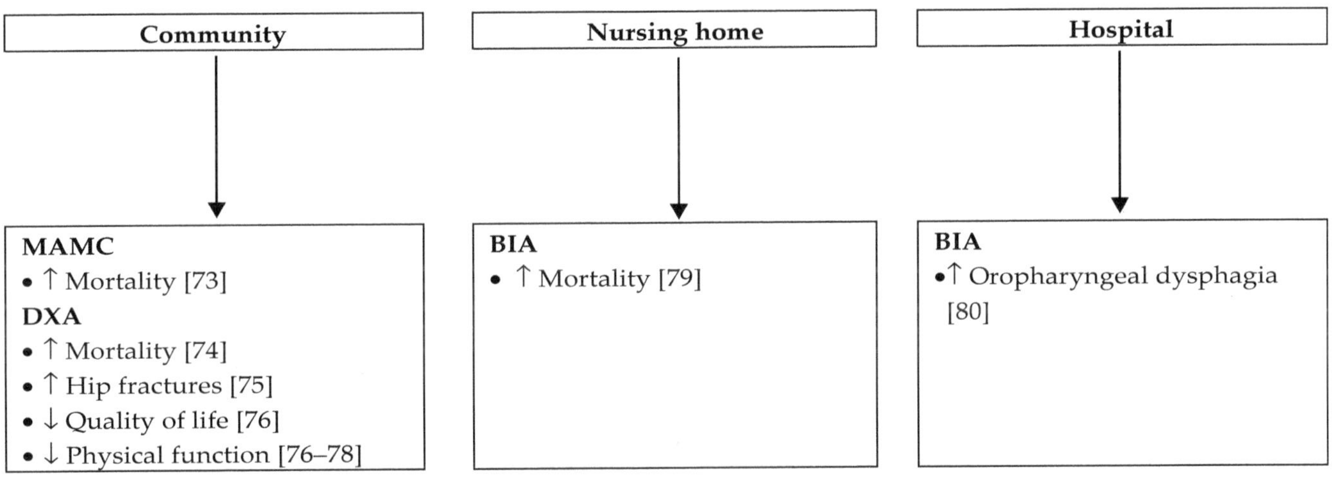


**Figure 2.** Impact of low muscle mass according to clinical setting [73–80]. MAMC: mid-arm muscle circumference; DXA: dual-energy X-ray absorptiometry; BIA: bioelectrical impedance analysis.

## 4. Improvement in Muscle Mass: Strategies and Clinical Benefits

Considering the negative effects of muscle mass loss, preserving or increasing muscle mass could lead to improvement of clinical outcomes. Therapeutic strategies to achieve this goal may include nutritional intervention, physical exercise, anabolic steroids, and growth hormone. Nutritional support is recommended for every malnourished patient, as defined by the GLIM [4]. Regular physical exercise is promoted for patients with COPD, chronic heart failure, and cancer as it improves cardiorespiratory fitness, muscle mass and strength, quality of life, and decreases COPD exacerbation and chemotherapy toxicity [81–84]. Anabolic steroids and growth hormone have been considered in malnourished patients, but no clinical practice guideline has been published yet [85,86]. These strategies are used either individually or as a multimodal treatment in clinical research with the aim to prevent muscle mass loss. In this section, we focused on non-pilot randomized controlled trials published during the last three years. We did not find new relevant studies with growth hormone supplementation.

### 4.1. Chronic Diseases

#### 4.1.1. Chronic Obstructive Pulmonary Disease

Calder et al. evaluated the benefits of a 12-week specific oral nutritional supplementation (~230 kcal, 10 g whey proteins, enriched with omega 3 and vitamin D) vs. milk comparator (~200 kcal, 10 g proteins) in moderate to severe COPD with a BMI between 16–18 kg/m$^2$ and involuntary weight loss [87]. Although improvement in dyspnea was demonstrated in the intervention group, no modification of muscle mass was observed in either group. In another study, Van de Bool et al. demonstrated the interest of a 4-month multimodal rehabilitation, including nutritional supplementation and physical activity in moderate airflow limitation COPD patients with low muscle mass [88]. Low muscle mass was defined as a lean soft tissue index measured by DXA, under the sex and age-specific 25th percentile values published by Schutz et al. [89]. The intervention group consumed each day two or three oral nutritional supplements enriched in leucine, omega 3 and vitamin D (1 unit = 187.5 kcal, 9.4 g proteins) and underwent a supervised endurance/resistance training two to three times a week. Patients in the control group were only assigned to a supervised exercise program. In both groups, improvement in ASMM, quadriceps muscle strength, and endurance performance were observed. Inspiratory muscle strength, physical activity level, plasma vitamin D, eicosapentaenoic, and docosahexaenoic acids were improved only in the intervention group.

#### 4.1.2. Chronic Heart Failure

Dos Santos et al. randomized CHF patients with testosterone deficiency in a 4-month exercise program, testosterone injection, or combined exercise program and testosterone injection groups [90]. The exercise program consisted of 60 min sessions, three times a week, with stretching, endurance and resistance exercises. Patients with testosterone injection received one testosterone intramuscular injection (1000 mg of testosterone undecyclate) at the beginning of the study. Lean mass was assessed by DXA before and at the end of the intervention. The exercise program, isolated or combined with testosterone injection, increased significantly lean mass ($p < 0.01$) while testosterone injection alone was associated with decreased lean mass ($p < 0.01$). Nutritional intake has not been evaluated.

#### 4.1.3. Cancer

Randomized controlled trials studying the effects of diverse interventions on muscle mass are presented in Table 2. Only randomized controlled trials with nutritional or physical exercise interventions were found. Results are heterogeneous, probably due to significant differences in types of intervention and population. However, most studies show an increase in muscle mass and other outcomes such as muscle strength.

Under different conditions, interventions such as nutrition, physical exercise, and anabolic steroids are efficient to prevent the decrease of muscle mass and improve functional and biological parameters. In clinical practice, a body composition assessment should be used to monitor the effects of these interventions.

### 4.2. Older Adults

Table 3 shows randomized controlled trials studying the effects of nutritional or combined nutritional and physical interventions on muscle mass in older adults. To limit the size of the table and facilitate the reading, we reported studies including over 100 participants, but the results were similar in studies with fewer participants. As for cancer patients, population and results are heterogeneous. However, most studies demonstrated positive effects of interventions on physical function but not on muscle mass. In older adults, muscle mass quality and cardiorespiratory capacities could be more essential than muscle mass quantity to improve physical function.

**Table 2.** Randomized controlled trials: effects of nutritional or physical interventions on muscle mass in patients with cancer.

| | Studies | Population | Intervention Group | Comparison Group | Muscle Mass | Significant Results |
|---|---|---|---|---|---|---|
| Nutrition | Ritch et al. 2019 [91] | Urothelial bladder carcinoma undergoing radical cystectomy INT = 31/CO = 30 | Daily oral nutritional supplement with ω-3 and HMB(700 kcal, 26 g proteins)<br>4 weeks before and after surgery | Oral micronutrients 2×/day | CT | 30 days post-operatively:<br>- ↓ patients with SMI loss<br>- No impact on hospital length of stay, postoperative complications, readmissions and mortality |
| | Burden et al. 2017 [92] | Colorectal cancer INT = 55/CO = 46 | Daily oral nutritional supplement (600 kcal, 24 g proteins)<br>≥5 days before surgery+ dietary advice | Dietary advice | BIA | 5–7 days post-operatively:<br>- No impact on FFMI and postoperative complications<br>- ↓ % weight loss and surgical site infection |
| Physical exercise | Galvao et al. 2018 [93] | Metastatic prostate cancer INT = 28/CO = 29 | Supervised endurance, resistance and flexibility exercises<br>3 months, 3×/week, 60 min | Usual physical activity | DXA | After 3-month intervention:<br>- No impact on lean soft tissue<br>- ↑ self reporting physical functioning and leg strength |
| | Taaffe et al. 2018 [94] | Prostate cancer with previous androgen deprivation therapy and radiotherapy INT = 50/CO = 50 | Supervised endurance and resistance exercises<br>6 months, 2×/week, 60 min followed by home-based endurance, resistance and flexibility exercises<br>6 months, 2×/week, 60 min | Recommendation for 150 min/week of moderate intensity physical exercise for 12 months based on educational material | DXA | After 6-month intervention:<br>- ↑ ASMM, chair rise time, leg and arm strength<br>- No impact on for lean soft tissue<br>After 12-month intervention:<br>- No impact on ASMM, leg strength and lean soft tissue<br>- ↑ chair rise time and arm strength |
| | Wall et al. 2017 [32] | Prostate cancer undergoing androgen deprivation therapy INT = 60/CO = 47 | Supervised endurance and resistance exercises<br>6 months, 2×/week, 60 min<br>+ home-based endurance exercise<br>6 months, 150 min/week | Usual physical activity | DXA | After 6-month intervention:<br>- ↑ lean soft tissue, $V0_{2max}$, fat oxidation<br>- No impact on resting metabolic rate, carbohydrate oxidation and body weight |
| | Adams et al. 2016 [95] | Breast cancer undergoing adjuvant chemotherapy INT endurance = 66<br>INT resistance = 64<br>CO = 70 | During chemotherapy:<br>INT endurance 3×/week, 105 min<br>INT resistance 3×/week | Usual physical activity | DXA | At the end of chemotherapy:<br>INT resistance VS CO:<br>- ↑ lean soft tissue index, leg and arm strengthINT endurance VS CO:<br>- No impact on lean soft tissue, leg and arm strength<br>INT resistance VS INT endurance:- No impact on lean soft tissue<br>- ↑ leg and arm strength |

INT: intervention group, CO: control group, ω-3: omega-3 fatty acids, HMB: β-hydroxy β-methyl butyrate, CT: computed tomography, BIA: bioelectrical impedance analysis, DXA: dual-energy X-ray absorptiometry, SMI: skeletal muscle index, FFMI: fat-free mass index, ASMM: appendicular skeletal muscle mass.

**Table 3.** Randomized controlled trials (>100 participants): effects of nutritional or combined nutritional and physical interventions on muscle mass in older adults.

| | Studies | Population | Intervention Group | Comparison Group | Muscle Mass | Significant Results |
|---|---|---|---|---|---|---|
| Nutrition | Cramer et al. 2016 [96] | Malnutrition and sarcopenia in the community<br>INT = 165/CO = 165 | Daily oral nutritional supplement with HMB<br>(660 kcal, 40 g proteins)<br>+<br>Usual diet<br>during 24 weeks | Daily oral nutritional supplement<br>(660 kcal, 28 g proteins)<br>+<br>Usual diet | DXA | After 24-week intervention, in both groups:<br>- No impact on lean soft tissue<br>- ↑ FM, handgrip strength, gait speed, muscle quality and isokenetic peak torque leg strength<br>- No outcome difference between groups |
| | Malafarina et al. 2017 [97] | Traumatic hip fracture in rehabilitation hospital<br>INT = 55/CO = 52 | Daily oral nutritional supplement with HMB<br>(660 kcal, 40 g proteins)<br>+<br>Standard diet<br>1500 kcal, 87.4 g protein<br>during rehabilitation stay | Standard diet<br>1500 kcal, 87.4 g protein | BIA | At the end of the rehabilitation:<br>- ↓ FFM, ASMM and BMI decrease<br>- No impact on handgrip strength, gait speed |
| Nutrition and physical exercise | Englund et al. 2017 [98]<br>Fielding et al. 2017 [99] | Mobility-limitation and vitamin D insufficiency in the community<br>INT = 74/CC = 75 | Daily oral nutritional supplement<br>(150 kcal, 20 g whey protein, 800UI vit D)<br>+<br>Supervised endurance, resistance, balance and flexibility exercises<br>3×/week, 60 min<br>during 6 months | Daily placebo<br>(30 kcal)<br>+<br>Supervised endurance, resistance, balance and flexibility exercises 3×/week, 60 min<br>during 6 months | DXA | After 6-month intervention, in both groups:<br>- No impact on ASMM<br>- ↑ muscle strength, thigh muscle composition, gait speed, short physical performance battery score<br>- ↓ FM<br>- ↑ lean soft tissue only for control group<br>- ↑ 25(OH)D only for intervention group<br>- No outcome difference between groups |

INT: Intervention group, CO: Control group, HMB: β-hydroxy β-methyl butyrate, DXA: dual-energy X-ray absorptiometry, BIA: bioelectrical impedance analysis, FM: fat mass, FFM: fat-free mass, ASMM: appendicular skeletal muscle mass, BMI: body mass index.

## 5. Use of Body Composition in Clinical Practice

Current trends towards the aging population and increased prevalence of chronic diseases will continue to rise in the next decades [100]. Malnutrition will thus likely become more problematic on a large scale and standardized care of this condition is needed. Although convenient and quick, BMI has shown limitations in the screening and the follow-up of malnutrition with a tendency to underestimate muscle mass [6–8]. The disparity between BMI and FFM raise the need for a precise quantitative evaluation of muscle mass or muscle function to both direct and validate the effects of clinical interventions in malnourished patients. Indeed, it has been established that a loss of muscle mass is associated with a decrease in physical function or muscle strength [101]. Thus, body composition evaluation should be used for the screening and diagnosis of malnutrition in clinical practice, but also for its follow-up, such as in investigation of weight loss composition following surgery or cancer therapy [4,72,84,102]. Repeated measurements of body composition will allow for the tailoring multimodal therapy. Examples of patient samples are presented in Figure 3. They highlight the clinical importance of body composition assessment to detect changes in muscle mass according to every specific patient event. Furthermore, these examples illustrate the advantage of body composition over BMI. For example, Figure 3a shows a stabilization of FFM but a decrease of total body weight and thus of BMI between July and September 2018. In Figure 3c, BMI tends to decrease as MAMC increases.

To date, MAMC, DXA, BIA, and CT at the L3 level seem to be more relevant to assess body composition in clinical practice. Figure 4 summarizes the best methods to evaluate muscle mass according to techniques availability, patient's hydration, and BMI. CT is highly precise, but, due to radiation exposure and the existence of less irradiating body composition methods, this technique should only be used in patients who undergo CT scan for other purposes such as diagnosis or follow-up [103]. Of note, deriving body composition from pre-existing clinical images is an opportunity to improve diagnosis and treatment without additional cost or patient burden. Clinical research in this area is warranted. The same applies to DXA, which can be performed without additional radiation, costs, and logistical constraints in patients who already benefit from repetitive measurement of bone density in routine care [11]. These two methods are, however, rarely used for body composition assessment in clinical routine, probably because clinical practitioners and radiologists lack information on these techniques. In other situations, BIA appears to be the most suitable method. Indeed, BIA is a portable non-invasive bedside method, quick, cheap, and reproducible [25]. Finally, MAMC will be useful especially in patients with variations in hydration level (e.g., ascites and edemas) or extreme BMI which are BIA limitations [104]. Furthermore, body composition should be integrated into routine clinical practice for a personalized nutritional support. FFM, including muscle mass, is the primary determinant of resting energy expenditure (REE) [105]. In clinical routine, indirect calorimetry is used to assess REE that reflects vital activities (cardiac, respiratory, secretory, cellular, basal muscle tone). The effect of FFM on REE depends on its quantity, assessed by body composition, and its metabolic activity [106]. Clinical conditions associated with muscle wasting, hypercatabolism and/or immobilization, lead to REE variations. Thus, in clinical practice, combining the measurement of body composition with indirect calorimetry may be useful to optimize the nutritional prescription and for the interpretation of feeding energy needs over time. Finally, clinicians should be trained to routinely use body composition in their practice, and interpreting the results should be included in pre- and post-graduate educational programs, as proposed by the European Society for Clinical Nutrition and Metabolism Life Long Learning (LLL) program. The awareness and the training of clinicians to body composition assessment may be a great opportunity to improve interdisciplinary care in the screening and management of malnutrition.

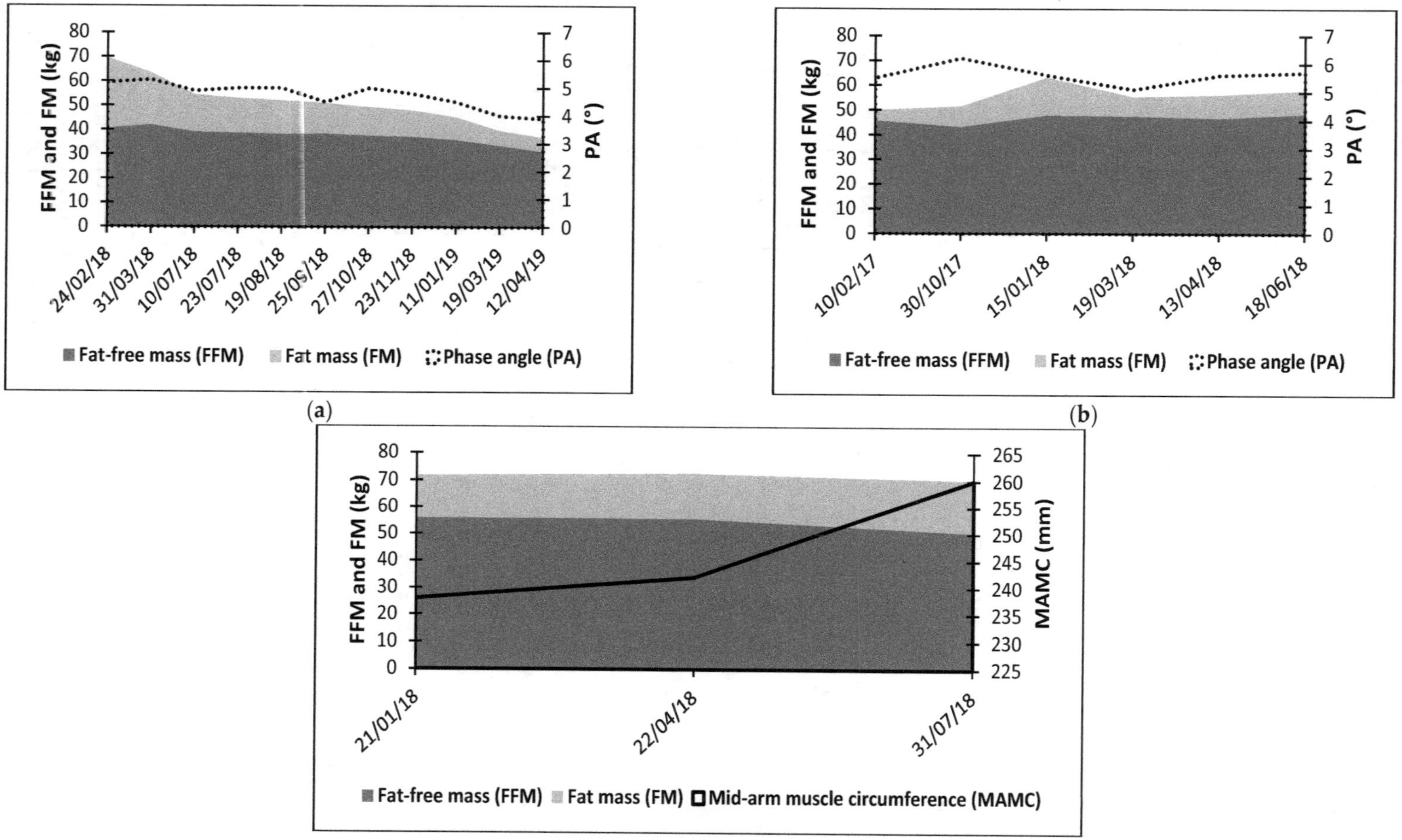


**Figure 3.** Patients samples (personal data). Evaluation of body composition by 50 kHz bioelectrical impedance analysis: (**a**) Obese patient with gastric cancer. February 2018: total gastrectomy. March to July 2018: severe diarrhea. October 2018: severe nausea. January 2019: tumor recurrence and beginning of a new cycle of chemotherapy until death in April 2019. A decrease in fat-free mass, fat mass and phase angle is observed for each new event and until patient's death. This example illustrates the association between muscle mass drop and mortality, (**b**) Malnourished COPD patient GOLD stage IV. October 2017: Start of multimodal therapy including enteral support, resistance and endurance physical training and anabolic steroids. An increase of fat-free mass, fat mass and phase angle is observed during the time of multimodal therapy. This example illustrates the importance of body composition assessment to monitor the effects of intervention(s). Evaluation of body composition by 50 kHz bioelectrical impedance analysis and mid-arm muscle circumference: (**c**) Cirrhotic patient with ascites. July 2018: Documented ascites. A decrease of fat-free mass but an increase of mid-arm muscle circumference are observed. This case illustrates BIA limitation in the presence of hydration level variations.

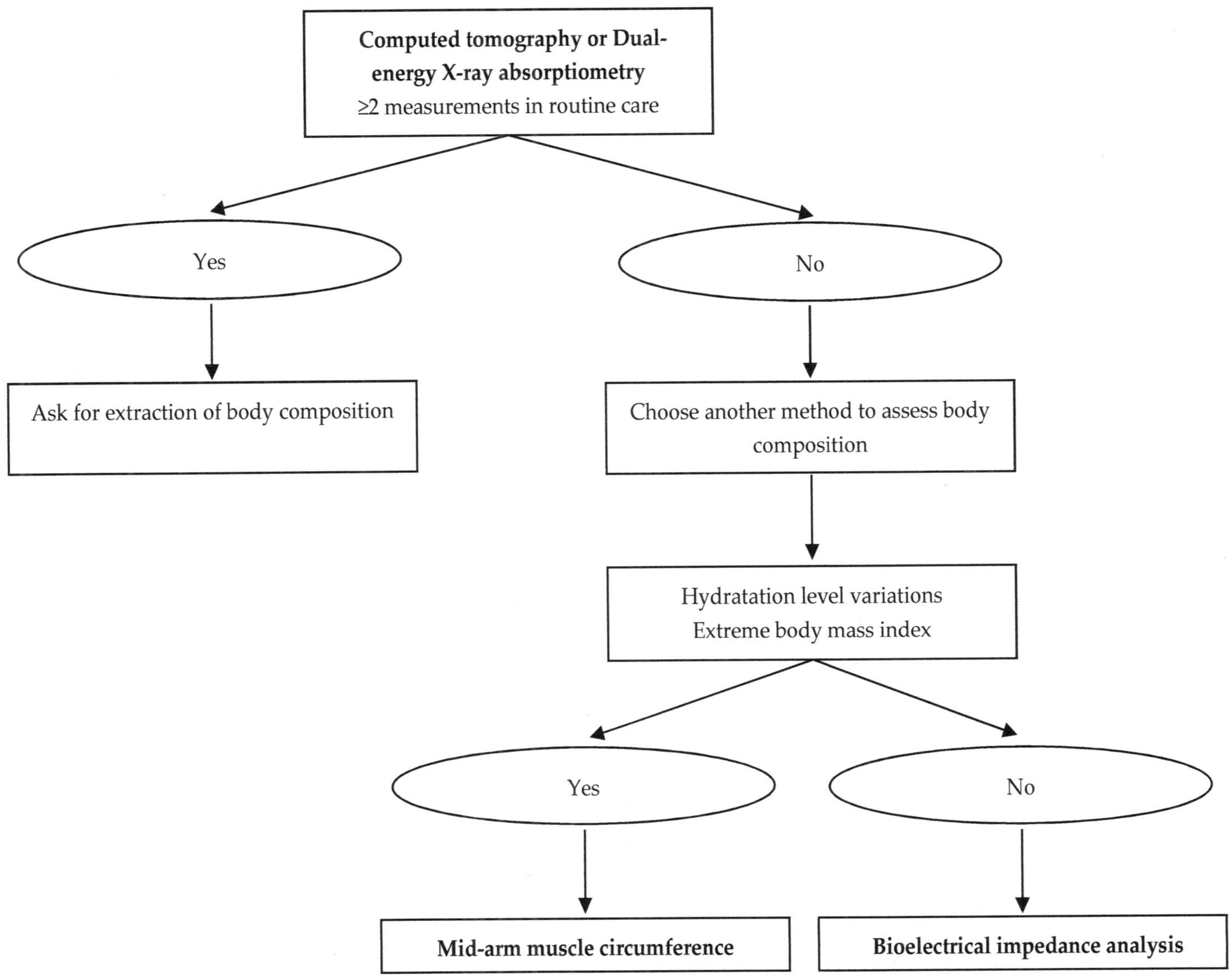


**Figure 4.** Muscle mass assessment in clinical practice: which method?

## 6. Conclusions

Available data suggest that precise assessment of body composition might be clinically relevant in the management of malnourished patients. Various methods have been validated to measure muscle mass. The method selection should be driven by the clinical situation, the patient's characteristics, and logistic and economic parameters. Standard measures of body composition such as BMI are valuable for their simplicity in daily practice. They do, however, not reflect body composition compartments. There is growing evidence in the literature that repartition of muscle mass is a more valuable tool in this assessment. Knowing this repartition allows a tailored approach to the nutritional treatment of malnourished patients and, according to the literature, led to improved clinical outcomes in various chronic diseases as well as in the older adult. Therefore, there is a need for more systematized data to orientate upcoming clinical guidelines of body composition assessment in malnourished patients.

**Author Contributions:** Conceptualization, J.M., N.A., K.N. and L.G.; methodology J.M. and L.G.; writing—original draft preparation, J.M.; writing—review and editing, N.A., K.N. and L.G.; supervision, L.G.

## Abbreviations

| | |
|---|---|
| GLIM | Global Leadership Initiative on Malnutrition |
| BMI | body mass index |
| MAMC | mid-arm muscle circumference |
| BIA | bioelectrical impedance analysis |
| DXA | dual-energy X-ray absorptiometry |
| CT | computed tomography |
| FFM | fat-free mass |
| ASMM | appendicular skeletal muscle mass |
| FFMI | fat-free mass index |
| ASMMI | appendicular skeletal muscle mass index |
| SMI | skeletal muscle index |
| COPD | chronic obstructive pulmonary disease |
| CHF | chronic heart failure |
| BNP | brain natriuretic peptide |
| GOLD | Global Initiative for Obstructive Lung Disease |
| BODE | Body mass index/Airflow obstruction/Dyspnea/Exercise capacity |
| REE | resting energy expenditure |

## References

1. Cederholm, T.; Barazzoni, R.; Austin, P.; Ballmer, P.; Biolo, G.; Bischoff, S.C.; Compher, C.; Correia, I.; Higashiguchi, T.; Holst, M.; et al. ESPEN guidelines on definitions and terminology of clinical nutrition. *Clin. Nutr.* **2017**, *36*, 49–64. [CrossRef] [PubMed]
2. Ljungqvist, O.; Van Gossum, A.; Sanz, M.L.; De Man, F. The European fight against malnutrition. *Clin. Nutr.* **2010**, *29*, 149–150. [CrossRef] [PubMed]
3. Norman, K.; Pichard, C.; Lochs, H.; Pirlich, M. Prognostic impact of disease-related malnutrition. *Clin. Nutr.* **2008**, *27*, 5–15. [CrossRef] [PubMed]
4. Cederholm, T.; Jensen, G.; Correia, M.; Gonzalez, M.; Fukushima, R.; Higashiguchi, T.; Baptista, G.; Barazzoni, R.; Blaauw, R.; Coats, A.; et al. GLIM criteria for the diagnosis of malnutrition—A consensus report from the global clinical nutrition community. *J. Cachexia Sarcopenia Muscle* **2019**, *10*, 207–217. [CrossRef] [PubMed]
5. Bigaard, J.; Frederiksen, K.; Tjønneland, A.; Thomsen, B.L.; Overvad, K.; Heitmann, B.L.; Sørensen, T.I. Body Fat and Fat-Free Mass and All-Cause Mortality. *Obes. Res.* **2004**, *12*, 1042–1049. [CrossRef] [PubMed]
6. Gonzalez, M.C.; Pastore, C.A.; Orlandi, S.P.; Heymsfield, S.B. Obesity paradox in cancer: New insights provided by body composition. *Am. J. Clin. Nutr.* **2014**, *99*, 999–1005. [CrossRef] [PubMed]

7. Kyle, U.G.; Janssens, J.-P.; Rochat, T.; Raguso, C.A.; Pichard, C. Body composition in patients with chronic hypercapnic respiratory failure. *Respir. Med.* **2006**, *100*, 244–252. [CrossRef] [PubMed]
8. Leal, V.O.; Moraes, C.; Stockler-Pinto, M.B.; Lobo, J.C.; Farage, N.E.; Velarde, L.G.; Fouque, D.; Mafra, D. Is a body mass index of 23 kg/m2 a reliable marker of protein–energy wasting in hemodialysis patients? *Nutrition* **2012**, *28*, 973–977. [CrossRef] [PubMed]
9. Scafoglieri, A.; Provyn, S.; Bautmans, I.; Van Roy, P.; Clarys, J.P. Direct relationship of body mass index and waist circumference with body tissue distribution in elderly persons. *J. Nutr. Health Aging* **2011**, *15*, 924–931. [CrossRef]
10. Seidell, J.C.; Oosterlee, A.; Thijssen, M.A.; Burema, J.; Deurenberg, P.; Hautvast, J.G.; Ruijs, J.H. Assessment of intra-abdominal and subcutaneous abdominal fat: Relation between anthropometry and computed tomography. *Am. J. Clin. Nutr.* **1987**, *45*, 7–13. [CrossRef]
11. Guglielmi, G.; Ponti, F.; Agostini, M.; Amadori, M.; Battista, G.; Bazzocchi, A. The role of DXA in sarcopenia. *Aging Clin. Exp. Res.* **2016**, *28*, 1047–1060. [CrossRef] [PubMed]
12. Antonelli Incalzi, R.; Landi, F.; Cipriani, L.; Bruno, E.; Pagano, F.; Gemma, A.; Capparella, O.; Carbonin, P. Nutritional assessment: A primary component of multidimensional geriatric assessment in the acute care setting. *J. Am. Geriatr. Soc.* **1996**, *44*, 166–174. [CrossRef] [PubMed]
13. Carnevale, V.; Castriotta, V.; Piscitelli, P.A.; Nieddu, L.; Mattera, M.; Guglielmi, G.; Scillitani, A. Assessment of Skeletal Muscle Mass in Older People: Comparison Between 2 Anthropometry-Based Methods and Dual-Energy X-ray Absorptiometry. *J. Am. Med. Dir. Assoc.* **2018**, *19*, 793–796. [CrossRef] [PubMed]
14. Noori, N.; Kopple, J.D.; Kovesdy, C.P.; Feroze, U.; Sim, J.J.; Murali, S.B.; Luna, A.; Gomez, M.; Luna, C.; Bross, R.; et al. Mid-Arm Muscle Circumference and Quality of Life and Survival in Maintenance Hemodialysis Patients. *Clin. J. Am. Soc. Nephrol.* **2010**, *5*, 2258–2268. [CrossRef] [PubMed]
15. Wijnhoven, H.A.; de Boer, M.R.; van Maanen, M.J.; van Dongen, D.M.; Kraaij, S.F.; Smit, T.; Visser, M. Reproducibility of measurements of mid-upper arm circumference in older persons. *J. Hum. Nutr. Diet.* **2013**, *26*, 24–31. [CrossRef] [PubMed]
16. Duren, D.L.; Sherwood, R.J.; Czerwinski, S.A.; Lee, M.; Choh, A.C.; Siervogel, R.M.; Chumlea, W.C. Body Composition Methods: Comparisons and Interpretation. *J. Diabetes Sci. Technol.* **2008**, *2*, 1139–1146. [CrossRef] [PubMed]
17. Kyle, U.G.; Bosaeus, I.; De Lorenzo, A.D.; Deurenberg, P.; Elia, M.; Gómez, J.M.; Heitmann, B.L.; Kent-Smith, L.; Melchior, J.-C.; Pirlich, M.; et al. Bioelectrical impedance analysis?part I: Review of principles and methods. *Clin. Nutr.* **2004**, *23*, 1226–1243. [CrossRef] [PubMed]
18. Kyle, U.G.; Genton, L.; Karsegard, L.; Slosman, D.O.; Pichard, C. Single prediction equation for bioelectrical impedance analysis in adults aged 20–94 years. *Nutr.* **2001**, *17*, 248–253. [CrossRef]
19. Kyle, U.; Genton, L.; Hans, D.; Pichard, C. Validation of a bioelectrical impedance analysis equation to predict appendicular skeletal muscle mass (ASMM). *Clin. Nutr.* **2003**, *22*, 537–543. [CrossRef]
20. Bosaeus, I.; Wilcox, G.; Rothenberg, E.; Strauss, B.J. Skeletal muscle mass in hospitalized elderly patients: Comparison of measurements by single-frequency BIA and DXA. *Clin. Nutr.* **2014**, *33*, 426–431. [CrossRef] [PubMed]
21. Peniche, D.B.R.; Giorguli, G.R.; Alemán-Mateo, H. Accuracy of a predictive bioelectrical impedance analysis equation for estimating appendicular skeletal muscle mass in a non-Caucasian sample of older people. *Arch. Gerontol. Geriatr.* **2015**, *61*, 39–43. [CrossRef] [PubMed]
22. Diaz, E.O.; Villar, J.; Immink, M.; Gonzales, T. Bioimpedance or anthropometry? *Eur. J. Clin. Nutr.* **1989**, *43*, 129–137. [PubMed]
23. Kyle, U.G.; Genton, L.; Slosman, D.O.; Pichard, C. Fat-free and fat mass percentiles in 5225 healthy subjects aged 15 to 98 years. *Nutrition* **2001**, *17*, 534–541. [CrossRef]
24. Norman, K.; Stobäus, N.; Pirlich, M.; Bosy-Westphal, A. Bioelectrical phase angle and impedance vector analysis—Clinical relevance and applicability of impedance parameters. *Clin. Nutr.* **2012**, *31*, 854–861. [CrossRef] [PubMed]
25. Kyle, U.G.; Bosaeus, I.; De Lorenzo, A.D.; Deurenberg, P.; Elia, M.; Gómez, J.M.; Heitmann, B.L.; Kent-Smith, L.; Melchior, J.-C.; Pirlich, M.; et al. Bioelectrical impedance analysis—part II: Utilization in clinical practice. *Clin. Nutr.* **2004**, *23*, 1430–1453. [CrossRef] [PubMed]
26. Andreoli, A.; Garaci, F.; Cafarelli, F.P.; Guglielmi, G. Body composition in clinical practice. *Eur. J. Radiol.* **2016**, *85*, 1461–1468. [CrossRef] [PubMed]

27. Deutz, N.E.; Ashurst, I.; Ballesteros, M.D.; Bear, D.E.; Cruz-Jentoft, A.J.; Genton, L.; Landi, F.; Laviano, A.; Norman, K.; Prado, C.M. The Underappreciated Role of Low Muscle Mass in the Management of Malnutrition. *J. Am. Med. Dir. Assoc.* **2019**, *20*, 22–27. [CrossRef]
28. Genton, L.; Hans, D.; Kyle, U.G.; Pichard, C. Dual-Energy X-ray absorptiometry and body composition: Differences between devices and comparison with reference methods. *Nutrition* **2002**, *18*, 66–70. [CrossRef]
29. Andreoli, A.; Scalzo, G.; Masala, S.A.; Tarantino, U.; Guglielmi, G. Body composition assessment by dual-energy X-ray absorptiometry (DXA). *La Radiol. Med.* **2009**, *114*, 286–300. [CrossRef]
30. Kelly, T.; Berger, N.; Richardson, T. DXA body composition: Theory and practice. *Appl. Radiat. Isot.* **1998**, *49*, 511–513. [CrossRef]
31. Bredella, M.A.; Ghomi, R.H.; Thomas, B.J.; Torriani, M.; Brick, D.J.; Gerweck, A.V.; Misra, M.; Klibanski, A.; Miller, K.K. Comparison of DXA and CT in the Assessment of Body Composition in Premenopausal Women with Obesity and Anorexia Nervosa. *Obesity* **2010**, *18*, 2227–2233. [CrossRef] [PubMed]
32. Amini, B.; Boyle, S.P.; Boutin, R.D.; Lenchik, L. Approaches to Assessment of Muscle Mass and Myosteatosis on Computed Tomography (CT): A Systematic Review. *J. Gerontol. Ser. A* **2019**. [CrossRef] [PubMed]
33. Fearon, K.; Strasser, F.; Anker, S.D.; Bosaeus, I.; Bruera, E.; Fainsinger, R.L.; Jatoi, A.; Loprinzi, C.; Macdonald, N.; Mantovani, G.; et al. Definition and classification of cancer cachexia: An international consensus. *Lancet Oncol.* **2011**, *12*, 489–495. [CrossRef]
34. Shen, W.; Punyanitya, M.; Wang, Z.; Gallagher, D.; St-Onge, M.P.; Albu, J.; Heymsfield, S.B.; Heshka, S. Total body skeletal muscle and adipose tissue volumes: Estimation from a single abdominal cross-sectional image. *J. Appl. Physiol.* **2004**, *97*, 2333–2338. [CrossRef] [PubMed]
35. Mattsson, S.; Thomas, B.J. Development of methods for body composition studies. *Phys. Med. Boil.* **2006**, *51*, R203–R228. [CrossRef] [PubMed]
36. Heymsfield, S.B.; Wang, Z.; Baumgartner, R.N.; Ross, R. Human Body Composition: Advances in Models and Methods. *Annu. Rev. Nutr.* **1997**, *17*, 527–558. [CrossRef] [PubMed]
37. Prado, C.M.; Heymsfield, S.B. Lean tissue imaging: A new era for nutritional assessment and intervention. *JPEN J. Parenter Enter. Nutr.* **2014**, *38*, 940–953. [CrossRef] [PubMed]
38. Prado, C.M.; Birdsell, L.A.; Baracos, V.E. The emerging role of computerized tomography in assessing cancer cachexia. *Curr. Opin. Support. Palliat. Care* **2009**, *3*, 269–275. [CrossRef]
39. Visser, M.; Fuerst, T.; Lang, T.; Salamone, L.; Harris, T.B. Validity of fan-beam dual-energy X-ray absorptiometry for measuring fat-free mass and leg muscle mass. Health, aging, and body composition study–dual-energy X-ray absorptiometry and body composition working group. *J. Appl. Physiol.* **1999**, *87*, 1513–1520. [CrossRef]
40. Hickson, M. Malnutrition and ageing. *Postgrad. Med. J.* **2006**, *82*, 2–8. [CrossRef]
41. Von Haehling, S.; Anker, M.S.; Anker, S.D. Prevalence and clinical impact of cachexia in chronic illness in Europe, USA, and Japan: Facts and numbers update 2016. *J. Cachexia Sarcopenia Muscle* **2016**, *7*, 507–509. [CrossRef] [PubMed]
42. Murray, C.J.; Lopez, A.D. Measuring the Global Burden of Disease. *N. Engl. J. Med.* **2013**, *369*, 448–457. [CrossRef] [PubMed]
43. Narumi, T.; Arimoto, T.; Funayama, A.; Kadowaki, S.; Otaki, Y.; Nishiyama, S.; Takahashi, H.; Shishido, T.; Miyashita, T.; Miyamoto, T.; et al. The prognostic importance of objective nutritional indexes in patients with chronic heart failure. *J. Cardiol.* **2013**, *62*, 307–313. [CrossRef] [PubMed]
44. Montes de Oca, M.; Talamo, C.; Perez-Padilla, R.; Jardim, J.R.; Muino, A.; Lopez, M.V.; Valdivia, G.; Pertuzé, J.; Moreno, D.; Halbert, R.J.; et al. Chronic obstructive pulmonary disease and body mass index in five Latin America cities: The PLATINO study. *Respir. Med.* **2008**, *102*, 642–650. [CrossRef] [PubMed]
45. Michallet, M.; De Montreuil, C.B.; Hébuterne, X.; Lemarié, E.; Schneider, S.M.; Goldwasser, F. Prevalence of Malnutrition and Current Use of Nutrition Support in Patients with Cancer. *J. Parenter. Enter. Nutr.* **2014**, *38*, 196–204. [CrossRef]
46. Costa, T.M.R.L.; Costa, F.M.; Jonasson, T.H.; Moreira, C.A.; Boguszewski, C.L.; Borba, V.Z.C. Body composition and sarcopenia in patients with chronic obstructive pulmonary disease. *Endocrine* **2018**, *60*, 95–102. [CrossRef]
47. Matkovic, Z.; Cvetko, D.; Rahelic, D.; Esquinas, C.; Zarak, M.; Miravitlles, M.; Tudoric, N. Nutritional Status of Patients with Chronic Obstructive Pulmonary Disease in Relation to their Physical Performance. *COPD J. Chronic Obstr. Pulm. Dis.* **2017**, *14*, 626–634. [CrossRef]

48. Celli, B.R.; Locantore, N.; Tal-Singer, R.; Riley, J.; Miller, B.; Vestbo, J.; Yates, J.C.; Silverman, E.K.; Owen, C.A.; Divo, M.; et al. Emphysema and extrapulmonary tissue loss in COPD: A multi-organ loss of tissue phenotype. *Eur. Respir. J.* **2018**, *51*. [CrossRef]
49. Bekfani, T.; Pellicori, P.; Morris, D.A.; Ebner, N.; Valentova, M.; Steinbeck, L.; Wachter, R.; Elsner, S.; Sliziuk, V.; Schefold, J.C.; et al. Sarcopenia in patients with heart failure with preserved ejection fraction: Impact on muscle strength, exercise capacity and quality of life. *Int. J. Cardiol.* **2016**, *222*, 41–46. [CrossRef]
50. Tsuchida, K.; Fujihara, Y.; Hiroki, J.; Hakamata, T.; Sakai, R.; Nishida, K.; Sudo, K.; Tanaka, K.; Hosaka, Y.; Takahashi, K.; et al. Significance of Sarcopenia Evaluation in Acute Decompensated Heart Failure. *Int. Heart J.* **2018**, *59*, 143–148. [CrossRef]
51. Sanada, K.; Miyachi, M.; Tanimoto, M.; Yamamoto, K.; Murakami, H.; Okumura, S.; Gando, Y.; Suzuki, K.; Tabata, I.; Higuchi, M. A cross-sectional study of sarcopenia in Japanese men and women: Reference values and association with cardiovascular risk factors. *Eur. J. Appl. Physiol.* **2010**, *110*, 57–65. [CrossRef] [PubMed]
52. Doust, J.A.; Pietrzak, E.; Dobson, A.; Glasziou, P. How well does B-type natriuretic peptide predict death and cardiac events in patients with heart failure: Systematic review. *BMJ* **2005**, *330*, 625. [CrossRef] [PubMed]
53. Bian, X.; Dai, H.; Feng, J.; Ji, H.; Fang, Y.; Jiang, N.; Li, W.; Liu, Y. Prognostic values of abdominal body compositions on survival in advanced pancreatic cancer. *Medicine* **2018**, *97*, e10988. [CrossRef] [PubMed]
54. Sjøblom, B.; Grønberg, B.H.; Wentzel-Larsen, T.; Baracos, V.E.; Hjermstad, M.J.; Aass, N.; Bremnes, R.M.; Fløtten, Ø.; Bye, A.; Jordhøy, M. Skeletal muscle radiodensity is prognostic for survival in patients with advanced non-small cell lung cancer. *Clin. Nutr.* **2016**, *35*, 1386–1393. [CrossRef] [PubMed]
55. Gu, W.; Wu, J.; Liu, X.; Zhang, H.; Shi, G.; Zhu, Y.; Ye, D. Early skeletal muscle loss during target therapy is a prognostic biomarker in metastatic renal cell carcinoma patients. *Sci. Rep.* **2017**, *7*, 7587. [CrossRef] [PubMed]
56. Otten, L.; Stobäus, N.; Franz, K.; Genton, L.; Müller-Werdan, U.; Wirth, R.; Norman, K. Impact of sarcopenia on 1-year mortality in older patients with cancer. *Age Ageing* **2019**, *48*, 413–418. [CrossRef] [PubMed]
57. El Amrani, M.; Vermersch, M.; Fulbert, M.; Prodeau, M.; Lecolle, K.; Hebbar, M.; Ernst, O.; Pruvot, F.-R.; Truant, S. Impact of sarcopenia on outcomes of patients undergoing pancreatectomy: A retrospective analysis of 107 patients. *Medicine* **2018**, *97*, e12076. [CrossRef]
58. Choi, M.H.; Kim, K.A.; Hwang, S.S.; Byun, J.Y.; Schaller, B. CT-quantified muscle and fat change in patients after surgery or endoscopic resection for early gastric cancer and its impact on long-term outcomes. *Medicine* **2018**, *97*, e13878. [CrossRef]
59. Kudou, K.; Saeki, H.; Nakashima, Y.; Edahiro, K.; Korehisa, S.; Taniguchi, D.; Tsutsumi, R.; Nishimura, S.; Nakaji, Y.; Akiyama, S.; et al. Prognostic Significance of Sarcopenia in Patients with Esophagogastric Junction Cancer or Upper Gastric Cancer. *Ann. Surg. Oncol.* **2017**, *24*, 1804–1810. [CrossRef]
60. Park, H.S.; Kim, H.S.; Beom, S.H.; Rha, S.Y.; Chung, H.C.; Kim, J.H.; Chun, Y.J.; Lee, S.W.; Choe, E.-A.; Heo, S.J.; et al. Marked Loss of Muscle, Visceral Fat, or Subcutaneous Fat After Gastrectomy Predicts Poor Survival in Advanced Gastric Cancer: Single-Center Study from the CLASSIC Trial. *Ann. Surg. Oncol.* **2018**, *25*, 3222–3230. [CrossRef]
61. Anandavadivelan, P.; Brismar, T.B.; Nilsson, M.; Johar, A.M.; Martin, L. Sarcopenic obesity: A probable risk factor for dose limiting toxicity during neo-adjuvant chemotherapy in oesophageal cancer patients. *Clin. Nutr.* **2016**, *35*, 724–730. [CrossRef] [PubMed]
62. Feliciano, E.M.C.; Lee, V.S.; Prado, C.M.; Meyerhardt, J.A.; Alexeeff, S.; Kroenke, C.H.; Xiao, J.; Castillo, A.L.; Caan, B.J. Muscle mass at diagnosis of non-metastatic colon cancer and early discontinuation of chemotherapy, delays and dose reductions on adjuvant FOLFOX: The C-SCANS Study. *Cancer* **2017**, *123*, 4868–4877. [CrossRef] [PubMed]
63. Pecorelli, N.; Capretti, G.; Sandini, M.; Damascelli, A.; Cristel, G.; De Cobelli, F.; Gianotti, L.; Zerbi, A.; Braga, M. Impact of sarcopenic obesity on failure to rescue from major complications following pancreaticoduodenectomy for cancer: Results from a multicenter study. *Ann. Surg. Oncol.* **2018**, *25*, 308–317. [CrossRef] [PubMed]
64. Zhou, C.-J.; Zhang, F.-M.; Zhang, F.-Y.; Yu, Z.; Chen, X.-L.; Shen, X.; Zhuang, C.-L.; Chen, X.-X. Sarcopenia: A new predictor of postoperative complications for elderly gastric cancer patients who underwent radical gastrectomy. *J. Surg. Res.* **2017**, *211*, 137–146. [CrossRef] [PubMed]
65. Elliott, J.A.; Doyle, S.L.; Murphy, C.F.; King, S.; Guinan, E.M.; Beddy, P.; Ravi, N.; Reynolds, J.V. Sarcopenia: Prevalence, and impact on operative and oncologic outcomes in the multimodal management of locally advanced esophageal cancer. *Ann. Surg.* **2017**, *266*, 822–830. [CrossRef] [PubMed]

66. Van Vugt, J.L.A.; Coebergh van den Braak, R.R.J.; Lalmahomed, Z.S.; Vrijland, W.W.; Dekker, J.W.T.; Zimmerman, D.D.E.; Vles, W.J.; Coene, P.-P.L.O.; IJzermans, J.N.M. Impact of low skeletal muscle mass and density on short and long-term outcome after resection of stage I-III colorectal cancer. *Eur. J. Surg. Oncol.* **2018**, *44*, 1354–1360. [CrossRef]
67. Reisinger, K.W.; Derikx, J.P.; Van Vugt, J.L.; Von Meyenfeldt, M.F.; Hulsewé, K.W.; Damink, S.W.O.; Stoot, J.H.; Poeze, M.; Information, P.E.K.F.C. Sarcopenia is associated with an increased inflammatory response to surgery in colorectal cancer. *Clin. Nutr.* **2016**, *35*, 924–927. [CrossRef] [PubMed]
68. Naito, T.; Okayama, T.; Aoyama, T.; Ohashi, T.; Masuda, Y.; Kimura, M.; Shiozaki, H.; Murakami, H.; Kenmotsu, H.; Taira, T.; et al. Skeletal muscle depletion during chemotherapy has a large impact on physical function in elderly Japanese patients with advanced non–small-cell lung cancer. *BMC Cancer* **2017**, *17*, 571. [CrossRef]
69. Huang, D.-D.; Ji, Y.-B.; Zhou, D.-L.; Li, B.; Wang, S.-L.; Chen, X.-L.; Yu, Z.; Zhuang, C.-L. Effect of surgery-induced acute muscle wasting on postoperative outcomes and quality of life. *J. Surg. Res.* **2017**, *218*, 58–66. [CrossRef]
70. Neefjes, E.C.; Hurk, R.M.V.D.; Blauwhoff-Buskermolen, S.; Van Der Vorst, M.J.; Becker-Commissaris, A.; De Van Der Schueren, M.A.; Buffart, L.M.; Verheul, H.M.; Vorst, M.J.; Schueren, M.A. Muscle mass as a target to reduce fatigue in patients with advanced cancer. *J. Cachexia Sarcopenia Muscle* **2017**, *8*, 623–629. [CrossRef]
71. Citak, E.; Tulek, Z.; Uzel, O. Nutritional status in patients with head and neck cancer undergoing radiotherapy: A longitudinal study. *Support. Care Cancer* **2019**, *27*, 239–247. [CrossRef] [PubMed]
72. Cruz-Jentoft, A.J.; Bahat, G.; Bauer, J.; Boirie, Y.; Bruyere, O.; Cederholm, T.; Cooper, C.; Landi, F.; Rolland, Y.; Aihie Sayer, A.; et al. Sarcopenia: Revised European consensus on definition and diagnosis. *Age Ageing* **2019**, *48*, 16–31. [CrossRef] [PubMed]
73. Landi, F.; Calvani, R.; Tosato, M.; Martone, A.M.; Bernabei, R.; Onder, G.; Marzetti, E. Impact of physical function impairment and multimorbidity on mortality among community-living older persons with sarcopaenia: Results from the ilSIRENTE prospective cohort study. *BMJ Open* **2016**, *6*, e008281. [CrossRef] [PubMed]
74. Kim, Y.H.; Kim, K.I.; Paik, N.J.; Kim, K.W.; Jang, H.C.; Lim, J.Y. Muscle strength: A better index of low physical performance than muscle mass in older adults. *Geriatr. Gerontol. Int.* **2016**, *16*, 577–585. [CrossRef] [PubMed]
75. Zaslavsky, O.; Li, W.; Going, S.; Datta, M.; Snetselaar, L.; Zelber-Sagi, S. Association between body composition and hip fractures in older women with physical frailty. *Geriatr. Gerontol. Int.* **2017**, *17*, 898–904. [CrossRef] [PubMed]
76. Verlaan, S.; Aspray, T.J.; Bauer, J.M.; Cederholm, T.; Hemsworth, J.; Hill, T.R.; McPhee, J.S.; Piasecki, M.; Seal, C.; Sieber, C.C.; et al. Nutritional status, body composition, and quality of life in community-dwelling sarcopenic and non-sarcopenic older adults: A case-control study. *Clin. Nutr.* **2017**, *36*, 267–274. [CrossRef] [PubMed]
77. Chiles Shaffer, N.; Ferrucci, L.; Shardell, M.; Simonsick, E.M.; Studenski, S. Agreement and predictive validity using less-conservative foundation for the national institutes of health sarcopenia project weakness cutpoints. *J. Am. Geriatr. Soc.* **2017**, *65*, 574–579. [CrossRef] [PubMed]
78. Resnick, B.; Hebel, J.R.; Gruber-Baldini, A.L.; Hicks, G.E.; Hochberg, M.C.; Orwig, D.; Eastlack, M.; Magaziner, J. The impact of body composition, pain and resilience on physical activity, physical function and physical performance at 2 months post hip fracture. *Arch. Gerontol. Geriatr.* **2018**, *76*, 34–40. [CrossRef]
79. Yalcin, A.; Aras, S.; Atmis, V.; Cengiz, O.K.; Cinar, E.; Atli, T.; Varli, M. Sarcopenia and mortality in older people living in a nursing home in Turkey. *Geriatr. Gerontol. Int.* **2017**, *17*, 1118–1124. [CrossRef]
80. Carrión, S.; Roca, M.; Costa, A.; Arreola, V.; Ortega, O.; Palomera, E.; Serra-Prat, M.; Cabré, M.; Clavé, P. Nutritional status of older patients with oropharyngeal dysphagia in a chronic versus an acute clinical situation. *Clin. Nutr.* **2017**, *36*, 1110–1116. [CrossRef]
81. Coats, A.J.S. Clinical utility of exercise training in chronic systolic heart failure. *Nat. Rev. Cardiol.* **2011**, *8*, 380–392. [CrossRef] [PubMed]
82. Maltais, F.; Decramer, M.; Casaburi, R.; Barreiro, E.; Burelle, Y.; Debigare, R.; Dekhuijzen, P.N.R.; Franssen, F.; Gayan-Ramirez, G.; Gea, J.; et al. An Official American Thoracic Society/European Respiratory Society Statement: Update on Limb Muscle Dysfunction in Chronic Obstructive Pulmonary Disease. *Am. J. Respir. Crit. Care Med.* **2014**, *189*, e15–e62. [CrossRef] [PubMed]

83. Fong, D.Y.T.; Ho, J.W.C.; Hui, B.P.H.; Lee, A.M.; Macfarlane, D.J.; Leung, S.S.K.; Cerin, E.; Chan, W.Y.Y.; Leung, I.P.F.; Lam, S.H.S.; et al. Physical activity for cancer survivors: Meta-analysis of randomised controlled trials. *BMJ* **2012**, *344*, e70. [CrossRef] [PubMed]
84. Arends, J.; Bachmann, P.; Baracos, V.; Barthelemy, N.; Bertz, H.; Bozzetti, F.; Fearon, K.; Hütterer, E.; Isenring, E.; Kaasa, S.; et al. ESPEN guidelines on nutrition in cancer patients. *Clin. Nutr.* **2017**, *36*, 11–48. [CrossRef] [PubMed]
85. Gullett, N.P.; Hebbar, G.; Ziegler, T.R. Update on clinical trials of growth factors and anabolic steroids in cachexia and wasting1234. *Am. J. Clin. Nutr.* **2010**, *91*, 1143S–1147S. [CrossRef] [PubMed]
86. Liu, H.; Bravata, D.M.; Olkin, I.; Nayak, S.; Roberts, B.; Garber, A.M.; Hoffman, A.R. Systematic Review: The Safety and Efficacy of Growth Hormone in the Healthy Elderly. *Ann. Internal Med.* **2007**, *146*, 104. [CrossRef]
87. Calder, P.C.; Laviano, A.; Lonnqvist, F.; Muscaritoli, M.; Ohlander, M.; Schols, A. Targeted medical nutrition for cachexia in chronic obstructive pulmonary disease: A randomized, controlled trial. *J. Cachexia Sarcopenia Muscle* **2018**, *9*, 28–40. [CrossRef]
88. Van De Bool, C.; Rutten, E.P.; Van Helvoort, A.; Franssen, F.M.; Wouters, E.F.; Schols, A.M.; Bool, C.; Helvoort, A. A randomized clinical trial investigating the efficacy of targeted nutrition as adjunct to exercise training in COPD. *J. Cachexia Sarcopenia Muscle* **2017**, *8*, 748–758. [CrossRef]
89. Schutz, Y.; Kyle, U.U.G.; Pichard, C. Fat-free mass index and fat mass index percentiles in Caucasians aged 18–98 y. *Int. J. Obes.* **2002**, *26*, 953–960. [CrossRef]
90. Dos Santos, M.R.; Sayegh, A.L.; Bacurau, A.V.; Arap, M.A.; Brum, P.C.; Pereira, R.M.; Takayama, L.; Barretto, A.C.P.; Negrão, C.E.; de Nazaré NunesAlves, M.L. Effect of exercise training and testosterone replacement on skeletal muscle wasting in patients with heart failure with testosterone deficiency. *Mayo Clin. Proc.* **2016**, *91*, 575–586. [CrossRef]
91. Ritch, C.R.; Cookson, M.S.; Clark, P.E.; Chang, S.S.; Fakhoury, K.; Ralls, V.; Thu, M.H.; Penson, D.F.; Smith, J.A.; Silver, H.J. Perioperative Oral Nutrition Supplementation Reduces Prevalence of Sarcopenia following Radical Cystectomy: Results of a Prospective Randomized Controlled Trial. *J. Urol.* **2019**, *201*, 470–477. [CrossRef] [PubMed]
92. Burden, S.T.; Gibson, D.J.D.J.; Lal, S.; Hill, J.; Pilling, M.; Soop, M.; Ramesh, A.; Todd, C.; Burden, S.T.S.T. Pre-operative oral nutritional supplementation with dietary advice versus dietary advice alone in weight-losing patients with colorectal cancer: Single-blind randomized controlled trial. *J. Cachexia Sarcopenia Muscle* **2017**, *8*, 437–446. [CrossRef] [PubMed]
93. Galvao, D.A.; Taaffe, D.R.; Spry, N.; Cormie, P.; Joseph, D.; Chambers, S.K.; Chee, P.; Peddle-Mcintyre, C.J.; Hart, N.H.; Baumann, F.T.; et al. Exercise preserves physical function in prostate cancer patients with bone metastases. *Med. Sci. Sports Exerc.* **2018**, *50*, 393–399. [CrossRef] [PubMed]
94. Taaffe, D.R.; Buffart, L.M.; Newton, R.U.; Spry, N.; Denham, J.; Joseph, D.; Lamb, D.; Chambers, S.K.; Galvão, D.A. Time on androgen deprivation therapy and adaptations to exercise: Secondary analysis from a 12-month randomized controlled trial in men with prostate cancer. *BJU Int.* **2018**, *121*, 194–202. [CrossRef] [PubMed]
95. Adams, S.C.; Segal, R.J.; McKenzie, D.C.; Vallerand, J.R.; Morielli, A.R.; Mackey, J.R.; Gelmon, K.; Friedenreich, C.M.; Reid, R.D.; Courneya, K.S. Impact of resistance and aerobic exercise on sarcopenia and dynapenia in breast cancer patients receiving adjuvant chemotherapy: A multicenter randomized controlled trial. *Breast Cancer Res. Treat.* **2016**, *158*, 497–507. [CrossRef] [PubMed]
96. Cramer, J.T.; Cruz-Jentoft, A.J.; Landi, F.; Hickson, M.; Zamboni, M.; Pereira, S.L.; Hustead, D.S.; Mustad, V.A. Impacts of High-Protein Oral Nutritional Supplements Among Malnourished Men and Women with Sarcopenia: A Multicenter, Randomized, Double-Blinded, Controlled Trial. *J. Am. Med. Dir. Assoc.* **2016**, *17*, 1044–1055. [CrossRef] [PubMed]
97. Malafarina, V.; Uriz-Otano, F.; Malafarina, C.; Martinez, J.A.; Zulet, M.A. Effectiveness of nutritional supplementation on sarcopenia and recovery in hip fracture patients. A multi-centre randomized trial. *Maturitas* **2017**, *101*, 42–50. [CrossRef]
98. Englund, D.A.; Kirn, D.R.; Koochek, A.; Zhu, H.; Travison, T.G.; Reid, K.F.; Von Berens, Å.; Melin, M.; Cederholm, T.; Gustafsson, T.; et al. Nutritional Supplementation with Physical Activity Improves Muscle Composition in Mobility-Limited Older Adults, The VIVE2 Study: A Randomized, Double-Blind, Placebo-Controlled Trial. *J. Gerontol. Ser. A* **2017**, *73*, 95–101. [CrossRef]

99. Fielding, R.A.; Travison, T.G.; Kirn, D.R.; Koochek, A.; Reid, K.F.; Von Berens, Å.; Zhu, H.; Folta, S.C.; Sacheck, J.M.; Nelson, M.E.; et al. Effect of structured physical activity and nutritional supplementation on physical function in mobility-limited older adults: Results from the VIVE2 randomized trial. *J. Nutr. Health Aging* **2017**, *21*, 936–942. [CrossRef]
100. Van Oostrom, S.H.; Gijsen, R.; Stirbu, I.; Korevaar, J.C.; Schellevis, F.G.; Picavet, H.S.J.; Hoeymans, N. Time trends in prevalence of chronic diseases and multimorbidity not only due to aging: Data from general practices and health surveys. *PLoS ONE* **2016**, *11*, e0160264. [CrossRef]
101. Health AgingBody Composition Study; Delmonico, M.J.; Harris, T.B.; Visser, M.; Park, S.W.; Conroy, M.B.; Velasquez-Mieyer, P.; Boudreau, R.; Manini, T.M.; Nevitt, M.; et al. Longitudinal study of muscle strength, quality, and adipose tissue infiltration. *Am. J. Clin. Nutr.* **2009**, *90*, 1579–1585. [CrossRef] [PubMed]
102. Kiyama, T.; Mizutani, T.; Okuda, T.; Fujita, I.; Tokunaga, A.; Tajiri, T.; Barbul, A. Postoperative Changes in Body Composition after Gastrectomy. *J. Gastrointest. Surg.* **2005**, *9*, 313–319. [CrossRef] [PubMed]
103. Mourtzakis, M.; Prado, C.M.; Lieffers, J.R.; Reiman, T.; McCargar, L.J.; Baracos, V.E. A practical and precise approach to quantification of body composition in cancer patients using computed tomography images acquired during routine care. *Appl. Physiol. Nutr. Metab.* **2008**, *33*, 997–1006. [CrossRef] [PubMed]
104. Raman, M.; Mourtzakis, M.; Merli, M.; Tandon, P. A practical approach to nutritional screening and assessment in cirrhosis. *Hepatology* **2017**, *65*, 1044–1057. [CrossRef]
105. Hopkins, M.; Finlayson, G.; Duarte, C.; Whybrow, S.; Ritz, P.; Horgan, G.W.; Blundell, J.E.; Stubbs, R.J. Modelling the associations between fat-free mass, resting metabolic rate and energy intake in the context of total energy balance. *Int. J. Obes.* **2016**, *40*, 312–318. [CrossRef]
106. Cunningham, J.J. Body composition as a determinant of energy expenditure: A synthetic review and a proposed general prediction equation. *Am. J. Clin. Nutr.* **1991**, *54*, 963–969. [CrossRef]

# 10

# Management of Malnutrition in Older Patients—Current Approaches, Evidence and Open Questions

**Dorothee Volkert [1,*], Anne Marie Beck [2,3], Tommy Cederholm [4,5], Emanuele Cereda [6], Alfonso Cruz-Jentoft [7], Sabine Goisser [8], Lisette de Groot [9], Franz Großhauser [1], Eva Kiesswetter [1], Kristina Norman [10,11,12], Maryam Pourhassan [13], Ilse Reinders [14], Helen C. Roberts [15], Yves Rolland [16], Stéphane M. Schneider [17], Cornel C. Sieber [1,18], Ulrich Thiem [19], Marjolein Visser [14], Hanneke A.H. Wijnhoven [14] and Rainer Wirth [13]**

1 Institute for Biomedicine of Aging, Friedrich-Alexander-Universität Erlangen-Nürnberg, 90408 Nuremberg, Germany
2 Department Nutrition and Health, University College Copenhagen, 2200 Copenhagen, Denmark
3 Herlev and Gentofte University Hospital, 2703 Herlev, Denmark
4 Clinical Nutrition and Metabolism, Department of Public Health and Caring Sciences, Uppsala University, 701 05 Uppsala, Sweden
5 Theme Ageing, Karolinska University Hospital, 171 76 Stockholm, Sweden
6 Clinical Nutrition and Dietetics Unit, Fondazione IRCCS Policlinico San Matteo, 27100 Pavia, Italy
7 Servicio de Geriatría, Hospital Universitario Ramón y Cajal (IRYCIS), 28034 Madrid, Spain
8 Heidelberg University Centre for Geriatric Medicine and Network Aging Research (NAR), University of Heidelberg, 69126 Heidelberg, Germany
9 Division of Human Nutrition, Wageningen University, 6708 WE Wageningen, The Netherlands
10 German Institute for Human Nutrition Potsdam-Rehbrücke, Department of Nutrition and Gerontology, 14558 Nuthetal, Germany
11 Research Group on Geriatrics, Charité Universitätsmedizin Berlin, corporate member of Freie Universität Berlin, Humboldt-Universität zu Berlin, and Berlin Institute of Health, 10117 Berlin, Germany
12 Institute of Nutritional Science, University of Potsdam, 14558 Nuthetal, Germany
13 Department for Geriatric Medicine, Marien Hospital Herne—University Hospital, Ruhr-Universität Bochum, 44625 Herne, Germany
14 Department of Health Sciences, Faculty of Science, and Amsterdam Public Health Research Institute, Vrije Universiteit Amsterdam, 1081 HV Amsterdam, The Netherlands
15 Southampton NIHR Biomedical Research Centre, University of Southampton, Southampton General Hospital, Southampton SO16 6YD, UK
16 Gérontopôle, Centre Hospitalo-Universitaire de Toulouse, 31059 Toulouse, France
17 Nutritional Support Unit, Centre Hospitalier Universitaire de Nice, Université Côte d'Azur, 06200 Nice, France
18 Department of Medicine, Kantonsspital Winterthur, 8401 Winterthur, Switzerland
19 Centre of Geriatrics and Gerontology, Albertinen-Haus, Hamburg, and Chair of Geriatrics and Gerontology, University Medical Centre Eppendorf, 20246 Hamburg, Germany
* Correspondence: dorothee.volkert@fau.de

**Abstract:** Malnutrition is widespread in older people and represents a major geriatric syndrome with multifactorial etiology and severe consequences for health outcomes and quality of life. The aim of the present paper is to describe current approaches and evidence regarding malnutrition treatment and to highlight relevant knowledge gaps that need to be addressed. Recently published guidelines of the European Society for Clinical Nutrition and Metabolism (ESPEN) provide a summary of the available evidence and highlight the wide range of different measures that can be taken—from the identification and elimination of potential causes to enteral and parenteral nutrition—depending on the patient's abilities and needs. However, more than half of the recommendations therein are based on expert consensus because of a lack of evidence, and only three are concern patient-centred outcomes. Future research should further clarify the etiology of malnutrition and identify the most relevant causes in order to prevent malnutrition. Based on limited and partly conflicting evidence and the limitations of existing studies, it remains unclear which interventions are most effective in which patient groups, and if specific situations, diseases or etiologies of malnutrition require specific approaches. Patient-relevant outcomes such as functionality and quality of life need more attention, and research methodology should be harmonised to allow for the comparability of studies.

**Keywords:** Geriatric patients; older persons; malnutrition; therapy; interventions

---

## 1. Malnutrition in Geriatric Patients

Although geriatric patients are usually at an advanced age, a geriatric patient is not defined by a specific age, but rather by a high degree of frailty and the presence of chronic disease. Functional reserves are reduced and vulnerability to stress increased as a consequence of a cumulative decline in many physiological systems during ageing. Limitations are, however, not restricted to physical functions, but may also affect mental and/or social integrity, leading to the need of comprehensive treatment to maintain or restore independence in everyday life as far as possible.

Among other typical geriatric syndromes, such as dementia, delirium, falls or incontinence, which are characterised by high prevalence, multifactorial origin and poor outcomes [1], malnutrition (i.e., protein-energy-malnutrition or undernutrition) merits attention.

### *1.1. Prevalence*

Malnutrition is reported in up to 50% of older adults, although prevalence estimates vary substantially depending on the population considered, the healthcare setting, and the tool used for its assessment [2–4]. A recent systematic review and meta-analysis of studies using the Mini Nutritional Assessment®— the most widespread malnutrition screening tool for older people—has summarised the following estimates according to the setting of care: community, 3%; outpatients, 6%; home-care services, 9%; nursing homes, 17.5%; hospital, 22%; long-term care, 29%; rehabilitation/sub-acute care, 29%. In addition, a high proportion of older adults are at risk of malnutrition, with estimates ranging between 27% (community/outpatients) and 50% (all other healthcare settings) [2]. These figures are in accordance with other studies and reviews, describing an increasing prevalence of malnutrition with decreasing health and functional status and increasing dependency and disability [5,6]. Prevalence rates may however vary widely between study samples even when using the same definition in the same health-care setting [2,7].

Since low muscle mass is now included as one important phenotypic criterion in the new global definition of malnutrition [8,9], and older adults are characterised by a decline of muscle mass not only due to ageing and poor physical activity but also to a poor adaptation to nutritional deficits [10], it is reasonable to argue that prevalence estimates may be even higher than previously reported.

### *1.2. Etiology*

Due to a variety of factors, older people and specifically in-patients are at increased risk of malnutrition. A decrease in food intake is common [11] and often associated with a disease, acute or chronic, which is increasing energy needs. The combination of a decrease in dietary intake and increased needs during an illness places the older person in a group of particular risk.

The decrease in food intake is often associated with a loss of the sensory abilities of taste and smell, that results in anorexia and is termed "anorexia of ageing" [12,13], but may also be caused by a poor oral health, difficulties in chewing and swallowing, side effects of pharmacological treatment, cognitive limitations, social isolation, loneliness or depression. Many acute conditions (e.g., infections, surgery) often occur on a background of chronic co-morbidities (e.g., heart failure, respiratory disease, cancer, renal failure) and increase energy needs and precipitate malnutrition in already vulnerable older people.

Besides these individual aspects, external factors such as the quality of meals, meal ambience, and the quality of (medical and nutritional) care may affect dietary intake and contribute to malnutrition, in particular in hospitals and care homes.

Many other factors may be involved [14–16], which may be of different relevance in different health-care settings, and may also differ from person to person. Thus, without doubt, the development of malnutrition in older persons is multifactorial and complex, and presently, only partly understood.

### *1.3. Consequences*

It is well established that malnutrition is associated with increased morbidity and mortality both in acute and chronic disease and has serious implications for recovery from disease, trauma and surgery [17]. Loss of body protein resulting from insufficient protein intake or increased requirements in disease is one hallmark of malnutrition, followed by an impaired immune status and loss of muscle mass, which contribute in large part to the increased morbidity observed in malnutrition. In old and sick individuals in particular, decreased muscle mass and strength, referred to as sarcopenia, in turn lead to impaired physical status, loss of independence and increased risk of falls and subsequent fractures which have a debilitating impact on quality of life [18]. Recovery from disease is delayed in malnutrition with longer convalescence periods. Not surprisingly, malnourished patients therefore have significantly longer hospital stays with more infectious and non-infectious complications, an increased rate of unplanned readmissions to hospital and higher health resource utilisation in the outpatient setting. These consequences not only increase the burden for the individuals concerned, but ultimately also increase the economic burden for the health care system [19]. A prospective study in adults aged over 70 recently showed that adjusted healthcare costs were 714 € per year greater in patients with malnutrition or malnutrition risk compared to well-nourished patients, mainly due to hospital admission costs [20].

In summary, malnutrition is widespread in older people and represents a major geriatric syndrome with multifactorial etiology and severe consequences. In the following section, we aim to describe current approaches and evidence regarding malnutrition treatment, and to highlight relevant knowledge gaps that need to be addressed.

## 2. Management of Malnutrition

### *2.1. General Aims and Options*

Nutritional interventions in the older adult may have several complementary aims [21]:

- Maintenance or improvement of nutritional status, which may replenish the protein and energy storage that is necessary to accommodate the needs induced by a metabolic stress;
- Maintenance or improvement of function and capacity for rehabilitation; this is mostly related to the muscle compartment including muscle mass. Activities of daily living but also community living may therefore be secondary aims;
- Maintenance or improvement of health-related quality of life, probably more important, compared to the reduction in mortality, than in younger adults; restoring food intake may play a direct role as being an important mediator of pleasure and well-being;
- Reduction of morbidity, including an improved outcome of underlying chronic diseases;
- Reduction of mortality as a consequence of morbidity reduction but also by increasing treatment tolerability of the underlying chronic disease (e.g., cancer);
- Reduction of malnutrition-associated costs (reduction of the hospital length of stay, the need for subacute care stays, reduction of nursing home admissions, the number of medical examinations and prescriptions).

Thus, the aims and approaches of malnutrition treatment in older patients do not generally differ from those in younger patients, but maintenance of function and quality of life gain in importance compared to reduction of mortality.

Nutritional interventions for older people cover a broad range of different measures, which all may contribute to support adequate intake and go far beyond just providing adequate amounts of energy and nutrients. As with any geriatric syndrome, the identification and management of multiple causes constitutes the basis of appropriate nutritional care. Furthermore, adequate intake may be supported by various strategies—first of all but not only by help with eating if required. Regarding direct nutritional measures, oral strategies are always the first choice. These include various modifications of usual foods as well as offering oral nutritional supplements. Moreover, enteral and parenteral nutrition are important options also for older patients, although less often indicated.

### *2.2. Current Recommendations and Evidence: ESPEN Guidelines 2019*

Current knowledge about the effectiveness of nutritional interventions is summarised in the updated 'ESPEN guidelines on clinical nutrition and hydration in geriatrics', which were developed in a multidisciplinary group of 13 experienced experts from 9 European countries [21]. In contrast to the previous guidelines from 2006 [22] and 2009 [23], they focus on systematic reviews, where available, and for the first time also cover the topic of dehydration, a very relevant, frequent and serious aspect of malnutrition in older persons.

Central recommendations of the ESPEN guideline for the management of malnutrition and corresponding evidence are summarised in Table 1 and described in the following Sections 2.2.1–2.2.7.

**Table 1.** Intervention strategies for the management of malnutrition (based on [21]).

| |
|---|
| **Basic recommendations** |
| • Routine screening for malnutrition with validated tool (GPP) followed by assessment, individualised intervention, monitoring and adjustment of interventions (GPP)<br>• Individualised and comprehensive nutritional care (A)<br>• Nutritional interventions as part of a multimodal and multidisciplinary team intervention (B)<br>• Identification and elimination of potential causes of malnutrition (GPP)<br>• Avoidance of dietary restrictions (GPP) |
| **Supportive interventions** |
| • Pleasant eating environment in institutions (A)<br>• Mealtime assistance in case of eating dependency (A in institutions, GPP in home-care)<br>• Sharing mealtimes with others (GPP)<br>• Energy-dense meals on wheels with additional meals (B)<br>• Nutritional information and education (B)<br>• Easy access to food * |
| **Nutritional counselling** |
| • for older persons/care givers—individualised (B)<br>• by a qualified person in several sessions (GPP) |
| **Food modification** |
| • food fortification (B)<br>• additional snacks/meals*, finger food (GPP)<br>• texture-modified, enriched foods (GPP)<br>• organoleptic enhancement (flavor/taste/visual appearance) *<br>• increasing variety of diet *<br>• considering individual preferences * |
| **Oral nutritional supplements (ONS)** (3 A, 3 GPP) |
| **Enteral/parenteral nutrition** (12 GPP) |

Grades of recommendation: A = based on strong evidence (at least one high-quality RCT), B = based on medium evidence (high quality case-control or cohort studies); GPP = good practice point/expert consensus: Recommended best practice based on the clinical experience of the guideline development group.* topic not addressed in the ESPEN Guideline 2019 [21]).

### 2.2.1. Basic Recommendations

It is common sense that, as a first step in the management of malnutrition, those affected and also those at risk need to be identified. Thus, routine-screening for (risk of) malnutrition is recommended in all older people in institutions and in the community (at admission/initial contact and at regular intervals) independent of their diagnosis and the presence of overweight or obesity [21]. The use of a validated tool is considered to be good clinical practice, confirmed by recent study results indicating an association of the use of validated tools with lower prevalence of malnutrition and better nutritional care in hospitals [24]. The most common screening tool developed and validated for older persons is the short-form of the Mini Nutritional Assessment (MNA), which can be applied in all geriatric settings [2,21,25]. There are, however, many other tools available. Among 48 tools used to screen for risk of malnutrition in older adults, and recently rated with respect to validation, parameters and practicability, the highest scoring tools were: i) DETERMINE your health checklist for the community setting; ii) the Nutritional Form for the Elderly (NUFFE) for the rehabilitation setting; iii) the Short Nutritional Assessment Questionnaire-Residential Care (SNAQ$^{RC}$) for residential care and iv) both the Malnutrition Screening Tool (MST) and the Mini Nutritional Assessment Short Form Version 1 (MNA-SF-V1) for the hospital setting [26].

In people with a positive screening result, a comprehensive nutritional assessment should follow as the basis for targeted interventions [21]. The assessment should focus on the identification of potential underlying causes of malnutrition as well as of individual preferences, resources and expectations, evaluation of the severity of the nutritional deficit, and a critical review of existing dietary prescriptions. To check whether intervention goals have been reached, a close monitoring is necessary in clinical practice [21].

Regarding interventions, due to the huge heterogeneity of older people and the multitude of potential causes of malnutrition [14,15], individualised and comprehensive approaches are recommended to optimally tackle malnutrition [21]. Beneficial effects on several outcomes are documented in quite a few randomised controlled trials, interestingly all reporting benefits with respect to quality of life [21].

It is recognised that identifying and eliminating potential causes as far as possible is fundamental, although scientific evidence for this recommendation is unfortunately lacking. In older patients, adequate medical treatment is certainly of central importance, preferably avoiding medication with potentially harmful side effects on appetite, taste and smell perception, salivation or cognition.

Comprehensive approaches and treatment focused on potential causes from all areas of life require the involvement of different professional disciplines namely dietitians, nurses, nurse-aids, kitchen staff, medical doctors including dentists, and all types of therapists (e.g., speech-/swallowing, occupational, physio- and psycho-). This team effort is regarded an important factor for successful nutrition interventions. Positive effects on body weight, functional and clinical outcome have been shown in several trials, although results are partly inconsistent [21].

### 2.2.2. Supportive Interventions

Several recommendations in the ESPEN guideline address supportive interventions, which were highlighted more than 15 years ago in the resolution of the Council of Europe on food and nutritional care in hospitals [27]. Beneficial effects of assistance with eating, as far as required, and of a pleasant eating environment in institutions on dietary intake of older persons with malnutrition or at risk of malnutrition are well documented in several systematic reviews. A home-like dining environment has been shown also to contribute to quality of life. Based on expert consensus, it is also recommended to encourage older persons to share their mealtimes with others, since eating in company is known to stimulate dietary intake and may also be an important aspect with respect to quality of life [21].

In addition, the ability to access the meal (in case of mobility limitations) and the food (e.g., in packages that are difficult to open) may be relevant [28]. Of course, food should be easily accessible—also between meals—and support with shopping and preparing meals, reaching the dining room and opening packages should be provided as needed. In individual cases, it may be sensible to provide specially adapted cutlery or cups with special shapes.

The need for education regarding nutrition among all staff groups and the need for knowledge among patients about the importance of a good nutritional status are well recognised [27]. Several systematic reviews document that older persons with malnutrition or who are at risk of malnutrition, as well as their care givers, should be offered nutritional information and education as part of a comprehensive intervention concept in order to improve awareness of and basic knowledge about nutritional problems, and thus promote adequate dietary intake, albeit based on partly conflicting and fragmentary evidence [21].

### 2.2.3. Nutritional Counselling

Nutritional counselling goes beyond information and education with the aim to develop a sound understanding of nutritional topics and to support sustainable health-promoting eating habits, and is regarded as the first line of nutrition therapy. Current guidelines recommend that older people with or at risk of malnutrition and/or their caregivers should be offered individualised nutritional counselling by a qualified dietician in several sessions to develop their understanding of the importance of nutrition and support healthy eating habits [21]. Individual sessions may be combined with group sessions, telephone contacts and written advice.

Counselling by a dietician or nutritionist is recommended, but in practice this may be impractical for all and reserved for those patients at highest risk. Many older people at risk of malnutrition live at home and will have initial contact with their primary healthcare team who could review their nutritional status and deliver appropriate advice, supported by local care pathways that include dietetic referral where appropriate [29]. However, it is unclear how to train these healthcare teams to best deliver the nutritional counselling. Group educational sessions for older people can be cost-effective but difficult to access for those with limited mobility. Older people may have difficulty accessing advice delivered in electronic formats but telephone consultations can effectively offer nutritional support for older people [30] and for family carers of those with dementia at risk of malnutrition [31].

### 2.2.4. Food Modification

Food modifications include adjustments of macro- and/or micronutrient content, or the avoidance of specific allergens as well as modifications of food texture or of flavor, taste and/or visual appearance (organoleptic enhancement). Nutrients or additional ingredients can be added to regular foods in order to increase energy and/or nutrient density (fortified or enriched food) or to yield specific beneficial health effects (functional food) [32].

It has been shown in several studies and summarised in two systematic reviews that food fortification—i.e., by means of natural foods (e.g., oil, cream, butter, eggs) and/or specific nutrient preparations (e.g., maltodextrin, protein powder)—can enable increased intake while eating similar amounts of food [21]. Snacks between meals and/or finger foods can also help to increase intake, in particular for people who have difficulties using cutlery or remaining at the table for the meal; this is, however, not well studied [21].

Texture-modified foods are available in various qualities (e.g., liquidised/thin puree, thick puree/soft and smooth, finely minced) [32] and intend to compensate for chewing and swallowing problems, which are widespread in older people and related to poor food intake [33]. Since evidence regarding the effects of texture-modified food is scarce [21], it was concluded that it is 'good clinical practice' to offer texture-modified, enriched foods to older persons with malnutrition or at risk of malnutrition and signs of oropharyngeal dysphagia and/or chewing problems as a compensatory strategy to support adequate dietary intake [21,34]. Based on positive effects of enrichment of regular texture diets it was assumed that enrichment could have similar effects in texture-modified diets for patients with chewing and/or swallowing problems [21]. Since insufficient dietary and fluid intake is described in older people receiving texture-modified diets, it seems reasonable to monitor nutritional intake closely [21].

Due to little expense and no risk of harm, these recommendations were made despite presently very limited scientific evidence [21].

In addition, it seems logical that increasing the variety of foods offered and considering individual food preferences could help to ensure adequate intake of older persons—this is however not studied up to now and not addressed in current guidelines.

#### 2.2.5. Oral Nutritional Supplements (ONS)

Several recommendations of the ESPEN guideline on clinical nutrition and hydration in geriatrics address whether older people with malnutrition or at risk of malnutrition should be offered ONS. Such supplements provide both macro- and micronutrients which are delivered as ready to drink liquids, or as semi-solids or powders that can be prepared as drinks or added to drinks or foods. According to a vast body of high-level evidence and strong consensus among experts, these supplements should provide at least 400 kcal and a minimum of 30 g of protein per day. They should be given to all older people with (risk of) malnutrition when nutritional goals cannot be met through dietary counselling for enhancing (fortified) food consumption, to improve dietary intake, body weight and to lower the risk of complications and readmission and to lower the risk of functional decline after discharge. Once offered, ONS should be given for at least one month with concurrent monthly assessment of presumed benefits and compliance evaluation, thereby tailoring ONS-type, flavour, texture and timing of supply to the older person's characteristics [21].

#### 2.2.6. Enteral and Parenteral Nutrition

Enteral nutrition (EN)—mostly via nasogastric tubes or percutaneous endoscopic gastrostomy (PEG)—and parenteral nutrition (PN) via central or peripheral veins are important options also for old and very old patients. These invasive measures should however be reserved for those who are unable to meet their nutritional requirements by the oral or enteral route, respectively, but have a reasonable prospect of general recovery or at least stabilisation of health and well-being. Twelve recommendations in the ESPEN guideline refer to this topic, all based on available descriptive studies and expert consensus, since randomised trials would be unethical in this field. Application of these techniques always requires careful weighing of expected individual benefits and risks [21].

#### 2.2.7. Relevance of the Refeeding Syndrome (RFS)

Based on recent research activities, management of malnutrition in older persons cannot be described without pointing out the RFS, a serious metabolic complication after reinitiating nutrition in malnourished patients [35,36]. If patients with RFS are not adequately treated, adverse effects may range from muscle weakness and peripheral oedema to multi-organ dysfunction and death [36].

The risk of developing RFS is suggested to be high especially among malnourished older patients, and is not restricted to enteral or parenteral nutrition. However, due to nonspecific initial symptoms [36] but also due to a lack of knowledge among many physicians [37], the RFS is frequently not diagnosed and consequently not treated in these patients [38]. A recent cross-sectional multicentre-study showed that nearly three-quarters of 342 geriatric hospitalised patients who were at risk of malnutrition demonstrated significant risk of RFS [39]. Like malnutrition, RFS remains a widely unrecognised and undertreated condition in clinical practice.

The key to improved patient care in this context is to raise awareness of RFS among physicians involved in nutritional care in order to identify at-risk patients and to recognise the occurrence of the RFS. In the ESPEN guideline, it is recommended to pay special attention during the first three days of EN and PN therapy in malnourished individuals to serum levels of phosphate, magnesium potassium and thiamine, which decline in RFS and should be supplemented where appropriate [21]. Accordingly, a recent review [38] also recommends close monitoring of vital parameters, fluid, serum electrolytes and thiamine in older patients at risk of RFS, whereas nutrition repletion should be started slowly and increased cautiously to reach nutritional goals after four to seven days. Using this strategy in a randomised clinical trial, mortality risk was reduced among critically ill patients [40].

### *2.3. New Evidence after the ESPEN Guidelines*

After the literature review for the ESPEN guideline was completed, a number of new systematic reviews and clinical trials addressing different nutritional interventions in different setting have been published.

A systematic review and meta-analysis considered studies that only included older persons with malnutrition and found no beneficial effects of ONS in changing body weight, body mass index, MNA score, muscle strength, activities of daily living, Timed Up&Go test, quality of life and mortality. Results of other interventions (dietary counselling and ONS, ONS combined with exercise, new ONS nutrition delivery systems) were inconsistent [41]. Another systematic review that explored the role of exercise added to oral nutritional support reported improvements in muscle strength but not in any other outcome, however mostly based on low or very low quality evidence [42]. An interesting analysis showed that nutritional support performed by a multidisciplinary team—as recommended in the ESPEN guideline—might fare better than simple interventions in reducing mortality risk and improving quality of life [43]. A systematic review looking at studies performed in nursing homes found an effect on handgrip strength only and not in other functional parameters [44]. A further recent review focused on various treatments for anorexia of ageing, also including pharmacologic approaches and flavour enhancement, suggests that some interventions may have an impact on energy intake and body weight, but calls for methodological improvements in the field [45]. Based on a systematic review and meta-analysis, the use of telehealth interventions seems to be a new, promising strategy also for malnutrition in older people. Improved protein intake and quality of life are reported, but further research is demanded [30].

Thus, the number of systematic reviews is rapidly increasing with only few remarkable original studies. Among these, a pooled analysis of individual data from nine RCTs in older adults at risk of malnutrition merits attention. Positive intervention effects on energy intake and body weight were found, whereby the combination of nutritional counselling and ONS showed the strongest effects [46]. Pooled data from studies targeting muscle strength and mortality, however, revealed no intervention effect [47]. In contrast, the recently published large multicentre EFFORT trial demonstrated beneficial effects on important clinical outcomes by routine malnutrition screening connected with individualised nutrition support in medical inpatients managed by a dietician during hospital stay [48].

## 3. Knowledge Gaps

### *3.1. Lacking Evidence in Many Fields*

Despite increasing numbers of systematic reviews on the topic, more than half of the recommendations in the ESPEN guideline are "good practice points", meaning that they are based on the clinical experience of the guideline development group because of a lack of studies [49]. The level of evidence of only 15 of the 82 recommendations justifies a grade A recommendation, and only three recommendations are directed towards patient-centered outcomes [21].

Regarding outcome parameters, most studies testing the effects of supportive interventions or food modification focus on dietary intake but do not include functional or clinical outcomes.

Most randomised clinical trials performed have examined the effects of ONS in (malnourished) older adults. Given the large number of studies and the generally quite good compliance (78%) [50], this study and intervention type currently provides the strongest evidence in the field. Besides positive effects on intake, positive effects on nutritional status are also reported, and a couple of studies also look at functional and clinical outcomes. Unfortunately, findings in this latter respect are inconsistent and often negative [21], and benefits were generally questioned just recently [41].

A general lack of scientific evidence on the effects of nutritional interventions on functional or clinical outcomes in malnourished older adults is also concluded in multiple systematic reviews [21,41,51–55].

### *3.2. Limitations of Existing Studies*

The conflicting evidence regarding effects of nutritional interventions on functional and clinical outcomes of malnourished older adults may be explained by various limitations of previous studies. The limitations frequently addressed in the literature are summarised in Figure 1, categorised according to sample selection, design of the study, adherence to the intervention, outcome assessment, and data analyses and reporting. Some of these limitations result in a high risk of bias [56,57], thereby reducing the internal validity of previous studies.

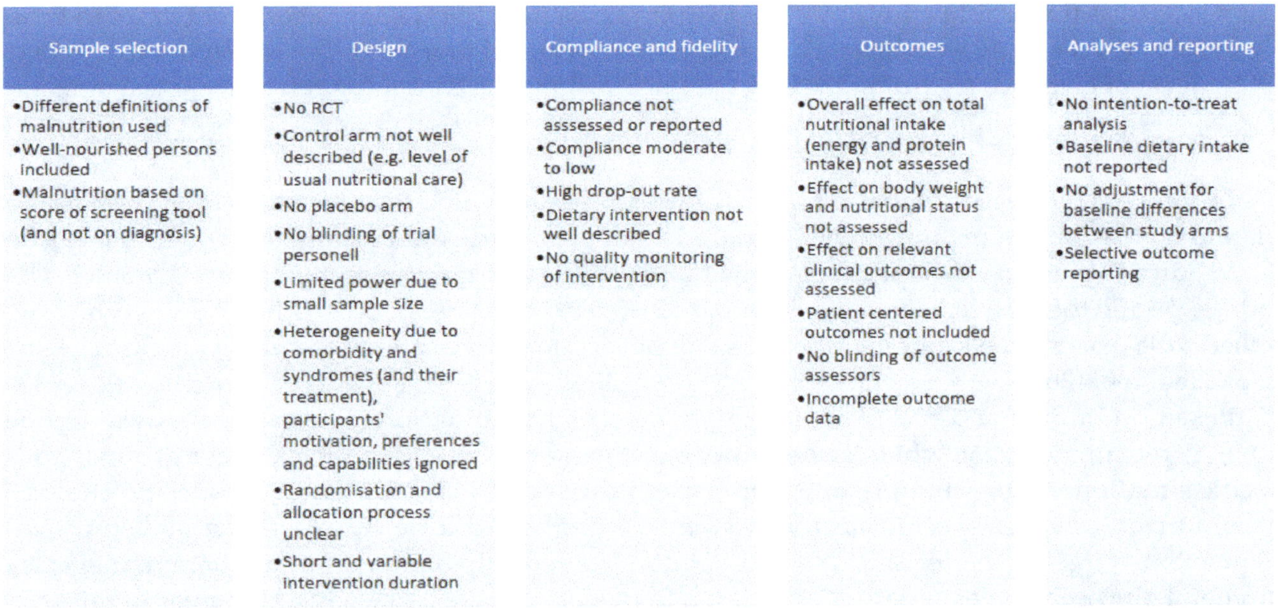


**Figure 1.** Limitations of previous studies investigating the effect of nutritional interventions in malnourished older people.

With regard to sample selection, some previous studies have not only included malnourished persons but older adults without malnutrition as well, which likely dilutes the potential effect of treatment on outcomes [55]. Different definitions of malnutrition were used to select participants, reducing comparability between studies. Among frequently occurring limitations of study design are a small sample size and/or lack of a proper power calculation based on a primary outcome variable, thus limiting the power to detect an effect. Baseline nutritional intake is usually not reported. In studies using 'usual care' in the control arm, the level of nutritional care is mostly not or only poorly described, and thus the contrast between control and intervention arm remains unclear. Hence, possible differences are not attributable to the specific intervention but rather to the difference in the overall quality of nutritional care. Further, participants and study personnel are often not blinded leading to performance bias. Even in situations where a placebo intervention appears possible (for example using a low caloric, similar looking supplement when ONS is being tested) placebo is rarely used. In most studies, a single intervention is used for all selected participants, without incorporating knowledge of participants' health and functional status, other treatments, and participants' motivation and preferences, which may reduce its effect. Details regarding compliance and intervention fidelity are sometimes not reported, while low compliance and poor fidelity will likely reduce potential effects. With regard to study outcomes, some studies lack the inclusion of clinically relevant or patient-centred parameters such as quality of life. Detection bias is often present due to non-blinding of the outcome assessors [56,57]. Moreover, studies often describe the provided amounts of energy and protein but do not report the net effect on the overall daily intake (which may have increased less due to energy compensation at other meal times) [46]. Finally, when analysing the results, several previous studies did not perform intention-to-treat analyses, but used complete case analysis only, possibly inducing further bias.

Overall, due to one or more of these limitations in most of the studies, the available evidence is mostly of only low or moderate quality. Moreover, due to large heterogeneity of inclusion criteria and study populations, intervention types and outcome assessments, the pooling of individual patient data and performing meta-analyses is currently seriously hampered [47,57]. Applying a fixed definition for malnutrition in future studies could importantly increase comparability between studies. The field could also benefit from establishing a minimum dataset (MDS) for clinically relevant outcome variables, per setting when deemed necessary, and defining the preferred method for assessing these outcome variables. This MDS would stimulate the incorporation of standardised outcome variables in future trials, and would enable the pooling of data and the performance of meta-analyses in order to obtain the highest level of evidence regarding the effect of nutritional interventions on relevant clinical outcomes.

### *3.3. Open Questions and Research Needs*

In view of the recent global malnutrition definitions, which also consider muscle mass and inflammation as part of malnutrition [8], an update of prevalence data using this definition is needed.

Validity of available screening tools remains unclear due to multiple methodological problems [58]. Setting-specific tools have been suggested based on a newly developed scoring system which was applied to 48 existing tools, but more work is still needed to derive sound recommendations regarding the optimal tool [26].

Based on limited and partly conflicting evidence and limitations of existing studies outlined above, it remains unclear which interventions are most effective in which patient groups, and if specific situations (e.g., acute malnutrition), specific diseases (e.g., dementia) or specific etiologies of malnutrition require specific approaches. Interestingly and for example, an animal study with an infection-triggered model of acute malnutrition has recently demonstrated differential effects of parenteral glucose supplementation in addition to free oral intake on survival: Whereas in mice with an experimental viral infection a significant survival benefit was observed, mortality was significantly higher in mice with an experimental bacterial infection [59]. Thus, it may be hypothesised that especially in acute malnutrition nutrition support is not always beneficial or might need a specific approach.

With regard to a causative treatment, the complex etiology of malnutrition needs further research. The etiologic relevance of the many different potential causes and therefore the priority of distinct diagnostic measures remains unclear, and a treatment, based on individually identified causative factors is probably only rarely performed. More knowledge about the most relevant causes and their common pathophysiology would increase the potential for causation-oriented treatment and could in addition contribute to enhance malnutrition awareness and preventive approaches in patients with the respective problems.

Regarding general intervention characteristics, individualised, multimodal and multi-disciplinary strategies seem to be promising and should be pursued further.

In terms of specific interventions, food fortification, additional snacks and finger food are promising options but need high-quality reassessment through further studies that provide reliable evidence. Possible beneficial effects of all different types of food modifications including also organoleptic enhancement or texture modifications need to be tested in explorative trials as well as in subsequent sufficiently powered high-quality trials.

Further research is also needed to determine which methods of delivering dietary counselling are appropriate and cost-effective for different participants and care settings. It is also unclear whether and if when the counselling should be repeated and followed up. Furthermore, the role of social care staff, such as domiciliary carers, in delivering nutritional advice and support should also be explored.

Moreover, RFS must be highlighted as an area that needs further high-quality research to develop the best preventive strategies as effective treatments for malnutrition.

Relevant outcomes for malnutrition intervention studies were recently agreed in a Delphi study among geriatric and nutrition experts [57], however more research is also needed in this regard. Clearly, patient-centred outcomes such as independence in activities of daily living and quality of life need much more attention than in the past and should be assessed using reliable and meaningful tools. Also, health and social care resource use and cost-effectiveness are important outcomes which need to be further addressed. Here, a comprehensive, cross-sectoral perspective is needed as treatment costs in one setting may only be offset by a larger cost saving in another setting.

As studies were mainly conducted in the hospital setting, further research in other health-care settings is needed.

Furthermore, the topic of dehydration urgently needs further research efforts. As one of the most frequent diagnoses of older patients, the issue of dehydration has been addressed in the current ESPEN guidelines [21], which however also uncovered many open questions and lacking evidence. For example, there is no uniform definition of dehydration, the diagnostic criteria remain vague and there is no accepted screening tool. Effective strategies to better prevent dehydration must be developed.

Last but not least, effective ways to implement current knowledge in clinical practice need to be explored.

These and other topics considered important by the authors are listed in Table 2.

**Table 2.** Open questions regarding management of malnutrition in older people.

| **Prevalence, screening and diagnosis** |
|---|
| • How are prevalence data affected by the new global definition of malnutrition (GLIM criteria)?<br>• Are the new GLIM criteria appropriate for older persons?<br>• Are different screening tools needed in different care settings?<br>• Which screening tools should be used in which setting?<br>• Are there biomarkers that could enhance screening and diagnosis of malnutrition? |
| **Determinants and multifactorial etiology of malnutrition** |
| • What are the most relevant causes of malnutrition in older patients?<br>• What are the etiologic mechanisms?<br>• What is the role of medication in malnutrition and reduced appetite?<br>• What are the essential aspects of assessment of the causes of malnutrition in an individual? |
| **Effectiveness and safety of interventions** |
| • Which interventions are most effective in which patient groups?<br>• Should specific interventions have priority?<br>• What are the best outcomes to assess the effect of interventions?<br>• Which interventions are most cost-effective?<br>• What is the optimal duration of interventions in each health-care setting?<br>• Do specific situations (e.g., acute malnutrition), specific diseases (e.g., dementia) or specific etiologies of malnutrition require specific intervention approaches?<br>• Are there situations, e.g., acute disease, where increasing energy intake could be harmful?<br>• Which strategies are most effective to prevent RFS but effectively treat malnutrition at the same time?<br>• Which types of food modifications are beneficial?<br>• Which methods of delivering nutritional counselling are appropriate and cost-effective for different participants and care settings?<br>• (When) should nutritional counselling be repeated and followed up?<br>• What is the role of social care staff in delivering nutritional advice and support?<br>• At what degree of malnutrition do patients benefit from interventions?<br>• At what degree of malnutrition do patients benefit from (par)enteral nutrition?<br>• Which interventions are effective with respect to patient-centred outcomes?<br>• Do malnourished obese patients need a specific approach? |

**Table 2.** *Cont.*

| |
|---|
| **Natural recovery** |
| • Are there patients who do not need treatment because of early natural recovery?<br>• Can early natural recovery be predicted? |
| **Role of protein and other specific nutrients** |
| • How much protein is required in specific situations (e.g., diseases, nutritional states, functional states)?<br>• How should protein intake be distributed over the day?<br>• Is there an optimal time of protein intake in relation to physical training?<br>• What is the relevance of different protein sources for meaningful outcomes?<br>• Which micronutrients are frequently deficient in malnourished older persons?<br>• Is supplementation of any micronutrient beneficial in malnourished older persons? |
| **Dehydration** |
| • What are reliable diagnostic criteria for dehydration?<br>• How could an effective screening for dehydration be performed?<br>• How is the overlap of dehydration with malnutrition?<br>• What are effective preventive approaches against dehydration? |
| **Knowledge transfer into clinical practice** |
| • How can knowledge about malnutrition and respective guidelines be effectively implemented in clinical practice?<br>• What are the effects of nutritional training for health care professionals? |

GLIM = Global Leadership Initiative on Malnutrition.

## 4. Conclusions

In conclusion, we are faced to a wide range of unresolved issues regarding the management of malnutrition in older persons which need to be addressed. Many of these questions cannot easily be answered, and it is an important next step to develop innovative strategies and well-conceived concepts for this purpose. Altogether, high-quality research is urgently required to develop effective strategies for the prevention and treatment of malnutrition in the increasing number of old and very old patients at risk.

**Author Contributions:** All authors contributed to writing the manuscript and to discussing and collecting the gaps regarding management of malnutrition in older people listed in Table 2. DV developed the structure of the manuscript and collated and harmonized the manuscript sections received from the co-authors. RW critically reviewed the final manuscript. All authors read and commented on the complete manuscript and approved the final version.

**Acknowledgments:** We are grateful to the BANSS foundation who enabled a two-day live-meeting of all authors in Biedenkopf an der Lahn, Germany, to discuss the topic without any obligation.

## References

1. Inouye, S.K.; Studenski, S.; Tinetti, M.E.; Kuchel, G.A. Geriatric Syndromes: Clinical, Research and Policy Implications of a Core Geriatric Concept. *J. Am. Geriatr. Soc.* **2007**, *55*, 780–791. [CrossRef] [PubMed]
2. Cereda, E.; Pedrolli, C.; Klersy, C.; Bonardi, C.; Quarleri, L.; Cappello, S.; Turri, A.; Rondanelli, M.; Caccialanza, R. Nutritional status in older persons according to healthcare setting: A systematic review and meta-analysis of prevalence data using MNA ®. *Clin. Nutr.* **2016**, *35*, 1282–1290. [CrossRef] [PubMed]
3. Lacau St. Guily, J.L.S.; Bouvard, É.; Raynard, B.; Goldwasser, F.; Maget, B.; Prevost, A.; Seguy, D.; Romano, O.; Narciso, B.; Couet, C.; et al. NutriCancer: A French observational multicentre cross-sectional study of malnutrition in elderly patients with cancer. *J. Geriatr. Oncol.* **2018**, *9*, 74–80. [CrossRef] [PubMed]
4. Cereda, E.; Veronese, N.; Caccialanza, R. The final word on nutritional screening and assessment in older persons. *Curr. Opin. Clin. Nutr. Metab. Care* **2018**, *21*, 24–29. [CrossRef] [PubMed]

5. Kaiser, M.J.; Bauer, J.M.; Rämsch, C.; Uter, W.; Guigoz, Y.; Cederholm, T.; Thomas, D.R.; Anthony, P.S.; Charlton, K.E.; Maggio, M.; et al. Frequency of Malnutrition in Older Adults: A Multinational Perspective Using the Mini Nutritional Assessment. *J. Am. Geriatr. Soc.* **2010**, *58*, 1734–1738. [CrossRef] [PubMed]
6. Clarke, D.M.; Strauss, B.J.G.; Wahlqvist, M.L. Undereating and undernutrition in old age: Integrating bio-psychosocial aspects. *Age Ageing* **1998**, *27*, 527–534. [CrossRef] [PubMed]
7. Wolters, M.; Volkert, D.; Streicher, M.; Kiesswetter, E.; Torbahn, G.; O'Connor, E.M.; O'Keeffe, M.; Kelly, M.; O'Herlihy, E.; O'Toole, P.W.; et al. Prevalence of malnutrition using harmonized definitions in older adults from different settings—A MaNuEL study. *Clin. Nutr.* **2018**. [CrossRef] [PubMed]
8. Cederholm, T.; Jensen, G.L.; Correia, M.I.T.D.; Gonzalez, M.C.; Fukushima, R.; Higashiguchi, T.; Baptista, G.; Barazzoni, R.; Blaauw, R.; Coats, A.; et al. GLIM criteria for the diagnosis of malnutrition–A consensus report from the global clinical nutrition community. *Clin. Nutr.* **2019**, *38*, 1–9. [CrossRef] [PubMed]
9. Cederholm, T.; Bosaeus, I.; Barazzoni, R.; Bauer, J.; Van Gossum, A.; Klek, S.; Muscaritoli, M.; Nyulasi, I.; Ockenga, J.; Schneider, S.; et al. Diagnostic criteria for malnutrition–An ESPEN Consensus Statement. *Clin. Nutr.* **2015**, *34*, 335–340. [CrossRef]
10. Schneider, S.M.; Al-Jaouni, R.; Pivot, X.; Braulio, V.B.; Rampal, P.; Hebuterne, X. Lack of adaptation to severe malnutrition in elderly patients. *Clin. Nutr.* **2002**, *21*, 499–504. [CrossRef]
11. Agarwal, E.; Miller, M.; Yaxley, A.; Isenring, E. Malnutrition in the elderly: A narrative review. *Maturitas* **2013**, *76*, 296–302. [CrossRef] [PubMed]
12. Malafarina, V.; Uriz-Otano, F.; Gil-Guerrero, L.; Iniesta, R. The anorexia of ageing: Physiopathology, prevalence, associated comorbidity and mortality. A systematic review. *Maturitas* **2013**, *74*, 293–302. [CrossRef] [PubMed]
13. Landi, F.; Picca, A.; Calvani, R.; Marzetti, E. Anorexia of Aging: Assessment and Management. *Clin. Geriatr. Med.* **2017**, *33*, 315–323. [CrossRef] [PubMed]
14. O'Keeffe, M.; Kelly, M.; O'Herlihy, E.; O'Toole, P.W.; Kearney, P.M.; Timmons, S.; O'Shea, E.; Stanton, C.; Hickson, M.; Rolland, Y.; et al. Potentially Modifiable Determinants of Malnutrition in Older Adults: A systematic review. Available online: https://www.sciencedirect.com/science/article/pii/S0261561418325755 (accessed on 28 June 219).
15. Van Der Pols-Vijlbrief, R.; Wijnhoven, H.A.; Schaap, L.A.; Terwee, C.B.; Visser, M. Determinants of protein–energy malnutrition in community-dwelling older adults: A systematic review of observational studies. *Ageing Res. Rev.* **2014**, *18*, 112–131. [CrossRef] [PubMed]
16. Volkert, D.; Kiesswetter, E.; Cederholm, T.; Donini, L.M.; Eglseer, D.; Norman, K.; Schneider, S.M.; Ströbele-Benschop, N.; Torbahn, G.; Rainer Wirth, R.; et al. Development of a model on Determinants of Malnutrition in Aged Persons (DoMAP) – a MaNuEL project. *Gerontol. Geriatr. Med.* **2019**, *5*, 1–8. [CrossRef]
17. Norman, K.; Pichard, C.; Lochs, H.; Pirlich, M. Prognostic impact of disease-related malnutrition. *Clin. Nutr.* **2008**, *27*, 5–15. [CrossRef] [PubMed]
18. Deutz, N.E.; Ashurst, I.; Ballesteros, M.D.; Bear, D.E.; Cruz-Jentoft, A.J.; Genton, L.; Landi, F.; Laviano, A.; Norman, K.; Prado, C.M. The Underappreciated Role of Low Muscle Mass in the Management of Malnutrition. *J. Am. Med Dir. Assoc.* **2019**, *20*, 22–27. [CrossRef] [PubMed]
19. Abizanda, P.; Sinclair, A.; Barcons, N.; Lizan, L.; Rodriguez-Manas, L. Costs of Malnutrition in Institutionalized and Community-Dwelling Older Adults: A Systematic Review. *J. Am. Med. Dir. Assoc.* **2016**, *17*, 17–23. [CrossRef]
20. Martínez-Reig, M.; Aranda-Reneo, I.; Peña-Longobardo, L.M.; Oliva-Moreno, J.; Barcons-Vilardell, N.; Hoogendijk, E.O.; Abizanda, P. Use of health resources and healthcare costs associated with nutritional risk: The FRADEA study. *Clin. Nutr.* **2018**, *37*, 1299–1305. [CrossRef]
21. Volkert, D.; Beck, A.M.; Cederholm, T.; Cruz-Jentoft, A.; Goisser, S.; Hooper, L.; Kiesswetter, E.; Maggio, M.; Raynaud-Simon, A.; Sieber, C.C.; et al. ESPEN guideline on clinical nutrition and hydration in geriatrics. *Clin. Nutr.* **2019**, *38*, 10–47. [CrossRef]
22. Volkert, D.; Berner, Y.N.; Berry, E.; Cederholm, T.; Coti Bertrand, P.; Milne, A.; Palmblad, J.; Schneider, S.; Sobotka, L.; Stanga, Z.; et al. ESPEN Guidelines on Enteral Nutrition: Geriatrics. *Clin. Nutr.* **2006**, *25*, 330–360. [CrossRef] [PubMed]
23. Sobotka, L.; Schneider, S.; Berner, Y.; Cederholm, T.; Krznaric, Z.; Shenkin, A.; Stanga, Z.; Toigo, G.; Vandewoude, M.; Volkert, D.; et al. ESPEN Guidelines on Parenteral Nutrition: Geriatrics. *Clin. Nutr.* **2009**, *28*, 461–466. [CrossRef] [PubMed]

24. Eglseer, D.; Halfens, R.J.; Lohrmann, C. Is the presence of a validated malnutrition screening tool associated with better nutritional care in hospitalized patients? *Nutrition.* **2017**, *37*, 104–111. [CrossRef] [PubMed]
25. Kaiser, M.J.; Bauer, J.M.; Uter, W.; Donini, L.M.; Stange, I.; Volkert, D.; Diekmann, R.; Drey, M.; Bollwein, J.; Tempera, S.; et al. Prospective Validation of the Modified Mini Nutritional Assessment Short-Forms in the Community, Nursing Home, and Rehabilitation Setting. *J. Am. Geriatr. Soc.* **2011**, *59*, 2124–2128. [CrossRef] [PubMed]
26. Power, L.; de van der Schueren, M.A.E.; Leij-Halfwerk, S.; Bauer, J.; Clarke, M.; Visser, M.; Volkert, D.; Bardon, L.; Gibney, E.; Corish, C.A. Development and application of a scoring system to rate malnutrition screening tools used in older adults in community and healthcare settings—A MaNuEL study. *Clin. Nutr.* **2018**. [CrossRef] [PubMed]
27. Council of Europe, Committee of ministers. Resolution ResAP(2003)3 on Food and Nutritional Care in Hospitals. Available online: https://www.nutritionday.org/cms/upload/pdf/11.resolution/Resolution_of_the_Council_of_Europe.pdf (accessed on 1 July 2019).
28. Keller, H.; Carrier, N.; Duizer, L.; Lengyel, C.; Slaughter, S.; Steele, C. Making the Most of Mealtimes (M3): Grounding mealtime interventions with a conceptual model. *J. Am. Med Dir. Assoc.* **2014**, *15*, 158–161. [CrossRef] [PubMed]
29. Roberts, H.C.; Lim, S.E.R.; Cox, N.J.; Ibrahim, K. The challenge of managing undernutrition in older people with Frailty. *Nutrition* **2019**, *11*, 808. [CrossRef] [PubMed]
30. Marx, W.; Kelly, J.T.; Crichton, M.; Craven, D.; Collins, J.; Mackay, H.; Isenring, E.; Marshall, S. Is telehealth effective in managing malnutrition in community—dwelling older adults? A systematic review and meta–analysis. *Maturitas* **2018**, *111*, 31–46. [CrossRef]
31. Marshall, S.; Agarwal, E.; Young, A.; Isenring, E. Role of domiciliary and family carers in individualised nutrition support for older adults living in the community. *Maturitas* **2017**, *98*, 20–29. [CrossRef]
32. Cederholm, T.; Barazzoni, R.; Austin, P.; Ballmer, P.; Biolo, G.; Bischoff, S.C.; Compher, C.; Correia, I.; Higashiguchi, T.; Holst, M.; et al. ESPEN guidelines on definitions and terminology of clinical nutrition. *Clin. Nutr.* **2017**, *36*, 49–64. [CrossRef]
33. Wirth, R.; Dziewas, R.; Beck, A.M.; Clave, P.; Hamdy, S.; Heppner, H.J.; Langmore, S.; Leischker, A.H.; Martino, R.; Pluschinski, P.; et al. Oropharyngeal dysphagia in older persons— from pathophysiology to adequate intervention: A review and summary of an international expert meeting. *Clin. Interv. Aging.* **2016**, *11*, 189–208. [CrossRef] [PubMed]
34. Beck, A.M.; Kjaersgaard, A.; Hansen, T.; Poulsen, I. Systematic review and evidence based recommendations on texture modified foods and thickened liquids for adults (above 17 years) with oropharyngeal dysphagia–An updated clinical guideline. *Clin. Nutr.* **2018**, *37*, 1980–1991. [CrossRef] [PubMed]
35. Friedli, N.; Stanga, Z.; Sobotka, L.; Culkin, A.; Kondrup, J.; Laviano, A.; Mueller, B.; Schuetz, P. Revisiting the refeeding syndrome: Results of a systematic review. *Nutrition* **2017**, *35*, 151–160. [CrossRef] [PubMed]
36. Friedli, N.; Stanga, Z.; Culkin, A.; Crook, M.; Laviano, A.; Sobotka, L.; Kressig, R.W.; Kondrup, J.; Mueller, B.; Schuetz, P. Management and prevention of refeeding syndrome in medical inpatients: An evidence-based and consensus—supported algorithm. *Nutrition* **2018**, *47*, 13–20. [CrossRef] [PubMed]
37. Janssen, G.; Pourhassan, M.; Lenzen-Großimlinghaus, R.; Jäger, M.; Schäfer, R.; Spamer, C.; Cuvelier, I.; Volkert, D.; Wirth, R.; on Behalf of the Working Group on Nutrition and Metabolism of the German Geriatric Society (DGG). The Refeeding Syndrome Revisited: You can only Diagnose What You Know. Available online: https://www.nature.com/articles/s41430-019-0441-x (accessed on 29 June 2019).
38. Aubry, E.; Friedli, N.; Schuetz, P.; Stanga, Z. Refeeding syndrome in the frail elderly population: Prevention, diagnosis and management. *Clin. Exp. Gastroenterol.* **2018**, *11*, 255–264. [CrossRef] [PubMed]
39. Pourhassan, M.; Cuvelier, I.; Gehrke, I.; Marburger, C.; Modreker, M.K.; Volkert, D.; Willschrei, H.P.; Wirth, R. Risk factors of refeeding syndrome in malnourished older hospitalized patients. *Clin. Nutr.* **2018**, *37*, 1354–1359. [CrossRef] [PubMed]
40. Doig, G.S.; Simpson, F.; Heighes, P.T.; Bellomo, R.; Chesher, D.; Caterson, I.D.; Reade, M.C.; Harrigan, P.W.J. Restricted versus continued standard caloric intake during the management of refeeding syndrome in critically ill adults: A randomised, parallel-group, multicentre, single-blind controlled trial. *Lancet Respir. Med.* **2015**, *3*, 943–952. [CrossRef]

41. Correa-Perez, A.; Abraha, I.; Cherubini, A.; Collinson, A.; Dardevet, D.; de Groot, L.; de van der Schueren, M.A.E.; Hebestreit, A.; Hickson, M.; Jaramillo-Hidalgo, J.; et al. Efficacy of non-pharmacological interventions to treat malnutrition in older persons: A systematic review and meta-analysis. The SENATOR project ONTOP series and MaNuEL knowledge hub project. *Ageing Res. Rev.* **2019**, *49*, 27–48. [CrossRef] [PubMed]
42. Wright, J.; Baldwin, C. Oral nutritional support with or without exercise in the management of malnutrition in nutritionally vulnerable older people: A systematic review and meta-analysis. *Clin. Nutr.* **2018**, *37*, 1879–1891. [CrossRef] [PubMed]
43. Rasmussen, N.M.; Belqaid, K.; Lugnet, K.; Nielsen, A.L.; Rasmussen, H.H.; Beck, A.M. Effectiveness of multidisciplinary nutritional support in older hospitalised patients: A systematic review and meta-analyses. *Clin. Nutr. ESPEN* **2018**, *27*, 44–52. [CrossRef] [PubMed]
44. Tsuboi, M.; Momosaki, R.; Vakili, M.; Abo, M. Nutritional supplementation for activities of daily living and functional ability of older people in residential facilities: A systematic review. *Geriatr. Gerontol. Int.* **2018**, *18*, 197–210. [CrossRef] [PubMed]
45. Perna, S.; Rondanelli, M.; Spadaccini, D.; Lenzi, A.; Donini, L.M.; Poggiogalle, E. Are the therapeutic strategies in anorexia of ageing effective on nutritional status? A systematic review with meta-analysis. *J. Hum. Nutr. Diet.* **2019**, *32*, 128–138. [CrossRef] [PubMed]
46. Reinders, I.; Volkert, D.; de Groot, L.C.P.G.M.; Beck, A.M.; Feldblum, I.; Jobse, I.; Neelemaat, F.; de van der Schueren, M.A.E.; Shahar, D.R.; Smeets, E.T.H.C.; et al. Effectiveness of nutritional interventions in older adults at risk of malnutrition across different health care settings: Pooled analyses of individual participant data from nine randomized controlled trials. *Clin. Nutr.* **2018**. [CrossRef] [PubMed]
47. van Zwienen-Pot, J.I.; Reinders, I.; de Groot, L.C.P.G.M.; Beck, A.M.; Feldblum, I.; Jobse, I.; Neelemaat, F.; de van der Schueren, M.A.E.; Shahar, D.R.; Smeets, E.T.H.C.; et al. The effect of nutritional intervention in older adults at risk of malnutrition on handgrip strength and mortality: Results from 9 pooled RCTs. *Clin. Nutr.* **2018**, *37*, S177.
48. Schuetz, P.; Fehr, R.; Baechli, V.; Geiser, M.; Deiss, M.; Gomes, F.; Kutz, A.; Tribolet, P.; Bregenzer, T.; Braun, N.; et al. Individualised nutritional support in medical inpatients at nutritional risk: A randomised clinical trial. *Lancet* **2019**, *393*, 2312–2321. [CrossRef]
49. Bischoff, S.C.; Singer, P.; Koller, M.; Barazzoni, R.; Cederholm, T.; Van Gossum, A. Standard operating procedures for ESPEN guidelines and consensus papers. *Clin. Nutr.* **2015**, *34*, 1043–1051. [CrossRef] [PubMed]
50. Hubbard, G.P.; Elia, M.; Holdoway, A.; Stratton, R.J. A systematic review of compliance to oral nutritional supplements. *Clin. Nutr.* **2012**, *31*, 293–312. [CrossRef] [PubMed]
51. Baldwin, C.; Weekes, C.E. Dietary advice with or without oral nutritional supplements for disease-related malnutrition in adults. *Cochrane Database Syst. Rev.* **2011**. [CrossRef] [PubMed]
52. Abbott, R.A.; Whear, R.; Thompson-Coon, J.; Ukoumunne, O.C.; Rogers, M.; Bethel, A.; Hemsley, A.; Stein, K. Effectiveness of mealtime interventions on nutritional outcomes for the elderly living in residential care: A systematic review and meta-analysis. *Ageing Res. Rev.* **2013**, *12*, 967–981. [CrossRef]
53. Collins, J.; Porter, J. The effect of interventions to prevent and treat malnutrition in patients admitted for rehabilitation: A systematic review with meta-analysis. *J. Hum. Nutr. Diet.* **2015**, *28*, 1–15. [CrossRef]
54. Poscia, A.; Milovanovic, S.; La Milia, D.I.; Duplaga, M.; Grysztar, M.; Landi, F.; Moscato, U.; Magnavita, N.; Collamati, A.; Ricciardi, W. Effectiveness of nutritional interventions addressed to elderly persons: Umbrella systematic review with meta-analysis. *Eur. J. Public Health* **2018**, *28*, 275–283. [CrossRef] [PubMed]
55. Milne, A.C.; Potter, J.; Vivanti, A.; Avenell, A. Protein and energy supplementation in elderly people at risk from malnutrition. *Cochrane Database Syst. Rev.* **2009**. [CrossRef] [PubMed]
56. Baldwin, C.; Weekes, C.E. Dietary counselling with or without oral nutritional supplements in the management of malnourished patients: A systematic review and meta-analysis of randomised controlled trials. *J. Hum. Nutr. Diet.* **2012**, *25*, 411–426. [CrossRef] [PubMed]
57. Correa-Pérez, A.; Lozano-Montoya, I.; Volkert, D.; Visser, M.; Cruz-Jentoft, A.J. Relevant outcomes for nutrition interventions to treat and prevent malnutrition in older people: A collaborative senator-ontop and manuel delphi study. *Eur. Geriatr. Med.* **2018**, *9*, 243–248. [CrossRef]

58. Power, L.; Mullally, D.; Gibney, E.R.; Clarke, M.; Visser, M.; Volkert, D.; Bardon, L.; De Van Der Schueren, M.A.; Corish, C.A. A review of the validity of malnutrition screening tools used in older adults in community and healthcare settings–A MaNuEL study. *Clin. Nutr. ESPEN* **2018**, *24*, 1–13. [CrossRef] [PubMed]
59. Wang, A.; Huen, S.C.; Luan, H.H.; Yu, S.; Zhang, C.; Gallezot, J.-D.; Booth, C.J.; Medzhitov, R. Opposing Effects of Fasting Metabolism on Tissue Tolerance in Bacterial and Viral Inflammation. *Cell* **2016**, *166*, 1512–1525.e12. [CrossRef] [PubMed]

11

# Nutritional Management and Outcomes in Malnourished Medical Inpatients: Anorexia Nervosa

**Cristina Cuerda [1,*], Maria F. Vasiloglou [2] and Loredana Arhip [1]**

1 Nutrition Unit, Instituto de Investigación Sanitaria Gregorio Marañón, Hospital General Universitario Gregorio Marañón, Calle del Dr. Esquerdo, 46, 28007 Madrid, Spain
2 Diabetes Technology Research Group, ARTORG Center for Biomedical Engineering Research, University of Bern, Murtenstrasse 50, 3008 Bern, Switzerland
* Correspondence: cuerda.cristina@gmail.com

**Abstract:** Background: Anorexia Nervosa (AN) is a psychiatric disorder characterised by a physical and psychosocial deterioration due to an altered pattern on the intake and weight control. The severity of the disease is based on the degree of malnutrition. The objective of this article is to review the scientific evidence of the refeeding process of malnourished inpatients with AN; focusing on the clinical outcome. Methods: We conducted an extensive search in Medline and Cochrane; on April 22; 2019; using different search terms. After screening all abstracts; we identified 19 papers that corresponded to our inclusion criteria. Results: The article focuses on evidence on the characteristics of malnutrition and changes in body composition; energy and protein requirements; nutritional treatment; physical activity programmes; models of organisation of the nutritional treatment and nutritional support related outcomes in AN patients. Conclusion: Evidence-based standards for clinical practice with clear outcomes are needed to improve the management of these patients and standardise the healthcare process.

**Keywords:** anorexia nervosa; refeeding syndrome; weight gain; mortality; length of stay

## 1. Introduction

AN is a psychiatric disorder characterised by a persistent restriction of energy intake leading to significantly low body weight, an intense fear of gaining weight or of becoming fat and a disturbance in the way one's body weight or shape is experienced.

The diagnostic criteria of AN according to the latest edition of the Diagnostic and Statistical Manual of Mental Disorders (DSM-5) is represented in Table 1 [1].

The prevalence of AN is estimated to be 1% [2], with a ratio between women and men of 9:1. The age of onset of AN is usually adolescence or youth, although some cases appear after 40 years or in childhood.

This disease has a great tendency to chronicity, it can produce serious medical complications, it can interfere with the individual's psychological and social development and it can even cause death. AN is associated with a high mortality rate (5%–10%) due to suicide, hydro-electrolyte alterations and arrhythmias, which places it at the head of psychiatric disorders [3].

Its aetiology is multifactorial and includes biological, psychological and cultural factors. Family and twin studies suggest a strong genetic component in AN. Within the biological factors are the neurochemical alterations [3,4]. The best known of these is the dysregulation of serotonin, which could also explain the high incidence of psychiatric comorbidities in these patients such as depression, anxiety and obsessive-compulsive disorders, which are associated with alterations in the serotonin system. Alterations have been found in these patients in some genes linked to different neurotransmitters (5HT2A receptor gene, MAOA monoamine oxidase gene, SERT serotonin transporter gene, NET noradrenaline transporter gene, among others) [4].

**Table 1.** Diagnostic criteria of anorexia nervosa according to DSM-5 classification.

| | | |
|---|---|---|
| Anorexia nervosa | A. | Restriction of energy intake relative to requirements leading to a significantly low body weight in the context of age, sex, developmental trajectory, and physical health. Significantly low weight is defined as a weight that is less than minimally normal or, for children and adolescents, less than that minimally expected. |
| | B. | Intense fear of gaining weight or becoming fat, or persistent behaviour that interferes with weight gain, even though at a significantly low weight. |
| | C. | Disturbance in the way in which one's body weight or shape is experienced, undue influence of body weight or shape on self-evaluation, or persistent lack of recognition of the seriousness of the current low body weight. |

In addition, there are usually psychological problems and family dynamics. Patients with AN are described as anxious, depressive, perfectionists and with low self-esteem. Cultural influences are also important with the emphasis on thinness in our society, exacerbated by the media. All these factors can conclude in the appearance of AN in a vulnerable adolescent [5].

The treatment of AN requires a multidisciplinary team in which specialised professionals (physicians, nurses, dietitians, psychiatrists, psychologists, among others) work together. The treatment is based on the nutritional rehabilitation, management of complications, as well as on psychotherapy and psychotropic drugs [6].

The clinical manifestations of AN are multisystemic. A summary of them is presented in Table 2. The treatment of these alterations can be found in the literature [7,8].

**Table 2.** Clinical manifestations of anorexia nervosa.

| | |
|---|---|
| Cardiovascular | Bradycardia and hypotension due to alterations in the autonomic nervous system.<br>Electrocardiographic alterations: Atrial, ventricular arrhythmias and alterations in the QTc space.<br>Myocardial alterations: decrease in cardiac mass, prolapse of the mitral valve and pericardial effusion. |
| Gastrointestinal | Delayed gastric emptying and constipation.<br>Alterations of liver function tests.<br>Parotid hypertrophy, loss of tooth enamel, gastroesophageal reflux, esophagitis, and oesophageal complications, Mallory–Weiss syndrome (especially in patients with purging habits, due to the chronicity of vomiting). |
| Neurological | Cortical atrophy and ventricular dilatation alterations.<br>Alterations in psychological and cognitive tests. |
| Renal and Hydro electrolytic | Decrease in glomerular filtration rate.<br>Hypokalaemia and hypochloremic metabolic alkalosis (vomit-induced)<br>Metabolic acidosis (laxative abuse).<br>Hyponatremia (diuretics abuse, potomania).<br>Hypophosphatemia, hypokalaemia, and hypomagnesemia (refeeding syndrome, RS). |
| Bone | Osteopenia.<br>Osteoporosis.<br>Osteomalacia. |
| Endocrinological | Hypogonadotropic hypogonadism.<br>Hypometabolism (resting energy expenditure, REE).<br>Hypercortisolism, without the stigmas of Cushing's syndrome.<br>Euthyroid sick syndrome (low-normal range of T4 and TSH, with low levels of T3 and an increase in rT3).<br>Hypoglycaemia.Growth and developmental delay in children |
| Haematological | Bone marrow hypoplasia with gelatinous transformation presenting variable degrees of anaemia, leukopenia, and thrombocytopenia. |
| Dermatological | Russell's sign.<br>Xerosis.<br>Lanugo.<br>Hypercarotenaemia. |

The objective of this article is to review the scientific evidence of the refeeding process of malnourished inpatients with AN, focusing on the clinical outcome.

## 2. Methods

We conducted an extensive search in Medline and Cochrane, on April 22nd 2019, using the following search terms: "Anorexia nervosa", "inpatients", "refeeding", "nutritional treatment", "tube-feeding", "energy expenditure", "physical activity", "exercise", "refeeding syndrome", "mortality", "weight gain", "rehospitalisation", "length of stay", in title and abstracts. We repeated the search using MeSH terms. We identified 259 papers. After screening all abstracts, we identified 19 papers that corresponded to our inclusion criteria. These were: (1) papers in English and Spanish in the last 15 years; (2) were performed in AN inpatients; (3) reported results on weight or body mass index (BMI) at admission and at discharge, length of stay, refeeding rate, type of nutritional treatment and outcome.

## 3. Results

As a result of the literature review, this article will cover the following topics: Characteristics of malnutrition and changes in body composition, energy and protein requirements, nutritional treatment, physical activity programmes, models of organisation of the nutritional treatment, and nutritional support related outcomes in AN patients.

### *3.1. Malnutrition and Body Composition in AN*

According to the Global Leadership Initiative on Malnutrition (GLIM) classification, the patients with AN present chronic disease related malnutrition without inflammation with different degrees of severity. This means that the main etiological factor of malnutrition is starvation. However, if these patients suffer from an acute illness, the inflammatory process will rapidly deteriorate their nutritional status, jeopardising their clinical outcome [9].

Based on DSM-5 severity definition, patients with AN can be classified into mild BMI (BMI ≥ 17.0 kg/m$^2$), moderate (BMI = 16.0–16.99 kg/m$^2$), severe (BMI = 15.0–15.99 kg/m$^2$) and extreme (BMI < 15.0 kg/m$^2$) malnutrition [1].

The patients with AN may present with a low-fat mass and fat-free mass, however they usually maintain plasmatic visceral proteins in the normal range. It has been shown that low prealbumin is a predictor of medical complications [10].

The body composition of these patients can be evaluated with anthropometry, Bioelectrical Impedance Analysis (BIA) and Dual-Energy X-ray Absorptiometry (DEXA) as the gold standard. BIA has proved to be one of the most useful in clinical practice, although in severely malnourished patients (BMI < 15.0 kg/m$^2$) may not be sufficiently accurate [11].

Phase angle is one of BIA measurements that has been associated with poor outcome in some diseases (HIV, cancer). In patients with low body weight, including healthy individuals, ballet dancers and AN patients, phase angle could be a useful marker of qualitative changes [12].

The use of BIA gives clinicians and researchers the advantage of monitoring the compartmental weight gain, ideally achieving an approximate 20/80%–25/75% fat/lean body mass ratio. Moreover, each patient can act as their own "control" that could potentially allow for a more effective, individualised nutrition regimen. Nevertheless, this information must be cautiously interpreted by qualified clinicians who understand this technique and its limitations [13].

The patients with AN present micronutrient deficiencies due to low food intake that can be aggravated in patients with purging habits and during the refeeding process. In a systematic review by Hanachi et al. including 374 patients with AN (restricting (AN-R) and binge-eating/purging (AN-BP) type), it was found that zinc deficiency had the highest prevalence (64.3%), followed by vitamin D (54.2%), copper (37.1%), selenium (20.5%), vitamin B1 (15%), vitamin B12 (4.7%), and vitamin B9 (8.9%).

The AN-BP subgroup had lower selenium ($p < 0.001$) and vitamin B12 plasma concentration ($p < 0.036$), whereas lower copper plasma concentration was observed in patients with AN-R type ($p < 0.022$) [14].

### 3.2. *Energy and Protein Requirements*

The refeeding process of patients with AN can be challenging since it must allow a weight gain without developing a refeeding syndrome (RS). On top of that, physicians must deal with the difficult personalities of a psychiatric disorder which in this case shows itself as a fear of weight gain.

In order to obtain the energy requirements, there are equations that estimate the resting energy expenditure (REE) or basal energy expenditure (BEE) and methods that directly measure REE with different types of indirect calorimetry. All of these are applicable to clinical practice as well as research. Additionally, the use of indirect calorimetry can be used to monitor the nutritional treatment in hospitalised patients. Sometimes this helps to uncover patients that are not gaining weight accordingly.

In the study conducted by Cuerda et al., 22 female inpatients were studied. REE was measured by indirect calorimetry (Deltatrac II MBM-200, Aldershot, UK) and was estimated by several predictive formulas (Fleisch, Harris–Benedict, FAO, Schofield–HW, Schebendach). All formulas overestimated REE compared to indirect calorimetry, except the Schebendach formula [15].

In another study by El Ghoch et al., the REE measured by indirect calorimetry by the Douglas bag method and FitMate method was compared to the Harris–Benedict and Müller et al. equations in 15 patients with AN. Using the Douglas Bag method as the gold standard (that measures VCO2/VO2), the authors found an accurate REE estimation with the FitMate method and the Müller et al. equation. Meanwhile, the Harris–Benedict equation overestimated the REE [16].

The literature regarding protein requirements is scarce. There is no evidence that these patients have specific requirements for protein intake. The refeeding process is based on the recommendations for the general population (0.8 g/kg of body weight/day; 10%–15% of energy requirements).

### 3.3. *Nutritional Treatment in AN*

Nutritional rehabilitation is probably the most important part of the treatment of patients with AN. Its objectives focus on [6]: Restore body weight; correct the physical complications of malnutrition; improve the patients' motivation to normalise their dietary habits and collaborate in the treatment; educate the patients about healthy nutrition and proper eating patterns; and correct wrong thoughts, attitudes, and feelings about the disorder.

Many of the cognitive and behavioural alterations of malnourished AN patients (food anxiety, taste alterations, binge eating, depression, obsessions, apathy, irritability) improve with the weight gain. Moreover, it increases the effectiveness of other treatments such as psychotherapy or psychotropic drugs [17].

Depending on the setting (outpatients, day hospital, inpatients), nutritional rehabilitation varies in terms of refeeding rate and type of nutritional treatment.

The restoration of body weight is done until the patient reaches a healthy weight in which women recover menstruation and ovulation, men normalise their sexual desire and hormone levels and children and adolescents normalise their growth and sexual development. This requires long treatments, sometimes with repeated hospitalisations followed by a continuity of care in the different settings.

The refeeding process is made according to the patient in a phased manner, agreeing on weight gains during hospitalisation and weight upon discharge. There are no clear criteria for hospitalisation. Some of the usual criteria are summarised in Table 3, even though this depends on the availability of a day hospital in the centre.

**Table 3.** Criteria for hospitalisation in anorexia nervosa.

| | Medical Indications |
|---|---|
| Adults | Bradycardia < 40 bpm or tachycardia > 110 bpm.<br>Blood pressure < 90/60 mmHg.<br>Symptomatic hypoglycaemia.<br>Hypokalaemia < 3 mmol/l.<br>Hypothermia < 36.1 °C.<br>Dehydration.<br>Uncontrolled vomiting or purging behaviour.<br>Weight < 75% of ideal body weight.<br>Rapid loss of weight (several kgs in a week).<br>Lack of improvement or worsening despite treatment as an outpatient. |
| Children and adolescents | Bradycardia < 50 bpm.<br>Orthostatic hypotension (increase of >20 bpm in heart rate or drop in blood pressure > 10–20 mmHg with orthostatism).<br>Blood pressure < 80/50 mmHg.<br>Hypokalaemia or hypophosphataemia<br>Rapid weight loss even if the weight is >75% of the ideal body weight.<br>Symptomatic hypoglycaemia.<br>Lack of improvement or worsening despite treatment as an outpatient. |
| | **Psychiatric Indications** |
| All ages | Suicidal ideation.<br>Serious concomitant psychiatric illness.<br>Impossibility to eat independently or needs tube feeding.<br>Unfavourable family environment.<br>Lack of cooperation despite treatment as an outpatient. |

Generally, a weight gain of 0.5–1.4 kg/week in hospitalised patients and 250–500 g/week in outpatients is established to avoid the appearance of RS [6,17,18].

Table 4 summarises the recommendations of different clinical guidelines on how to perform the refeeding in malnourished AN patients. Since very few high evidence level studies (RCT) are available, these recommendations are based mainly on clinical experience [6,19–23]. These guidelines differ in the number of calories administered at the beginning of the refeeding (from the most conservative ones that recommend 5–20 kcal/kg at hospital admission [24], to the most permissive ones that begin with 30–40 kcal/kg) [6]. The caloric intake will increase progressively to allow adequate weight gain, sometimes being necessary to reach 70–100 kcal/kg. Patients who have higher caloric requirements usually present inappropriate behaviours (throwing or hiding food, vomiting, intense exercise, etc.).

**Table 4.** Guidelines for the refeeding of malnourished anorexia nervosa patients.

| Guideline | Population | Kcal/kg |
|---|---|---|
| United Kingdom: National Institute for Health and Clinical Excellence (NICE), 2017 [24] | Adults | 5–20 |
| United Kingdom: MARSIPAN: Management of Really Sick Patients with Anorexia Nervosa, 2014 [20] | Adults | 5–20 |
| United Kingdom: Junior MARSIPAN: Management of Really Sick Patients under 18 with Anorexia Nervosa, 2012 [21] | <18 years | 15–20 |
| American Psychiatric Association (APA), 2006 [6] | Adults | 30–40 |
| American Dietetic Association (ADA), 2006 [22] | Adults | 30–40 |
| Australia and New Zealand, 2004 [23] | Adults | 15–20 (600–800 kcal/d) |

An example of the progressive refeeding of macronutrients and micronutrients in hospitalised patients is shown in Table 5 [19].

**Table 5.** Example of a refeeding process in terms of macronutrient and micronutrient intake [19].

| Days | Recommendations |
|---|---|
| Day 1–3 | • Start with 10–15 kcal/kg (600–1000 kcal/day).<br>• Prophylactic electrolyte supplementation (P, K, Mg).<br>• Thiamine (200–300 mg/day).<br>• Vitamins (200% RDI).<br>• Minerals and trace elements (100% RDI).<br>• Restrict the contribution of fluids to a zero balance.<br>• Restrict sodium to <1 mmol/kg/day.<br>• Glucose and electrolyte levels and the appearance of oedema should be adequately monitored, since the highest risk of RS occurs in these early days. |
| Day 4–10 | • Calorie intake will increase to allow weight gain, continuing with electrolyte, vitamin and mineral supplementation and close monitoring. |

In the last decades, many studies have been published regarding nutritional treatment in AN inpatients following different rates of refeeding. Some of them favour the side of "start slow, advance slow", which translates to a slow rate of refeeding especially in patients with very low BMI at admission. On the other hand, some groups follow the "start higher, advance faster", which means a more aggressive refeeding process generally in patients with moderate malnutrition with additional phosphate supplements. This usually conducts to a shorter hospital stay. In general, the results of these studies show that the refeeding is safe and effective in these patients if the supervision is adequate and follows a specific protocol [25–40].

By following any of the above recommendations the weight gain is progressive, and it avoids the appearance of RS (especially in patients weighing less than 70% of their ideal body weight). An algorithm of the nutritional treatment is shown in Figure 1.

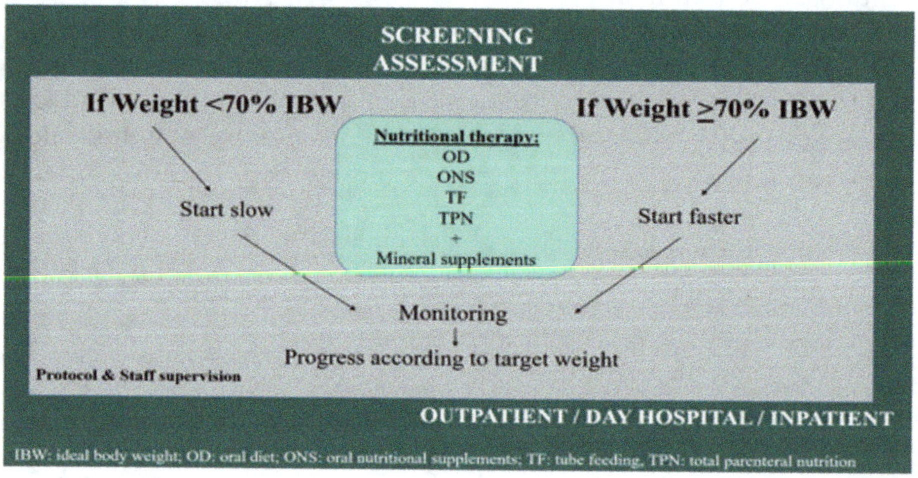


**Figure 1.** Algorithm of the nutritional treatment in AN.

The refeeding process can include oral diet (OD) as well as medical nutritional therapy.

OD should be the first option for the refeeding, even though there is no evidence of the best food choices and macronutrients distribution in the diet of these patients. The dietary plan should follow a healthy diet model, in which the portion size is personalised according to the patient's requirements and weight gain. Standardisation against personalised caloric prescriptions may confer advantages by facilitating accelerated early weight gain and lower the incidence of bed rest without increasing the incidence of RS [41].

No association between different nutrient contents (e.g. high-protein diet, diets with higher omega-3 polyunsaturated fatty-acid content, low-sodium versus normal-sodium diets) and refeeding outcome has been identified [18,42].

According to each protocol, oral nutritional supplements (ONS) is added if the patients' nutritional requirements are not met, or their weight is stagnating. However, some groups use ONS since the first day of hospital admission in order to shorten the hospital stay. Complete hypercaloric polymeric diets, with a caloric density of 1.5 kcal/ml or even higher, are generally used [27,29,34,38–40].

Tube feeding (TF) is indicated in those patients with severe malnutrition who refuse to eat [36]. Some patients with AN may reject this treatment, especially in the beginning, considering it as an aggression that increases their sense of lack of control over their own diet. Usually, polymeric, lactose free and fibre-enriched formulas are employed. The administration rate is progressively increased to favour tolerance. The use of infusion pumps allows a better control and it impedes the manipulation of the treatment by the patient.

Percutaneous endoscopic gastrostomy (PEG) remains a limited choice of refeeding, however, it may be necessary in patients who need a prolonged treatment. In a study conducted by Born et al. there was no increase in the rate of complications reported for patients using PEG feedings in comparison with those receiving TF [43].

Parenteral nutrition (PN) is used even less in patients with AN, although, it could be a solution in patients with severe malnutrition in whom the digestive tract is not functional (digestive haemorrhage, intestinal obstruction, intestinal perforation, ileus, etc.) [44]. PN is associated with more severe complications than TF, and there is a need to tailor the formulas with special emphasis on volume, macronutrient distribution, micronutrients, and minerals supplementation. There have been published cases with patients treated with home PN [45].

In any of the refeeding modalities, a close supervision by the ward staff is required. A detailed protocol of the steps to follow improves the daily management of the treatment of these patients and may facilitate the weight gain process.

### *3.4. Physical Activity Programmes*

The addition of physical activity in the treatment of patients with AN is exponentially growing, even though these programmes have been characterised as controversial [46–48]. Excessive exercise is often suggested as a causal factor in AN [47], and thus, it is not often prescribed in their clinical management [48]. However, prolonged restraint from physical activity may contribute to decreased bone mass, increased risk of atherosclerosis, and decreasing compliance with the treatment programme [49]. An increasing body of literature demonstrates that individuals suffering from AN could benefit from supervised exercise sessions in combination with nutritional assistance.

Several studies that integrated exercise programmes in the treatment of AN did not interfere with weight gain [50–53] or body fat [49] progression. Different types of exercises have been suggested as beneficial. For example, individualised yoga treatment resulted in reduced food preoccupation after each session [53]. A light resistance exercise programme for a period of 8 weeks showed positive effects on physical strength, body composition, and psychological well-being of hospitalised patients with

AN [54]. Furthermore, a high-intensity resistance exercise training programme effectively and safely improved participants' muscular strength as well as their ability to execute daily tasks [47]. In general, a programme incrementally going from mild to moderate exercise speed should be implemented, followed by the interrogation of emotions and thoughts after exercise [46].

Other benefits included less obligatory attitudes and distorted feelings towards exercise [51], less irregular or disorganised eating patterns [55], less drive for thinness, and reduction of the frequency of dangerous eating behaviours such as laxative abuse [56]. In addition, advantages include increased compliance with treatment [49], improved body satisfaction, positive mood states, and quality of life [52]. Physical strength [54] and cardiovascular fitness [48] also improve.

Notably, patients should only undertake physical training once weight stabilisation and nutritional status have progressed sufficiently in caloric and nutritional consumption in order to be able to support the chosen activities [46,54].

To date, there is no consensus or guideline for use of exercise in the treatment of AN [57]. The majority of studies were of small sample size and suggested training programmes varied, thus restricting generalisability of the findings. Moreover, the interventions are relatively short; there is limited follow-up, and most lack an assessment of the participants' fitness.

Nonetheless, when performed in a therapeutic setting, where training is supervised, exercise is safe and may improve treatment outcomes in some AN patients.

### *3.5. Models of Organisation of the Nutritional Treatment*

There is a need for a multidisciplinary team in the organisation model that may differ between centres. Regardless of this, having a written protocol may help to standardise treatment and improve clinical outcome. The protocol should establish the functions of each member of the team and it will determine the options each step of the way.

Close staff supervision is needed during hospitalisation, especially during mealtimes. Some authors have identified two main types of patterns: Rule adherence and rule bending when describing how staff choose how to intervene in different situations [58].

In the day hospital, the patients receive care without being hospitalised, including medical treatment, nutritional therapy, psychiatric and psychological care in individual and/or group modality, occupational therapy and social support. This resource of treatment may be indicated in some outpatients prior or after hospitalisation [59].

Continuity of care has proven to be useful to improve long term outcomes in these patients [60].

### *3.6. Nutritional Support Related Outcomes*

The main clinical outcomes related to the refeeding process in patients with AN are weight gain, the length of hospitalisation and rehospitalisation rate, RS, and mortality. A summary of the nutritional support related outcomes published in different studies is shown in Table 6.

**Table 6.** Studies in patients with anorexia nervosa reporting clinical outcomes of the nutritional treatment.

| Study | Study Type | N° Patients | Mean Age (years) | Weight (kg) or BMI (kg/m$^2$) at Admission | Weight (kg) or BMI (kg/m$^2$) at Discharge | Length of Stay (days) | Kcal/kg or kcal/day at Admission | Type of Nutritional Treatment | Outcome |
|---|---|---|---|---|---|---|---|---|---|
| Rigaud et al., 2007 [25] | RCT<br>a: TF<br>b: control | a: 41<br>b: 40 | a: 22.5<br>b: 24.2 | a: 12.1<br>b: 12.8 | a: 17.9<br>b: 15.9 | 60 | a: 1000 (D0)–2450 (D14)<br>b: 1000 (D0)–1850 (D14) | a: OD + TF<br>b: OD | No RS<br>1-year relapse:<br>a: 44%<br>b: 52% |
| Diamanti et al., 2008 [44] | Retrospective | a: 104<br>b: 94 | 15 | a: 36.3<br>b: 41 | a: 39.6<br>b: 41.5 | a: 30.7<br>b: 15.6 | 40 kcal/kg | a: OD + PN<br>b: OD | No RS<br>a: Hypophosphataemia (6 cases), Hypopotassaemia (3 cases) |
| Gentile et al., 2010 [26] | Retrospective | 33 | 22.8 | 11.3 | 13.5 | 60 | 1408 | OD + TF + iv. glucose | No RS |
| Vignaud et al., 2010 [33] | Retrospective | 68 | 31 | 12 | - | 7.6 (in ICU) | 22.3 kcal/kg | OD + TF + TPN | RS (10%)<br>Mortality (10%) |
| Whitelaw et al., 2010 [34] | Retrospective | 29 | 15.7 | 72.9% IBW | - | - | 1900–2200 (89% of patients) | OD + ONS + TF (7 patients) | Mild hypophosphataemia (37%) |
| Garber et al., 2012 [35] | Prospective | 35 | 16.2 | 16.3 | - | 17 | 1205 | OD | No RS<br>Hypophosphataemia (20%) |
| Gentile et al., 2012 [36] | Retrospective | 10 | 22 | 11.2 | 17.3 | 90 | 1199 | OD + TF + iv. glucose | No RS |
| Agostino et al., 2013 [37] | Retrospective cohort study:<br>a: Nasogastric cohort<br>b: bolus-fed cohort | 165 | 14.9 | a: 16.6<br>b: 16.7 | - | a: 33.8<br>b: 50.9 | a: 1617<br>b: 1069 | a: 31 patients<br>b: 134 patients | No RS<br>a: Hypopotassaemia (1 case); readmissions at 6 months (12.9%)<br>b: Hypopotassaemia (1 case); mild-moderate hypophosphataemia (8 cases); readmissions at 6 months (23%) |
| Garber et al., 2013 [38] | Prospective cohort:<br>a: high calorie<br>b: low calorie | 56 | 16.2 | a: 16.6<br>b: 15.8 | - | 14.9 | a: 1700<br>b: 1093 | OD + ONS | No RS<br>Hypophosphataemia (45%)<br>Length of stay:<br>a: 11.9 days<br>b: 17.6 days |
| Golden et al., 2013 [39] | Retrospective<br>a: low calorie<br>b: high calorie | a: 88<br>b: 222 | 16.1 | a: 15.9<br>b: 16.1 | a: 17.2<br>b: 17.1 | a: 16.6<br>b: 13 | a: 1163<br>b: 1557 | OD + ONS + TF (occasionally) | No RS<br>Hypophosphataemia (15.8%)<br>Hypomagnesaemia (15.2%)<br>Hypopotassaemia (20%) |
| Leclerc et al., 2013 [40] | Retrospective | 29 | 14.7 | 16.4 | - | 35.8 | 1500 | OD + ONS | Hypophosphataemia (3.5%) |
| Hofer et al., 2014 [27] | Retrospective | 65 | 27.9 | 13.7 | 15 | 49.5 | 10 kcal/kg | OD (mostly)<br>OD + ONS (8.1%)<br>OD + TF (8.1%)<br>TF (5%)<br>OD + TPN (1.2%) | Mild RS (10.5%)<br>Severe hypopotassaemia (4.7%) |

**Table 6.** *Cont.*

| Study | Study Type | N° Patients | Mean Age (years) | Weight (kg) or BMI (kg/m$^2$) at Admission | Weight (kg) or BMI (kg/m$^2$) at Discharge | Length of Stay (days) | Kcal/kg or kcal/day at Admission | Type of Nutritional Treatment | Outcome |
|---|---|---|---|---|---|---|---|---|---|
| Brown et al., 2015 [28] | Retrospective case-control | 123 | 28 | 13 | 13.9 | 13 | 1200 | OD | Hypophosphataemia (33%) |
| O'Connor et al., 2016 [61] | RCT<br>a: intervention<br>b: control | a: 18<br>b: 18 | 13.8 | a: 32.4<br>b: 34.6 | a: 34.1<br>b: 35.6 | 10 | a: 38 kcal/kg/d<br>b: 16 kcal/kg/d | OD + TF | a: Hypophosphataemia (28%)<br>b: Hypophosphataemia (11%) |
| Marugán et al., 2016 [29] | Retrospective | 50 | 14.5 | 15.45 | 17.58 | 44.54 | 1000 | OD<br>ONS (16%)<br>TF (8%) | No symptoms of RS |
| Kameoka et al., 2016 [30] | Retrospective | 99 | 30.9 | <17.5 | - | 82.7 | Low calorie diet | OD | Hypophosphataemia (21.2%) |
| Smith et al., 2016 [62] | Retrospective | 129 | 15.8 | 15.8 | 17.1 | 14.9 | 1585 | OD + ONS | No RS<br>Hypophosphataemia (47.3%)<br>Hypokalaemia (12%) |
| Davies et al., 2017 [31] | Retrospective | 65 | 24 | 12.8 | 14.4 | 60 | 20-30 | OD, ONS (infrequently) | Mild hypophosphataemia (<0.8 mmol/L) (6.5%)<br>Hypokalaemia (1 case).<br>No RS |
| Peebles et al., 2017 [32] | Retrospective | 215 | 15.3 | 17.1 | 18.2 | 11 | 1466 | OD, TF (10%) | No RF.<br>Hypophosphataemia (14%)<br>3.8% and 17.2% rehospitalisations after 30 days and 1 year, respectively |

TF: Tube Feeding, OR: Oral Diet, ONS: Oral Nutritional Supplements, RS: Refeeding Syndrome, PN: Parenteral Nutrition, TPN: Total Parenteral Nutrition, RCT: Randomised Controlled Trial.

### *3.7. Weight Gain*

The weight gain is the main objective in the nutritional rehabilitation of patients with AN. Achieving this is possible with any of the modalities of nutritional treatment. Some studies show that the greater the weight achieved by the patient up to hospital discharge, the lower the likelihood of relapse. This usually translates to a longer hospitalisation stay [6,63].

In a systematic review which included 10 studies with TF in AN patients, this treatment was considered safe and well tolerated, and effectively enhanced caloric intake and rate of weight gain in patients with AN [64].

In another systematic review, which included 7 observational studies with a total of 403 patients (children and adolescents), the prescribed calorie range varied between 1000–1900 kcal/day with progressive increase during hospitalisation. Additional TF increased the maximum energy intake and led to greater interim or discharge weight; however, this was also associated with a higher incidence of adverse effects [65].

Lastly, in the most recent systematic review by Hale et al., 19 out of 22 studies reported that significant short-term weight gain was achieved when TF was used for refeeding malnourished AN patients; however, results varied in the long-term weight gain, maintenance and recovery [66].

### *3.8. Hospital Stay and Rehospitalisation*

Hospital stay as an outcome is closely related to the weight gain. In many cases, the length of hospitalisation is carefully monitored by the hospital management. One of the strategies to shorten the hospitalisation period in patients with AN includes the use of more aggressive refeeding consisting of diets with lower carbohydrate load (<40% total calories), in continuous administration, accompanied by an adequate supplementation of phosphate and potassium [37,67].

In a retrospective study including 2015 children and adolescents with AN, the authors refer a rehospitalisation rate of 3.8% and 17.2% after 30 days and 1 year after discharge, respectively [32].

In an RCT study with TF versus OD in AN, the results in terms of weight gain and rehospitalisation rate were better in patients with enteral nutrition [25].

In another RCT aimed to compare the effectiveness of hospitalisation for weight restoration to medical stabilisation in adolescent AN patients, the number of rehospitalisations and their respective length of stay (after the first hospital admission), within 12 months, were similar in the two groups when the treatment included family-based therapy [68].

### *3.9. Refeeding Syndrome*

RS has been described in malnourished patients with AN and mainly involves mineral deficiencies (hypophosphataemia, hypokalaemia and hypomagnesaemia), as well as vitamin (thiamine) deficiencies, and volume overload. It can be presented as a symptomatic or asymptomatic clinical case, which implies that a close monitoring of laboratory parameters is necessary, especially during the first week of refeeding. The RS has been described with all feeding modalities (OD, TF, and PN) [66].

Table 7 summarises the main risk factors for developing a RS. There is no clear consensus on supplementing phosphorus in all patients starting refeeding, just in those who develop hypophosphataemia or in those severely malnourished [67].

Hypophosphataemia has been described as a hallmark in studies on RS. In a systematic review of 17 publications, an incidence of hypophosphataemia of 14% (0–38%) was reported, with the degree of malnutrition at admission being the main risk factor, without finding correlation with the refeeding rate (kcal/day) [34,69].

**Table 7.** Identification of patients with high risk of refeeding syndrome.

| | |
|---|---|
| Patients with 1 or more of the following: | • BMI < 16 kg/m$^2$<br>• Unintentional weight loss of >15% in the previous 3–6 months.<br>• Minimum or no intake for >10 days.<br>• Low levels of K, P, or Mg before refeeding. |
| Or, patients with 2 or more of the following: | • BMI < 18.5 kg/m$^2$<br>• Unintentional weight loss of >10% in the previous 3–6 months<br>• Minimum or no intake for >5 days.<br>• History of alcohol abuse, drugs, insulin treatment, chemotherapy, antacids, or diuretics. |

In a case-control study with 123 AN patients, the prevalence of hypophosphataemia was 33%, with the nadir occurring at the second day of admission. In this study, higher haemoglobin was the only risk factor associated with higher odds of developing hypophosphataemia; meanwhile a higher BMI, a higher serum potassium, and a higher serum prealbumin were protective factors against the development of hypophosphatemia [28].

### 3.10. Mortality

Classically, AN has been associated with a high mortality within the psychiatric disorders. In a series of 484 patients followed for 13 years, the authors refer a mortality rate of 1.2% [63].

In most of the revised articles in inpatients, the authors do not refer mortality rates during the refeeding process, even though the patients were severely malnourished [25–28,31,34,36,44].

On the other hand, in a retrospective study performed in France in 30 randomly selected ICUs including 68 patients with AN (average BMI at admission of 12 ± 3 kg/m$^2$), the authors mention a RS rate of 10% and a mortality rate of 10%. The causes included acute respiratory distress syndrome and multiorgan-failure associated with major hydro-electrolytic problems [33].

As exemplified in the refeeding of other malnourished patients, a higher awareness of the risk associated with refeeding may decrease the risk of mortality [70,71].

## 4. Discussion

The treatment of AN patients is challenging, especially regarding weight gain recovery, which is the most important part of it. In severely malnourished patients, closely related to the weight gain is the risk of RS, which must be accordingly monitored. Moreover, there are factors that interfere with the recovery process, which are mainly related to the patient´s attitudes and fears.

There is a high variability in the treatment between centres, both in the feeding rate and type of nutritional treatment. One of the reasons is the lack of good scientific evidence in this topic.

There are two established pathways when feeding the patients: "start low, advance slow" versus "start higher, advance faster". Both ways have proven to be safe and effective in terms of the in appearance of RS and weight recovery, respectively [25,27,29,40,44]. However, the main difference between them is the length of hospital stay and costs. On this basis, some centres prefer the "start higher, advance faster" method in patients without severe malnutrition.

Regarding the refeeding process, all modalities of feeding (mainly OD, ONS, and TF) can be used in a safe and effective way. In a recent systematic review, no significant differences were found between TF and oral refeeding cohorts regarding gastrointestinal disturbance, RS, or electrolyte abnormalities. However, TF has proved a slight superiority achieving a higher weight at discharge and in the short term [66].

The reviewed literature does not show a high rate of RS during the treatment of these patients, probably due to a close supervision of the feeding process. However, hydro-electrolytic alterations especially hypophosphataemia is frequently reported and up to 40%. Moreover, these studies show that the degree of malnutrition at hospitalisation is the main risk factor for developing hypophosphatemia and it is not related to the refeeding rate [34,69]. Hypophosphatemia is mainly reported in the first days of refeeding. There is no agreement on the use of phosphate supplement as a prophylactic option or after an already established hypophosphatemia.

Patients with less than 70% of IBW, may benefit out of a slow refeeding process with additional mineral supplements because of their potential high risk of RS. However, in patients with higher body weight a faster refeeding rate could be an option in order to rapidly improve weight gain and shorten the hospital stay.

Even though mortality during hospitalisation is rarely reported, this fatal outcome cannot be neglected in the short term nor in the long-term [33].

As a novelty in the management of these patients, physical activity may play an important role. Supervised exercise seems to be safe and may improve treatment outcomes in some patients.

This article contains a large number of studies and systematic reviews focused on the refeeding process of AN patients; however, the main limitation of the review is the quality of the studies. Most of them were observational, case-control, and only two were RCTs. This lowers the strength of recommendation of the results.

Evidence-based standards for clinical practice with clear outcomes (weight gain rate, hospital stay and rehospitalisation, RS, mortality) are needed to improve the management of these patients and standardise the healthcare process.

## 5. Conclusions

This review focuses on evidence of the refeeding process of malnourished inpatients with AN with emphasis on the clinical outcome (weight gain, hospital stay and rehospitalisation, RS and mortality). Firstly, patients with AN frequently present malnutrition and usually are at high risk of RS. Secondly, literature shows that RS risk mostly depends on the baseline nutritional status and is not associated with the refeeding rate and the type of nutritional treatment. Thirdly, TF seems to have better outcomes, especially in the short-term, though more studies are needed. Lastly, evidence-based standards for clinical practice with coherent outcomes are required to improve the management of these patients and standardise the healthcare process.

**Author Contributions:** Conceptualization, C.C., M.F.V., and L.A.; Writing—original draft Preparation, C.C., M.F.V., and L.A.; Writing—review and editing, C.C., M.F.V., and L.A.

## References

1. American Psychiatric Association. *Diagnostic and Statistical Manual of Mental Disorders*; American Psychiatric Association: Washington, DC, USA, 2013; ISBN 9780890425572.
2. Ozier, A.D.; Henry, B.W. Position of the American dietetic association: Nutrition intervention in the treatment of eating disorders. *J. Am. Diet. Assoc.* **2011**, *111*, 1236–1241. [CrossRef] [PubMed]
3. Baker, J.H.; Schaumberg, K.; Munn-Chernoff, M.A. Genetics of anorexia nervosa. *Curr. Psychiatry Rep.* **2017**, *19*, 84. [CrossRef] [PubMed]
4. Urwin, R.E.; Nunn, K.P. Epistatic interaction between the monoamine oxidase A and serotonin transporter genes in anorexia nervosa. *Eur. J. Hum. Genet.* **2005**, *13*, 370–375. [CrossRef]
5. Kaye, W.H.; Wierenga, C.E.; Bailer, U.F.; Simmons, A.N.; Bischoff-Grethe, A. Nothing tastes as good as skinny feels: The neurobiology of anorexia nervosa. *Trends Neurosci.* **2013**, *36*, 110–120. [CrossRef] [PubMed]

6. Yager, J.; Michael Devlin, C.J.; Halmi, K.A.; Herzog, D.B.; Mitchell, J.E., III; Powers, P.; Zerbe, K.J.; McIntyre, J.S.; Anzia, D.J.; Cook, I.A.; et al. *Practice Guideline for the Treatment of Patients with Eating Disorders*, 3rd ed.; Work Group on Eating Disorders, American Psychiatric Association Steering Committee on Practice Guidelines Area and Component Liaisons Staff: Washington, DC, USA, 2006.
7. Mehler, P.S.; Krantz, M.J.; Sachs, K.V. Treatments of medical complications of anorexia nervosa and bulimia nervosa. *J. Eat. Disord.* **2015**, *3*, 15. [CrossRef] [PubMed]
8. Støving, R.K. Anorexia nervosa and endocrinology: A clinical update. *Eur. J. Endocrinol.* **2019**, *180*, R9–R27. [CrossRef] [PubMed]
9. Cederholm, T.; Jensen, G.L.; Correia, M.I.T.D.; Gonzalez, M.C.; Fukushima, R.; Higashiguchi, T.; Baptista, G.; Barazzoni, R.; Blaauw, R.; Coats, A.; et al. GLIM criteria for the diagnosis of malnutrition—A consensus report from the global clinical nutrition community. *Clin. Nutr.* **2019**, *38*, 1–9. [CrossRef]
10. Gaudiani, J.L.; Sabel, A.L.; Mehler, P.S. Low prealbumin is a significant predictor of medical complications in severe anorexia nervosa. *Int. J. Eat. Disord.* **2014**, *47*, 148–156. [CrossRef]
11. Piccoli, A.; Codognotto, M.; di Pascoli, L.; Boffo, G.; Caregaro, L. Body mass index and agreement between bioimpedance and anthropometry estimates of body compartments in anorexia nervosa. *JPEN J. Parenter. Enteral Nutr.* **2005**, *29*, 148–156. [CrossRef]
12. Marra, M.; Sammarco, R.; de Filippo, E.; de Caprio, C.; Speranza, E.; Contaldo, F.; Pasanisi, F. Resting energy expenditure, body composition and phase angle in anorectic, ballet dancers and constitutionally lean males. *Nutrients* **2019**, *11*, 502. [CrossRef]
13. Saladino, C.F. The efficacy of bioelectrical impedance analysis (BIA) in monitoring body composition changes during treatment of restrictive eating disorder patients. *J. Eat. Disord.* **2014**, *2*, 34. [CrossRef] [PubMed]
14. Hanachi, M.; Dicembre, M.; Rives-Lange, C.; Ropers, J.; Bemer, P.; Zazzo, J.-F.; Poupon, J.; Dauvergne, A.; Melchior, J.-C. Micronutrients deficiencies in 374 severely malnourished anorexia nervosa inpatients. *Nutrients* **2019**, *11*, 792. [CrossRef] [PubMed]
15. Cuerda, C.; Ruiz, A.; Velasco, C.; Bretón, I.; Camblor, M.; García-Peris, P. How accurate are predictive formulas calculating energy expenditure in adolescent patients with anorexia nervosa? *Clin. Nutr.* **2007**, *26*, 100–106. [CrossRef] [PubMed]
16. El Ghoch, M.; Alberti, M.; Capelli, C.; Calugi, S.; Dalle Grave, R. Resting energy expenditure in anorexia nervosa: Measured versus estimated. *J. Nutr. Metab.* **2012**, *2012*, 1–6. [CrossRef] [PubMed]
17. Mehler, P.S.; Winkelman, A.B.; Andersen, D.M.; Gaudiani, J.L. Nutritional rehabilitation: Practical guidelines for refeeding the anorectic patient. *J. Nutr. Metab.* **2010**, *2010*, 1–7. [CrossRef] [PubMed]
18. Bargiacchi, A.; Clarke, J.; Paulsen, A.; Leger, J. Refeeding in anorexia nervosa. *Eur. J. Pediatr.* **2019**, *178*, 413–422. [CrossRef] [PubMed]
19. Stanga, Z.; Brunner, A.; Leuenberger, M.; Grimble, R.F.; Shenkin, A.; Allison, S.P.; Lobo, D.N. Nutrition in clinical practice—The refeeding syndrome: Illustrative cases and guidelines for prevention and treatment. *Eur. J. Clin. Nutr.* **2008**, *62*, 687–694. [CrossRef]
20. MARSIPAN. *Management of Really Sick Patients with Anorexia Nervosa*, 2nd ed.; Royal College Psychiatrists and Royal College of Physicians London: London, UK, 2014.
21. Marsipan, J. *Management of Really Sick Patients under 18 with Anorexia Nervosa*; Royal College Psychiatrists and Royal College of Physicians London: London, UK, 2012.
22. American Dietetic Association Position of the American Dietetic Association. Nutrition intervention in the treatment of anorexia nervosa, bulimia nervosa, and other eating disorders. *J. Am. Diet. Assoc.* **2006**, *106*, 2073–2082. [CrossRef]
23. Beumont, P.; Hay, P.; Beumont, D.; Birmingham, L.; Derham, H.; Jordan, A.; Kohn, M.; McDermott, B.; Marks, P.; Mitchell, J.; et al. Australian and New Zealand clinical practice guidelines for the treatment of anorexia nervosa. *Aust. N. Z. J. Psychiatry* **2004**, *38*, 659–670.
24. National Institute for Health and Care Excellence (NICE). *Eating Disorders: Recognition and Treatment*; National Institute for Health and Care Excellence (NICE): London, UK, 2017.
25. Rigaud, D.; Brondel, L.; Poupard, A.T.; Talonneau, I.; Brun, J.M. A randomized trial on the efficacy of a 2-month tube feeding regimen in anorexia nervosa: A 1-year follow-up study. *Clin. Nutr.* **2007**, *26*, 421–429. [CrossRef]

26. Gentile, M.G.; Pastorelli, P.; Ciceri, R.; Manna, G.M.; Collimedaglia, S. Specialized refeeding treatment for anorexia nervosa patients suffering from extreme undernutrition. *Clin. Nutr.* **2010**, *29*, 627–632. [CrossRef] [PubMed]
27. Hofer, M.; Pozzi, A.; Joray, M.; Ott, R.; Hähni, F.; Leuenberger, M.; von Känel, R.; Stanga, Z. Safe refeeding management of anorexia nervosa inpatients: An evidence-based protocol. *Nutrition* **2014**, *30*, 524–530. [CrossRef] [PubMed]
28. Brown, C.A.; Sabel, A.L.; Gaudiani, J.L.; Mehler, P.S. Predictors of hypophosphatemia during refeeding of patients with severe anorexia nervosa. *Int. J. Eat. Disord.* **2015**, *48*, 898–904. [CrossRef] [PubMed]
29. De Marugán Miguelsanz, J.M.; Torres Hinojal, M.D.C.; Geijo Uribe, M.S.; Redondo Del Río, M.P.; Mongil López, B.; de Brito García-Sousa, I.; Caballero Sanz, I.; Eiros Bouza, J.M. Abordaje nutricional de pacientes ingresados con anorexia nerviosa. *Nutr. Hosp.* **2016**, *33*, 258. [CrossRef]
30. Kameoka, N.; Iga, J.; Tamaru, M.; Tominaga, T.; Kubo, H.; Watanabe, S.-Y.; Sumitani, S.; Tomotake, M.; Ohmori, T. Risk factors for refeeding hypophosphatemia in Japanese inpatients with anorexia nervosa. *Int. J. Eat. Disord.* **2016**, *49*, 402–406. [CrossRef]
31. Davies, J.E.; Cockfield, A.; Brown, A.; Corr, J.; Smith, D.; Munro, C. The medical risks of severe anorexia nervosa during initial re-feeding and medical stabilisation. *Clin. Nutr. ESPEN* **2017**, *17*, 92–99. [CrossRef]
32. Peebles, R.; Lesser, A.; Park, C.C.; Heckert, K.; Timko, C.A.; Lantzouni, E.; Liebman, R.; Weaver, L. Outcomes of an inpatient medical nutritional rehabilitation protocol in children and adolescents with eating disorders. *J. Eat. Disord.* **2017**, *5*, 7. [CrossRef]
33. Vignaud, M.; Constantin, J.-M.; Ruivard, M.; Villemeyre-Plane, M.; Futier, E.; Bazin, J.-E.; Annane, D.; AZUREA group (AnorexieRea Study Group). Refeeding syndrome influences outcome of anorexia nervosa patients in intensive care unit: An observational study. *Crit. Care* **2010**, *14*, R172. [CrossRef]
34. Whitelaw, M.; Gilbertson, H.; Lam, P.-Y.; Sawyer, S.M. Does aggressive refeeding in hospitalized adolescents with anorexia nervosa result in increased hypophosphatemia? *J. Adolesc. Health* **2010**, *46*, 577–582. [CrossRef]
35. Garber, A.K.; Michihata, N.; Hetnal, K.; Shafer, M.-A.; Moscicki, A.-B. A prospective examination of weight gain in hospitalized adolescents with anorexia nervosa on a recommended refeeding protocol. *J. Adolesc. Health* **2012**, *50*, 24–29. [CrossRef]
36. Gentile, M.G. Enteral Nutrition for feeding severely underfed patients with anorexia nervosa. *Nutrients* **2012**, *4*, 1293–1303. [CrossRef] [PubMed]
37. Agostino, H.; Erdstein, J.; di Meglio, G. Shifting paradigms: Continuous nasogastric feeding with high caloric intakes in anorexia nervosa. *J. Adolesc. Health* **2013**, *53*, 590–594. [CrossRef] [PubMed]
38. Garber, A.K.; Mauldin, K.; Michihata, N.; Buckelew, S.M.; Shafer, M.-A.; Moscicki, A.-B. Higher calorie diets increase rate of weight gain and shorten hospital stay in hospitalized adolescents with anorexia nervosa. *J. Adolesc. Health* **2013**, *53*, 579–584. [CrossRef] [PubMed]
39. Golden, N.H.; Keane-Miller, C.; Sainani, K.L.; Kapphahn, C.J. Higher caloric intake in hospitalized adolescents with anorexia nervosa is associated with reduced length of stay and no increased rate of refeeding syndrome. *J. Adolesc. Health* **2013**, *53*, 573–578. [CrossRef] [PubMed]
40. Leclerc, A.; Turrini, T.; Sherwood, K.; Katzman, D.K. Evaluation of a nutrition rehabilitation protocol in hospitalized adolescents with restrictive eating disorders. *J. Adolesc. Health* **2013**, *53*, 585–589. [CrossRef] [PubMed]
41. Haynos, A.F.; Snipes, C.; Guarda, A.; Mayer, L.E.; Attia, E. Comparison of standardized versus individualized caloric prescriptions in the nutritional rehabilitation of inpatients with anorexia nervosa. *Int. J. Eat. Disord.* **2016**, *49*, 50–58. [CrossRef]
42. Garber, A.K.; Sawyer, S.M.; Golden, N.H.; Guarda, A.S.; Katzman, D.K.; Kohn, M.R.; le Grange, D.; Madden, S.; Whitelaw, M.; Redgrave, G.W. A systematic review of approaches to refeeding in patients with anorexia nervosa. *Int. J. Eat. Disord.* **2016**, *49*, 293–310. [CrossRef]
43. Born, C.; de la Fontaine, L.; Winter, B.; Müller, N.; Schaub, A.; Früstück, C.; Schüle, C.; Voderholzer, U.; Cuntz, U.; Falkai, P.; et al. First results of a refeeding program in a psychiatric intensive care unit for patients with extreme anorexia nervosa. *BMC Psychiatry* **2015**, *15*, 57. [CrossRef]
44. Diamanti, A.; Basso, M.S.; Castro, M.; Bianco, G.; Ciacco, E.; Calce, A.; Caramadre, A.M.; Noto, C.; Gambarara, M. Clinical efficacy and safety of parenteral nutrition in adolescent girls with anorexia nervosa. *J. Adolesc. Health* **2008**, *42*, 111–118. [CrossRef]

45. Hotta, M.; Araki, M.; Urano, A.; Ohwada, R. Home parenteral nutrition therapy in seven patients with anorexia nervosa: The role and indications. *Intern. Med.* **2014**, *53*, 2695–2699. [CrossRef]
46. Cook, B.J.; Wonderlich, S.A.; Mitchell, J.E.; Thompson, R.; Sherman, R.; McCallum, K. Exercise in eating disorders treatment: Systematic review and proposal of guidelines. *Med. Sci. Sports Exerc.* **2016**, *48*, 1408–1414. [CrossRef] [PubMed]
47. Fernandez-del-Valle, M.; Larumbe-Zabala, E.; Villaseñor-Montarroso, A.; Cardona Gonzalez, C.; Diez-Vega, I.; Lopez Mojares, L.M.; Perez Ruiz, M. Resistance training enhances muscular performance in patients with anorexia nervosa: A randomized controlled trial. *Int. J. Eat. Disord.* **2014**, *47*, 601–609. [CrossRef] [PubMed]
48. Ng, L.W.C.; Ng, D.P.; Wong, W.P. Is supervised exercise training safe in patients with anorexia nervosa? A meta-analysis. *Physiotherapy* **2013**, *99*, 1–11. [CrossRef] [PubMed]
49. Thien, V.; Thomas, A.; Markin, D.; Birmingham, C.L. Pilot study of a graded exercise program for the treatment of anorexia nervosa. *Int. J. Eat. Disord.* **2000**, *28*, 101–106. [CrossRef]
50. Danielsen, M.; Rø, Ø.; Bjørnelv, S. How to integrate physical activity and exercise approaches into inpatient treatment for eating disorders: Fifteen years of clinical experience and research. *J. Eat. Disord.* **2018**, *6*, 34. [CrossRef]
51. Calogero, R.M.; Pedrotty, K.N. The practice and process of healthy exercise: An investigation of the treatment of exercise abuse in women with eating disorders. *Eat. Disord.* **2004**, *12*, 273–291. [CrossRef] [PubMed]
52. Hausenblas, H.A.; Cook, B.J.; Chittester, N.I. Can exercise treat eating disorders? *Exerc. Sport Sci. Rev.* **2008**, *36*, 43–47. [CrossRef]
53. Carei, T.R.; Fyfe-Johnson, A.L.; Breuner, C.C.; Brown, M.A. Randomized controlled clinical trial of yoga in the treatment of eating disorders. *J. Adolesc. Health* **2010**, *46*, 346–351. [CrossRef]
54. Chantler, I.; Szabo, C.P.; Green, K. Muscular strength changes in hospitalized anorexic patients after an eight week resistance training program. *Int. J. Sports Med.* **2006**, *27*, 660–665. [CrossRef]
55. Bakland, M.; Rosenvinge, J.H.; Wynn, R.; Sundgot-Borgen, J.; Fostervold Mathisen, T.; Liabo, K.; Hanssen, T.A.; Pettersen, G. Patients' views on a new treatment for Bulimia nervosa and binge eating disorder combining physical exercise and dietary therapy (the PED-t). A qualitative study. *Eat. Disord.* **2019**, 1–18. [CrossRef]
56. Sundgot-Borgen, J.; Rosenvinge, J.H.; Bahr, R.; Schneider, L.S. The effect of exercise, cognitive therapy, and nutritional counseling in treating bulimia nervosa. *Med. Sci. Sports Exerc.* **2002**, *34*, 190–195. [CrossRef] [PubMed]
57. Bratland-Sanda, S.; Andersson, E.; Best, J.; Høegmark, S.; Roessler, K.K. The use of physical activity, sport and outdoor life as tools of psychosocial intervention: The Nordic perspective. *Sport Soc.* **2019**, *22*, 654–670. [CrossRef]
58. Hage, T.W.; Rø, Ø.; Moen, A. To bend or not to bend? Rule adherence among staff at an eating disorder unit. *Eat. Disord.* **2017**, *25*, 134–150. [CrossRef]
59. Gómez-Candela, C.; Palma Milla, S.; Miján-de-la-Torre, A.; Rodríguez Ortega, P.; Matía Martín, P.; Loria Kohen, V.; Campos Del Portillo, R.; Martín-Palmero, Á.; Virgili Casas, M.A.N.; Martínez Olmos, M.; et al. Consenso sobre la evaluación y el tratamiento nutricional de los trastornos de la conducta alimentaria: Anorexia nerviosa. *Nutr. Hosp.* **2018**, *35*, 11–48. [CrossRef] [PubMed]
60. Long, C.G.; Fitzgerald, K.-A.; Hollin, C.R. Treatment of chronic anorexia nervosa: A 4-year follow-up of adult patients treated in an acute inpatient setting. *Clin. Psychol. Psychother.* **2012**, *19*, 1–13. [CrossRef] [PubMed]
61. O'Connor, G.; Nicholls, D.; Hudson, L.; Singhal, A. Refeeding low weight hospitalized adolescents with anorexia nervosa: A multicenter randomized controlled trial. *Nutr. Clin. Pract.* **2016**, *31*, 681–689. [CrossRef] [PubMed]
62. Smith, K.; Lesser, J.; Brandenburg, B.; Lesser, A.; Cici, J.; Juenneman, R.; Beadle, A.; Eckhardt, S.; Lantz, E.; Lock, J.; et al. Outcomes of an inpatient refeeding protocol in youth with anorexia nervosa and atypical anorexia nervosa at children's hospitals and clinics of minnesota. *J. Eat. Disord.* **2016**, *4*, 35. [CrossRef]
63. Rigaud, D.; Pennacchio, H.; Bizeul, C.; Reveillard, V.; Vergès, B. Outcome in an adult patients: A 13 year follow-up in 484 patients. *Diabetes Metab.* **2011**, *37*, 305–311. [CrossRef]
64. Rizzo, S.M.; Douglas, J.W.; Lawrence, J.C. enteral nutrition via nasogastric tube for refeeding patients with anorexia nervosa: A systematic review. *Nutr. Clin. Pract.* **2019**, *34*, 359–370. [CrossRef]
65. Rocks, T.; Pelly, F.; Wilkinson, P. Nutrition therapy during initiation of refeeding in underweight children and adolescent inpatients with anorexia nervosa: A systematic review of the evidence. *J. Acad. Nutr. Diet.* **2014**, *114*, 897–907. [CrossRef]

66. Hale, M.D.; Logomarsino, J.V. The use of enteral nutrition in the treatment of eating disorders: A systematic review. *Eat. Weight Disord. Stud. Anorex. Bulim. Obes.* **2019**, *24*, 179–198. [CrossRef] [PubMed]
67. Leitner, M.; Burstein, B.; Agostino, H. Prophylactic phosphate supplementation for the inpatient treatment of restrictive eating disorders. *J. Adolesc. Health* **2016**, *58*, 616–620. [CrossRef] [PubMed]
68. Madden, S.; Miskovic-Wheatley, J.; Wallis, A.; Kohn, M.; Lock, J.; Le Grange, D.; Jo, B.; Clarke, S.; Rhodes, P.; Hay, P.; et al. A randomized controlled trial of in-patient treatment for anorexia nervosa in medically unstable adolescents. *Psychol. Med.* **2015**, *45*, 415–427. [CrossRef] [PubMed]
69. O'Connor, G.; Nicholls, D. Refeeding hypophosphatemia in adolescents with anorexia nervosa: A systematic review. *Nutr. Clin. Pract.* **2013**, *28*, 358–364. [CrossRef] [PubMed]
70. Schuetz, P.; Zurfluh, S.; Stanga, Z. Mortality due to refeeding syndrome? You only find what you look for, and you only look for what you know. *Eur. J. Clin. Nutr.* **2018**, *72*, 307–308. [CrossRef] [PubMed]
71. Matthews, K.L.; Capra, S.M.; Palmer, M.A. Throw caution to the wind: Is refeeding syndrome really a cause of death in acute care? *Eur. J. Clin. Nutr.* **2018**, *72*, 93–98. [CrossRef] [PubMed]

# 12

# Gastroparesis and Dumping Syndrome: Current Concepts and Management

**Stephan R. Vavricka [1,2,*] and Thomas Greuter [2]**

1 Center of Gastroenterology and Hepatology, CH-8048 Zurich, Switzerland
2 Department of Gastroenterology and Hepatology, University Hospital Zurich, CH-8091 Zurich, Switzerland
* Correspondence: stephan.vavricka@hin.ch

**Abstract:** Gastroparesis and dumping syndrome both evolve from a disturbed gastric emptying mechanism. Although gastroparesis results from delayed gastric emptying and dumping syndrome from accelerated emptying of the stomach, the two entities share several similarities among which are an underestimated prevalence, considerable impairment of quality of life, the need for a multidisciplinary team setting, and a step-up treatment approach. In the following review, we will present an overview of the most important clinical aspects of gastroparesis and dumping syndrome including epidemiology, pathophysiology, presentation, and diagnostics. Finally, we highlight promising therapeutic options that might be available in the future.

**Keywords:** gastroparesis; dumping syndrome; pathophysiology; clinical presentation; treatment

---

## 1. Introduction

Gastroparesis and dumping syndrome both evolve from a disturbed gastric emptying mechanism. While gastroparesis results from significantly delayed gastric emptying, dumping syndrome is a consequence of increased flux of food into the small bowel [1,2]. The two entities share several important similarities: (i) gastroparesis and dumping syndrome are frequent, but also frequently overlooked; (ii) they affect patient's quality of life considerably due to possibly debilitating symptoms; (iii) patients should be taken care of within a multidisciplinary team setting; and (iv) treatment should follow a step-up approach from dietary modifications and patient education to pharmacological interventions and, finally, surgical procedures and/or enteral feeding. Most importantly, the two diagnoses have to be considered by one of the treating specialists, regardless of whether this is the endocrinologist, nutritional specialist or gastroenterologist, when symptoms are present. Pre-test probability based on comorbidities (such as diabetes in case of gastroparesis or surgical history for dumping syndrome) together with the presence of typical symptoms should lead to a high degree of clinical suspicion. However, for both disorders, diagnostic evaluations should follow in order to confirm the diagnosis before initiation of treatment. Firstly, because treatment options might be invasive and require proper diagnostic evaluations beforehand. Secondly, several differential diagnoses might show a similar presentation. Such diagnoses are peptic ulcer disease, gastric cancer, celiac disease, abdominal angina for gastroparesis, anastomotic ulcers, internal herniation and gallbladder disease for early dumping syndrome and insulinoma, surreptitious use of glucose-lowering medication for late dumping [2–5]. In the following review, we will present an overview of the most important clinical aspects of gastroparesis and dumping syndrome including epidemiology, pathophysiology, presentation, diagnostics and treatment. Finally, we highlight promising therapeutic options that might be available in the future.

## 2. Definitions and Epidemiology

Gastroparesis and dumping syndrome are frequent, but their prevalence and incidence vary depending on definitions and studied populations. Therefore, heterogenous results have been reported in the literature.

### 2.1. Gastroparesis

Gastroparesis is a syndrome characterized by an objectively delayed gastric emptying in the absence of a mechanical gastric outlet obstruction and the presence of cardinal symptoms such as early satiety, postprandial fullness and nausea-vomiting [6]. The prevalence of gastroparesis in the general population is uncertain. A wide range in different at-risk populations has been reported. In addition, gastroparesis is likely significantly under diagnosed. While an epidemiological study from Olmsted county revealed a prevalence of 24.2/100,000 for definite gastroparesis and 50.5/100,000 for definite, probable or possible gastroparesis [7], prevalence might be as high as 1.8% [8]. Patients with type 1 diabetes are at particular risk. Here, 10-year incidence rates of 5.2% have been reported (in contrast to a rate of 1% for type 2 diabetes and 0.2% for non-diabetic patients [9]. Other studies demonstrate even higher rates for diabetics with 58% for type 1 and 30% for type 2 [10,11]. However, most of the performed studies have a considerable selection bias with inclusion of patients from tertiary referral centers only. Still, there might be a large proportion of undetected gastroparesis patients, because either the patient does not seek medical attention or the treating doctors are reluctant to evaluate symptoms and/or further diagnostics. The incidence of postsurgical gastroparesis after gastrectomy is approximately 0.4% to 5.0% [12]. Overall, the incidence of gastroparesis after surgery depends on the surgical procedure and the surgical site. In the early postoperative period after pylorus-preserving pancreatoduodenectomy, postsurgical gastroparesis occurs in up to 20% to 50% of patients [12]. In one study, 67% of patients who underwent pancreatic cancer cryoablation were found to suffer from gastroparesis [13]. There seems to be a gender-specific differences with women accounting for up to 70% of the affected population. Interestingly, elderly patients (>65 years old) are at particular risk [14].

### 2.2. Dumping Syndrome

Dumping syndrome is a frequently encountered postsurgical complication that can be divided into an early and late subtype [2]. Alterations in gastric anatomy after esophageal, gastric and bariatric surgery result in rapid passage of food into the small intestine, which leads to early gastrointestinal and vasomotor symptoms (within 1 h) and late hypoglycemia (1 to 3 h after meal ingestion) [15,16]. Reliable population-based prevalence data for dumping syndrome are still lacking. As of yet, the frequency of postsurgical dumping syndrome is estimated at 25%–50% with 5 to 10% of patients experiencing a severe disabling form [17]. These rates vary depending on type of surgery prodecure [2]. While 20% of patients suffer from symptoms of dumping syndrome after vagotomy and pyloroplasty, these rates rise to 40% after Roux-en-Y bypass and sleeve gastrectomy, and peak at 50% after esophagectomy [18–22]. The incidence and prevalence of dumping syndrome has been increasing due to the current obesity epidemics and the consecutive climb in gastric bypass surgeries [23]. Early dumping represents the most common type, while isolated late dumping is observed in only 25% [2,22]. Due to considerable overlap in clinical presentation it is, however, sometimes difficult to differentiate between the two and co-occurrence is frequently encountered.

## 3. Pathophysiology and Clinical Presentation

The occurrence of cardinal symptoms after ingestion of a meal in a patient with high pre-test probability should rise suspicion for the presence of gastroparesis or dumping syndrome. The symptoms per se are rather non-specific and might occur with many other diseases. However, the existence of risk factors such as diabetes for gastroparesis or bariatric surgery for dumping makes the diagnoses more likely (Tables 1 and 2).

### 3.1. Gastroparesis

Several aspects contribute to a delayed gastric emptying in gastroparesis patients. Among these are extrinsic denervation of the stomach, impaired inhibitory input to smooth muscles due to loss of nitric oxide in enteric nerves, loss of interstitial cells of Cajal (ICC, "pacemaker cells), smooth muscle atrophy and altered function of immune cells [1]. ICC generate electrical slow waves in the stomach, and disrupted ICC networks and gastric dysrhythmias have been associated with gastroparesis [24]. For details see Figure 1. The most frequent etiologies are diabetes and surgery [25]. In a high proportion of patients, the underlying cause remains unknown (so called idiopathic gastroparesis) [25]. This form is found in particular in younger women and appears to be associated with viral infection (in up to 20%) [26–28]. Less frequent etiologic factors are Parkinson's disease, amyloid, tumors (paraneoplastic gastroparesis), scleroderma, or mesenteric ischemia [29]. Importantly, medication-induced gastroparesis has to be considered in all patients. Typically here are opioids, ciclosporine, anticholinergics and glucagon-like peptide 1 (GLP1)-agonists [30–32]. The latter should be particularly suspected in diabetic patients before considering the gastroparesis to be caused by diabetes and poor control of blood glucose. From a clinical perspective, the simplest classification of gastroparesis is into the two categories diabetic vs. non-diabetic. Delayed gastric emptying can be observed in 28% to 65% of unselected patients with diabetes [33,34]. Patients with type 1 diabetes have a higher incidence of gastroparesis as compared with type 2 (5.25 vs. 1%) and an earlier age at onset [7,9,29]. Type 2 diabetics, however, have more serious symptoms. Gastroparesis in diabetic patients usually occurs 10 years after the onset of diabetes and it parallels other forms of diabetic microvascular disease, including neuropathy and retinopathy. Severe symptoms of diabetic gastroparesis cause poor glycemic control and poor nutritional status, and increase the risk of hypoglycaemia [35].

Gastroparesis is often a debilitating disease associated with significant morbidity and mortality [36,37]. The most frequently reported symptoms are: early satiety, postprandial fullness, nausea-vomiting, bloating and upper abdominal pain [38]. The latter is somewhat neglected by physicians, but appear to occur in up to 72%–90% of patients. Pain is often experienced after meals (72%), but can also occur during night time (74%) [29,39]. The presence of non-prandial abdominal pain can, therefore, not be used to rule out the diagnosis. It rather appears to be another piece in the wide presentation of the disease. Weight loss is not a typical feature of gastroparesis patients. Symptoms can vary depending on the specific etiology. Nausea, at least, is similar in all patients with gastroparesis, irrespectively of the underlying cause. Both nausea and vomiting significantly correlate with a reduced quality of life [40]. It should be kept in mind that the presence of symptoms is a sine qua non for the diagnosis of gastroparesis.

### 3.2. Dumping Syndrome

In early dumping syndrome, rapid transition of food into the small intestine results in a fluid shift (due to hyperosmolarity) and release of gastrointestinal hormones such as vasoactive substances (neurostatin, vasoactive intestinal peptide (VIP), incretins (gastric inhibitory polypeptide (GIP), GLP1) and glucose-modulators (insulin, glucagon) [2,15,41–43]. This results in gastrointestinal and vasomotor symptoms; the latter is characterized by hypotension (due to the above mentioned fluid shift) and a consecutive sympathetic nerve system response [15,16]. In late dumping, rapid absorption of glucose (due to the presence of undigested carbohydrates in the small intestine) increases incretin release (GLP1), which exaggerates insulin response [2,44–46]. This ultimately leads to hypoglycaemia within 1 to 3 h after meal intake (so called incretin-driven hyperinsulinemic response) [15,16]. Although these mechanisms are typically and frequently seen as a postsurgical complication, dumping can also occur in the absence of previous surgery [47]. While in these cases, there is no alteration in gastric anatomy, gastric emptying is accelerated due to a disturbed intrinsic gastric innervation [2]. Diabetes is the main contributor [47,48]. Thus, diabetes can be associated with both delayed (see gastroparesis) and increased gastric emptying. The latter is particularly seen in early diabetes and more so in type 2 than 1. Due to overlapping symptoms, it might be difficult to distinguish gastroparesis from dumping syndrome in diabetic patients. Vomiting makes gastroparesis more probable, while dumping should be considered in particular in the presence of diarrhea [49]. Idiopathic forms of dumping have been described also. Similarly to gastroparesis, viral infections are a possible cause [50]. About 50% of patients with idiopathic dumping syndrome report a history of gastroenteritis symptoms [50].

Symptoms of early and late dumping are quite different. Early dumping includes the following symptoms that occur within 1 h, typically 30 min after a meal ingestion [15]: abdominal pain, bloating, borborygmi, nausea, diarrhea (gastrointestinal symptoms); and fatigue, desire to lie down, flushing, palpitations/perspiration, tachycardia, hypotension and rarely syncope (vasomotor symptoms). For late dumping, typical symptoms can be divided into neuroglycopenia and autonomic reactivity [17]. While the first group comprises fatigue, weakness, confusion, hunger and syncope, the latter includes perspiration, palpitations, tremor and irritability. Dumping syndrome can result in significant weight loss (30%) and considerably affects quality of life [51]. It may lead to hospitalizations due to hypoglycemia, episodes of confusion, seizures and even epilepsy [52].

**Table 1.** Symptoms and causes of gastroparesis.

| **Symptoms and Causes of Gastroparesis** |
|---|
| Symptoms: |
| Postprandial fullness, early satiety, bloating, abdominal distension, nausea, and vomiting, abdominal pain, and dysphagia |
| Causes: |
| Diabetes |
| Non-diabetic causes |
| Surgery (such as gastrectomy with vagotomy, vagal nerve injury, Roux-en-Y, pancreatectomy, anti-reflux operations, lung transplant) |
| Gastrointestinal disorders: gastroesophageal reflux, gastric ulcer disease, gastritis, atrophic gastritis, pancreatitis |
| Diseases of the nervous system (such as parkinsonism) |
| Connective tissue diseases (such as scleroderma) |
| Unknown ("idiopathic gastroparesis") |
| Paraneoplastic |
| Mesenteric ischemia |
| Viral infections: e.g., CMV |
| Side effect of medications |
| Metabolic and endocrine disorders: hypothyroidism, pregnancy, uremia |

**Table 2.** Symptoms and causes of dumping syndrome.

| **Symptoms and Causes of Dumping Syndrome** |
|---|
| Symptoms: |
| Early dumping syndrome (within 1 h after meal ingestion) |
| Gastrointestinal symptoms: Abdominal pain, epigastric fullness, diarrhea, nausea, vomiting, borborygmi, and bloating |
| Vasomotor symptoms: desire to lie down, palpitations and tachycardia, fatigue, faintness, syncope, perspiration, headache, light-headedness, hypotension, flushing, and pallor |
| Late dumping syndrome (1–3 h after meal ingestion) |
| Neuroglycopenia: fatigue, weakness, confusion, hunger and syncope |
| Autonomic reactivity: perspiration, palpitations, tremor and irritability |
| Causes: |
| Surgery: gastrojejunostomy, antrectomy, pylorectomy, pyloroplasty, esophagectomy, vagotomy, Roux-en Y bypass, Nissen fundoplication |
| Not-surgery related: diabetes mellitus, viral illness, unkown ("idiopathic") |

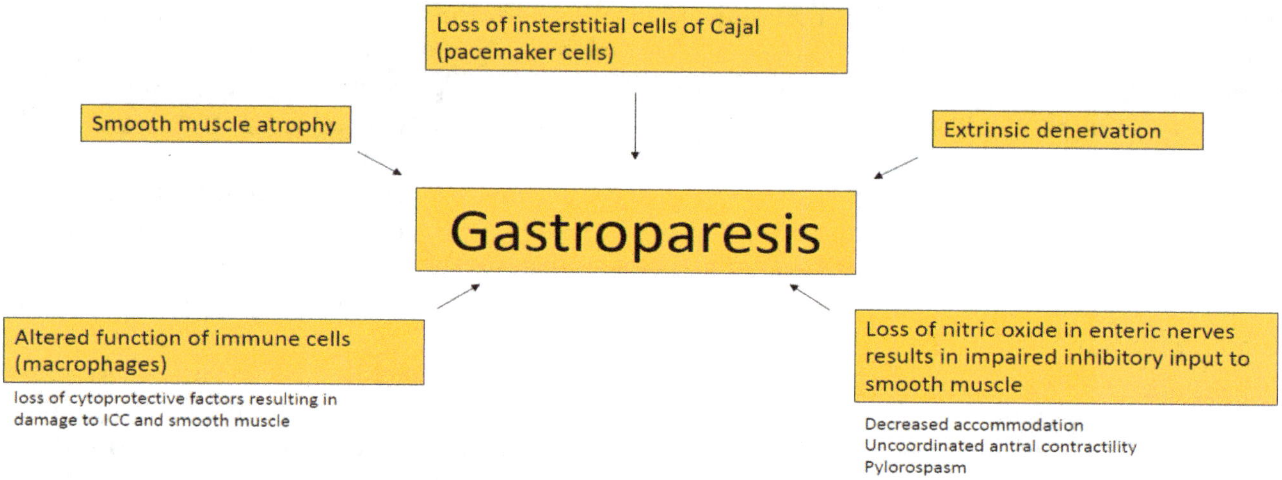


**Figure 1.** Pathophysiology of gastroparesis. ICC, interstitial cells of Cajal.

## 4. Diagnostic Evaluations

Gastroparesis and dumping syndrome have to be distinguished from several organic and functional diseases. Distinction between irritable bowel syndrome, functional dyspepsia and gastroparesis, dumping syndrome might be particularly difficult [29,53]. Many cardinal symptoms are shared between these entities. Diagnostic evaluations are therefore key to clearly establish the diagnosis of gastroparesis and dumping syndrome [54].

### *4.1. Gastroparesis*

Gastroparesis is diagnosed by a thorough history and physical examination, which help to identify the presence of characteristic symptoms of gastroparesis and exclude alternative diagnoses. Once the syndrome is suspected, an upper endoscopy is necessary to rule out mechanical gastric obstruction. Although an upper gastrointestinal series may suggest the diagnosis, there is a limited role for imaging in the workup for gastroparesis and delayed emptying should be confirmed by gastric transit testing such as gastric scintigraphy, breath testing, and wireless motility capsule [55,56]. Gastroparesis is diagnosed if typical symptoms are present, a delayed gastric emptying is documented and a correlation of symptoms with food intake is observed [29]. This definition of gastroparesis highlights two key points: (1) objective measures of delayed gastric emptying are needed to establish the diagnosis; and (2) symptoms are a sine-qua-non [29]. A test that is positive for delayed gastric emptying does not make the diagnosis if a patient is asymptomatic. Scintigraphy is the gold-standard to establish decreased gastric emptying and the most widely used technique. However, there are regional differences. Some European centers use breath tests more often because there are simply to handle and have been shown to correlate nicely with scintigraphy results [57]: A test meal (usually white bread, butter, water and an egg omelette with 13C octanoic acid) is ingested and 13C measured using expired breath gas analysis [58]. Magnetic resonance imaging (MRI) assesses gastric physiology by simultaneously measuring gastric emptying and motility without the need of ionizing radiation [59]. There is increasing evidence that MRI is a reliable non-invasive tool in the diagnostic evaluation of gastroparesis [59]. Given the importance of disrupted ICC networks in the pathophysiology of gastroparesis, slow wave measurements are another potential diagnostic test. In fact, a combination of electrogastrogram and magnetogastrogram is able to distinguish gastroparesis patients from controls [60].

### *4.2. Dumping Syndrome*

Increased pre-test probability such as a past surgical history and the presence of typical symptoms result in a high clinical suspicion for the presence of dumping syndrome. Two questionnaires have been established for the identification of clinically relevant symptoms of dumping syndrome, the Sigstad's score and the Arts' dumping questionnaire [2,51]. A simple visual analogue scale might also be used [61]. Objective measurements are less established compared to gastroparesis. Measuring glucose has a low diagnostic yield, but might be considered when symptoms of late dumping syndrome are present [2]. Importantly, glucose should be measured in the plasma and not in the capillary blood, since low glucose levels are less reliable in the latter. Suggested cut-offs are 2.8 and 3.3 mmol/L [62]. Provocation tests might have higher predictive values. Two options are available, oral glucose tolerance test (OGTT) and the mixed meal tolerance test [2,63]. For OGTT, 50 or 75 g sugar is ingested and blood glucose, haematocrit, pulse and blood pressure are measured every 30 min for 3 h [15]. An increase in the haematocrit by 3% and/or pulse acceleration by 10 min suggest early dumping syndrome, while development of hypoglycemia suggests late dumping syndrome [15]. In the mixed meal tolerance test, carbohydrates, fats and proteins are ingested, and glucose, insulin are checked every 30 min [44,64]. The ordering physician should keep in mind that even healthy individuals can show a drop in their blood sugar levels after meal intake and that therefore the test has a high false positive rate [65]. Gastric emptying studies are potential alternatives, but their specificity and sensitivity is rather low [2].

## 5. Treatment of Gastroparesis

Treatment strategies are quite similar in gastroparesis and dumping syndrome. In a multidisciplinary setting, a step-wise approach should be followed, where dietary modifications and patient education represent the first step, pharmacological interventions the second, and surgical interventions the last option (Figure 2). In the acute setting of gastroparesis, dehydration and electrolyte abnormalities should be corrected by oral or intravenous routes, as appropriate [66]. In severe cases, gastric decompression by insertion of a nasogastric tube might be necessary [29]. In a more chronic setting, the first step in the management of gastroparesis are nutritional counselling and dietary modifications. The patient should be educated to eat small, low-fat, low-fibre meals [29]. Counselling by a nutritional expert is of paramount importance, because gastroparesis can lead to considerable malnutrition due to inadequate oral intake and vomiting [67,68]. In case of underlying diabetes, controlling blood glucose levels should be aimed for [29]. Epidemiological studies have linked poor diabetes control with gastroparesis [69]. As of yet, there are no randomized controlled trials proving that lowering HbA1c indeed improves gastroparesis symptoms. Nonetheless, controlling diabetes makes sense for numerous reasons. When these initial steps do not lead to clinical improvement, pharmacological interventions are needed. The armamentarium is limited, but at least a few drugs are available [70]. Among those are the prokinetics metoclopramide and domperidone that act as dopamine 2 receptor antagonists. Their efficacy has been demonstrated in several randomized trials [71,72]. However, their efficacy appears to be independent of their potential for accelerating gastric emptying, since gastric emptying has been shown to poorly correlate with symptomatic response [73]. Other mechanisms such as affecting gastric hypersensivity or gastric accommodation may be responsible for their effect [74]. Data about their long-term effects are sparse, and several potentially deleterious side-effects limit their use in clinical practice. Metoclopramide imposes a risk for tardive dyskinesia in 1% of patients, while domperidone has been linked to serious cardiac side-effects. Use of metoclopramide should, therefore, be restricted to a maximum of 3 months, at the lowest possible dose [75]. Erythromycin, a macrolide antibiotic, improves gastric emptying through stimulating the motilin receptor and represents an option for short-term treatment, when metoclopramide and domperidone have failed [76]. Nausea, a frequent and bothersome symptom in gastroparesis, can be treated with antiemetics such as prochlorperazine, diphenhydramine, or a 5-HT3 antagonist [66]. Aprepitant can also be considered given its effects on nausea, vomiting and overall symptoms in gastroparesis patients [77]. Iberogast, an over-the-counter herbal preparation is frequently used in functional dyspepsia. Despite having no effect on gastric emptying, iberogast has been shown to positively affect gastroparesis symptoms in a placebo-controlled crossover trial [78]. Several interventional approaches have been developed and hyped in the past with different outcomes.

The injection of botulinum toxin during upper endoscopy into the pyloric muscle might be effective, albeit only in the short term [79–82]. However, the two only randomized controlled trials failed to show efficacy of pyloric botox [83,84]. Whether this was due to small sample size and consecutive lack of power has yet to be determined. Another therapy option is gastric electrical stimulation (GES), where electric current is delivered to gastric smooth muscles via implanted electrodes with a positive impact on gastroparesis symptoms and gastric emptying [85]. GES has been proposed as an alternative for patients with intractable gastroparesis, but a double-blind controlled trial showed only minor improvement with a significant complication rate [86]. A meta-analysis, including 10 studies, suggested that diabetic gastroparesis patients seem to benefit the most, whereas idiopathic gastroparesis patients and postsurgical patients are less responsive and need further research [87]. Another technique, the gastric peroral endoscopic pyloromyotomy (G-POEM) showed some efficacy in gastroparesis patients but further studies are needed [88–93]. Esoflip is currently the newest kid on the block. It is a balloon catheter that was developed for dilations in the gastrointestinal tract. Non-controlled studies revealed high rates of technical success with increased distensibility and symptomatic improvement after pyloric dialation [94]. Esoflip might have its role in difficult to treat patients before considering surgical interventions, but more data, particularly randomized controlled trials are needed first. Surgery should be seen as treatment of last resort and should be discussed individually in a multidisciplinary team setting due to the sparse clinical data. At least, a recent case series including 28 patients suggested improvement of symptoms, gastric emptying and a consecutive reduction in the need for prokinetic treatment 3 months after surgery [95]. However, surgery clearly has its role when oral nutritional intake is compromised. In these cases, jejunostomy feeding should be considered. A percutaneous or surgical placement of a gastrostomy-jejunostomy tube enables decompression of the stomach and permits enteral feeding [96].

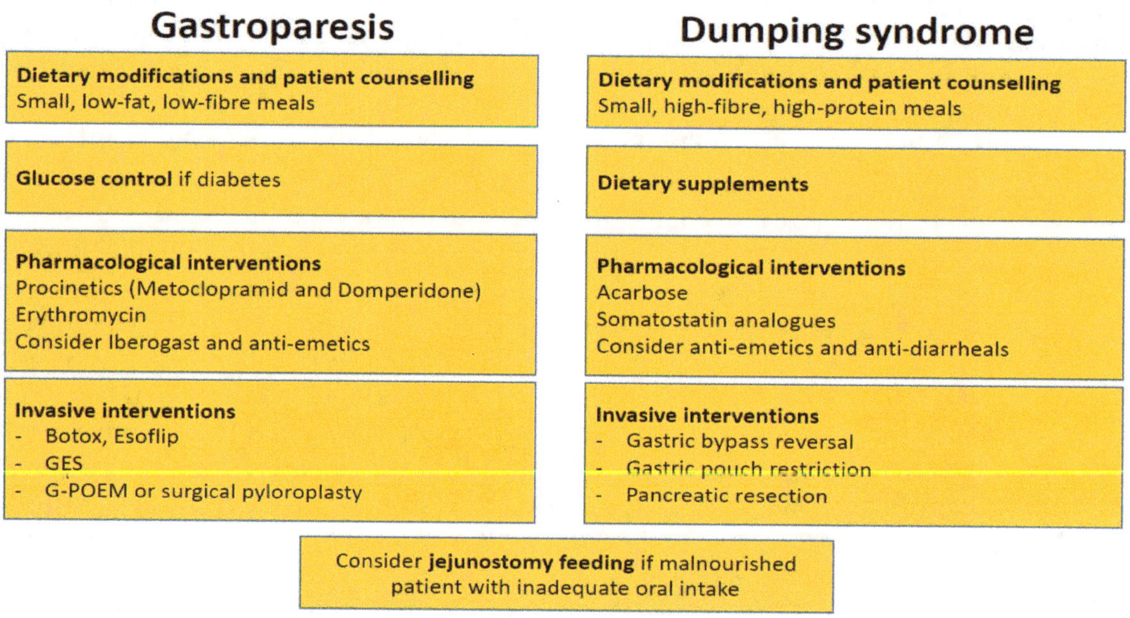


**Figure 2.** Treatment algorithm for gastroparesis and dumping syndrome. GES, gastric electrical stimulation; G-POEM, gastric peroral endoscopic pyloromyotomy.

## 6. Treatment of Dumping Syndrome

Similarly to gastroparesis, dietary modifications and patient education by a nutritional expert are the first steps in the treatment of dumping syndrome [2,97–100]. Smaller and more frequent meals (around six per day) are recommended [2]. Intake of fluids should be delayed by at least 30 min. Rapidly absorbable carbohydrates and alcoholic beverages should be avoided, while intake of high-fibre, high-protein food is recommended [2]. The rationale behind is that liquids further accelerate gastric emptying. Lying down after a meal for 30 min may further delay emptying of the stomach [15,101]. As a second step, dietary supplements such as guar gum, pectin or glucomannan can be added to enhance food viscosity [102–104]. However, most patients do not tolerate these agents due to frequent side-effects such as gas formation and bloating [2]. Pharmacological interventions are the third step in the therapeutic ladder. However, it should be kept in mind that as of yet no treatment has been approved for dumping syndrome. The currently available options are (1) acarbose and (2) for severe cases somatostatin analogues. Acarbose is an alpha-glucosidase inhibitor that decreases intraluminal digestion of carbohydrates in the duodenum. Therefore, it is used to treat postprandial hypoglycemia in late dumping syndrome [105–108]. However, as seen for the dietary supplements, acarbose is associated with side-effects such as flatulence occurring in a high proportion of patients [109]. Somatostatin analogues can improve dumping syndrome by affecting several disease mechanisms: (i) delaying gastric emptying; (ii) slowering small intestine transit; (iii) decreasing release of gastrointestinal hormones including insulin secretion; and (iv) inhibition of postprandial vasodilation [2,51]. Somatostatin analogues such as octreotide can be applied either subcutaneously three times a day or intramuscularly every 2 to 4 weeks [51,110–112]. The latter is probably preferred by the majority of patients. Most important side-effects are steatorrhea, diarrhea, nausea, gallstone formation, pain at injection site and weight gain. Due to these side-effects daily applied doses should start as low as 25 mcg and then titrated up to a maximum of 100 mcg. Treatment should be stopped after 2 weeks (subcutaneous application) or 2 months (intramuscular application) if no improvement is observed [2]. Non-specific symptoms such as nausea and diarrhea may be symptomatically treated with antiemetics (meclizine, promethazine) and antidiarrheals (tincture of opium, loperamide). Anticholinergics like dicyclomine, hyoscyamine, and propantheline slow gastric emptying and are antispasmotic. Diazoxide is a potassium channel activator, which influences hypoglycaemia and is used in late dumping [113]. However, these drugs have been studied in only few patients with dumping syndrome. As for gastroparesis, surgical interventions (revision surgery) should be discussed on a case to case basis, since data for their efficacy are limited [2].

## 7. Conclusions

Gastroparesis and dumping syndrome are frequent disorders, particularly in diabetic and postsurgical patients. Since symptoms are non-specific, these two entities have to be distinguished from several differential diagnoses and require objective measures that document delayed or accelerated gastric emptying. A multidisciplinary team approach including nutritional experts, endocrinologists and gastroenterologists is key to success. Within this setting, optimal treatment strategies can be discussed and individually tailored to each patient. This is particularly important in cases that are difficult to treat, where possible treatment options are limited and data for their efficacy conflicting.

**Author Contributions:** Conceptualization, S.R.V. and T.G.; methodology, S.R.V. and T.G.; writing—original draft preparation, S.R.V. and T.G., writing—review and editing, S.R.V. and T.G.; visualization, T.G.; supervision, S.R.V. and T.G.; project administration, S.R.V.

## References

1. Camilleri, M.; Bharucha, A.E.; Farrugia, G. Epidemiology, mechanisms, and management of diabetic gastroparesis. *Clin. Gastroenterol. Hepatol.* **2011**, *9*, 5–12. [CrossRef] [PubMed]
2. van Beek, A.P.; Emous, M.; Laville, M.; Tack, J. Dumping syndrome after esophageal, gastric or bariatric surgery: Pathophysiology, diagnosis, and management. *Obes. Rev.* **2017**, *18*, 68–85. [CrossRef] [PubMed]
3. Talley, N.J.; Vakil, N.B.; Moayyedi, P. American gastroenterological association technical review on the evaluation of dyspepsia. *Gastroenterology* **2005**, *129*, 1756–1780. [CrossRef] [PubMed]

4. Mulla, C.M.; Storino, A.; Yee, E.U.; Lautz, D.; Sawnhey, M.S.; Moser, A.J.; Patti, M.E. Insulinoma After Bariatric Surgery: Diagnostic Dilemma and Therapeutic Approaches. *Obes. Surg.* **2016**, *26*, 874–881. [CrossRef] [PubMed]
5. Mathur, A.; Gorden, P.; Libutti, S.K. Insulinoma. *Surg. Clin. N. Am.* **2009**, *89*, 1105–1121. [CrossRef] [PubMed]
6. Bharucha, A.E. Epidemiology and natural history of gastroparesis. *Gastroenterol. Clin. N. Am.* **2015**, *44*, 9–19. [CrossRef] [PubMed]
7. Jung, H.K.; Choung, R.S.; Locke, G.R.; Schleck, C.D.; Zinsmeister, A.R.; Szarka, L.A.; Mullan, B.; Talley, N.J. The incidence, prevalence, and outcomes of patients with gastroparesis in Olmsted County, Minnesota, from 1996 to 2006. *Gastroenterology* **2009**, *136*, 1225–1233. [CrossRef] [PubMed]
8. Rey, E.; Choung, R.S.; Schleck, C.D.; Zinsmeister, A.R.; Talley, N.J.; Locke, G.R. Prevalence of hidden gastroparesis in the community: The gastroparesis "iceberg". *J. Neurogastroenterol. Motil.* **2012**, *18*, 34–42. [CrossRef]
9. Choung, R.S.; Locke, G.R.; Schleck, C.D.; Zinsmeister, A.R.; Melton, L.J.; Talley, N.J. Risk of gastroparesis in subjects with type 1 and 2 diabetes in the general population. *Am. J. Gastroenterol.* **2012**, *107*, 82–88. [CrossRef]
10. Horowitz, M.; Harding, P.E.; Maddox, A.F.; Wishart, J.M.; Akkermans, L.M.; Chatterton, B.E.; Shearman, D.J. Gastric and oesophageal emptying in patients with type 2 (non-insulin-dependent) diabetes mellitus. *Diabetologia* **1989**, *32*, 151–159. [CrossRef]
11. Horowitz, M.; Maddox, A.F.; Wishart, J.M.; Harding, P.E.; Chatterton, B.E.; Shearman, D.J. Relationships between oesophageal transit and solid and liquid gastric emptying in diabetes mellitus. *Eur. J. Nucl. Med.* **1991**, *18*, 229–234. [CrossRef] [PubMed]
12. Dong, K.; Yu, X.J.; Li, B.; Wen, E.G.; Xiong, W.; Guan, Q.L. Advances in mechanisms of postsurgical gastroparesis syndrome and its diagnosis and treatment. *Chin. J. Dig. Dis.* **2006**, *7*, 76–82. [CrossRef] [PubMed]
13. Dong, K.; Li, B.; Guan, Q.L.; Huang, T. Analysis of multiple factors of postsurgical gastroparesis syndrome after pancreaticoduodenectomy and cryotherapy for pancreatic cancer. *World J. Gastroenterol.* **2004**, *10*, 2434–2438. [CrossRef] [PubMed]
14. Nusrat, S.; Bielefeldt, K. Gastroparesis on the rise: Incidence vs awareness? *Neurogastroenterol. Motil.* **2013**, *25*, 16–22. [CrossRef] [PubMed]
15. Tack, J.; Arts, J.; Caenepeel, P.; De Wulf, D.; Bisschops, R. Pathophysiology, diagnosis and management of postoperative dumping syndrome. *Nat. Rev. Gastroenterol. Hepatol.* **2009**, *6*, 583–590. [CrossRef]
16. Tack, J.; Deloose, E. Complications of bariatric surgery: Dumping syndrome, reflux and vitamin deficiencies. *Best Pract. Res. Clin. Gastroenterol.* **2014**, *28*, 741–749. [CrossRef] [PubMed]
17. Eagon, J.C.; Miedema, B.W.; Kelly, K.A. Postgastrectomy syndromes. *Surg. Clin. N. Am.* **1992**, *72*, 445–465. [CrossRef]
18. Vecht, J.; Masclee, A.A.; Lamers, C.B. The dumping syndrome. Current insights into pathophysiology, diagnosis and treatment. *Scand. J. Gastroenterol. Suppl.* **1997**, *223*, 21–27.
19. McLarty, A.J.; Deschamps, C.; Trastek, V.F.; Allen, M.S.; Pairolero, P.C.; Harmsen, W.S. Esophageal resection for cancer of the esophagus: Long-term function and quality of life. *Ann. Thorac. Surg.* **1997**, *63*, 1568–1572. [CrossRef]
20. Banerjee, A.; Ding, Y.; Mikami, D.J.; Needleman, B.J. The role of dumping syndrome in weight loss after gastric bypass surgery. *Surg. Endosc.* **2013**, *27*, 1573–1578. [CrossRef]
21. Papamargaritis, D.; Koukoulis, G.; Sioka, E.; Zachari, E.; Bargiota, A.; Zacharoulis, D.; Tzovaras, G. Dumping symptoms and incidence of hypoglycaemia after provocation test at 6 and 12 months after laparoscopic sleeve gastrectomy. *Obes. Surg.* **2012**, *22*, 1600–1606. [CrossRef] [PubMed]
22. Tzovaras, G.; Papamargaritis, D.; Sioka, E.; Zachari, E.; Baloyiannis, I.; Zacharoulis, D.; Koukoulis, G. Symptoms suggestive of dumping syndrome after provocation in patients after laparoscopic sleeve gastrectomy. *Obes. Surg.* **2012**, *22*, 23–28. [CrossRef] [PubMed]
23. Berg, P.; McCallum, R. Dumping Syndrome: A Review of the Current Concepts of Pathophysiology, Diagnosis, and Treatment. *Dig. Dis. Sci.* **2016**, *61*, 11–18. [CrossRef]
24. O'Grady, G.; Angeli, T.R.; Du, P.; Lahr, C.; Lammers, W.J.E.P.; Windsor, J.A.; Abell, T.L.; Farrugia, G.; Pullan, A.J.; Cheng, L.K. Abnormal initiation and conduction of slow-wave activity in gastroparesis, defined by high-resolution electrical mapping. *Gastroenterology* **2012**, *143*, 589–598.e583. [CrossRef] [PubMed]

25. Hyett, B.; Martinez, F.J.; Gill, B.M.; Mehra, S.; Lembo, A.; Kelly, C.P.; Leffler, D.A. Delayed radionucleotide gastric emptying studies predict morbidity in diabetics with symptoms of gastroparesis. *Gastroenterology* **2009**, *137*, 445–452. [CrossRef] [PubMed]
26. Chen, J.D.; Lin, Z.; Pan, J.; McCallum, R.W. Abnormal gastric myoelectrical activity and delayed gastric emptying in patients with symptoms suggestive of gastroparesis. *Dig. Dis. Sci.* **1996**, *41*, 1538–1545. [CrossRef] [PubMed]
27. Oh, J.J.; Kim, C.H. Gastroparesis after a presumed viral illness: Clinical and laboratory features and natural history. *Mayo Clin. Proc.* **1990**, *65*, 636–642. [CrossRef]
28. Bityutskiy, L.P.; Soykan, I.; McCallum, R.W. Viral gastroparesis: A subgroup of idiopathic gastroparesis–clinical characteristics and long-term outcomes. *Am. J. Gastroenterol.* **1997**, *92*, 1501–1504.
29. Camilleri, M.; Parkman, H.P.; Shafi, M.A.; Abell, T.L.; Gerson, L. Clinical guideline: Management of gastroparesis. *Am. J. Gastroenterol.* **2013**, *108*, 18–37. [CrossRef]
30. Mittal, R.K.; Frank, E.B.; Lange, R.C.; McCallum, R.W. Effects of morphine and naloxone on esophageal motility and gastric emptying in man. *Dig. Dis. Sci.* **1986**, *31*, 936–942. [CrossRef]
31. Salehi, M.; Aulinger, B.A.; D'Alessio, D.A. Targeting beta-cell mass in type 2 diabetes: Promise and limitations of new drugs based on incretins. *Endocr. Rev.* **2008**, *29*, 367–379. [CrossRef] [PubMed]
32. Maes, B.D.; Vanwalleghem, J.; Kuypers, D.; Ghoos, Y.; Rutgeerts, P.J.; Vanrenterghem, Y.F. Differences in gastric motor activity in renal transplant recipients treated with FK-506 versus cyclosporine. *Transplantation* **1999**, *68*, 1482–1485. [CrossRef] [PubMed]
33. Samsom, M.; Vermeijden, J.R.; Smout, A.J.; Van Doorn, E.; Roelofs, J.; Van Dam, P.S.; Martens, E.P.; Eelkman-Rooda, S.J.; Van Berge-Henegouwen, G.P. Prevalence of delayed gastric emptying in diabetic patients and relationship to dyspeptic symptoms: A prospective study in unselected diabetic patients. *Diabetes Care* **2003**, *26*, 3116–3122. [CrossRef]
34. Jones, K.L.; Russo, A.; Stevens, J.E.; Wishart, J.M.; Berry, M.K.; Horowitz, M. Predictors of delayed gastric emptying in diabetes. *Diabetes Care* **2001**, *24*, 1264–1269. [CrossRef] [PubMed]
35. Horváth, V.J.; Izbéki, F.; Lengyel, C.; Kempler, P.; Várkonyi, T. Diabetic gastroparesis: Functional/morphologic background, diagnosis, and treatment options. *Curr. Diabetes Rep.* **2014**, *14*, 527. [CrossRef] [PubMed]
36. Woodhouse, S.; Hebbard, G.; Knowles, S.R. Psychological controversies in gastroparesis: A systematic review. *World J. Gastroenterol.* **2017**, *23*, 1298–1309. [CrossRef] [PubMed]
37. Bielefeldt, K. Gastroparesis: Concepts, controversies, and challenges. *Scientifica (Cairo)* **2012**, *2012*, 424802. [CrossRef]
38. Liu, N.; Abell, T. Gastroparesis Updates on Pathogenesis and Management. *Gut Liver* **2017**, *11*, 579–589. [CrossRef]
39. Cherian, D.; Sachdeva, P.; Fisher, R.S.; Parkman, H.P. Abdominal pain is a frequent symptom of gastroparesis. *Clin. Gastroenterol. Hepatol.* **2010**, *8*, 676–681. [CrossRef]
40. Cherian, D.; Parkman, H.P. Nausea and vomiting in diabetic and idiopathic gastroparesis. *Neurogastroenterol. Motil.* **2012**, *24*, 217–222. [CrossRef]
41. Tack, J. Gastric motor disorders. *Best Pract. Res. Clin. Gastroenterol.* **2007**, *21*, 633–644. [CrossRef] [PubMed]
42. Mayer, E.A.; Thompson, J.B.; Jehn, D.; Reedy, T.; Elashoff, J.; Meyer, J.H. Gastric emptying and sieving of solid food and pancreatic and biliary secretion after solid meals in patients with truncal vagotomy and antrectomy. *Gastroenterology* **1982**, *83 Pt 2*, 184–192.
43. Lawaetz, O.; Blackburn, A.M.; Bloom, S.R.; Aritas, Y.; Ralphs, D.N. Gut hormone profile and gastric emptying in the dumping syndrome. A hypothesis concerning the pathogenesis. *Scand. J. Gastroenterol.* **1983**, *18*, 73–80. [CrossRef] [PubMed]
44. Salehi, M.; Gastaldelli, A.; D'Alessio, D.A. Blockade of glucagon-like peptide 1 receptor corrects postprandial hypoglycemia after gastric bypass. *Gastroenterology* **2014**, *146*, 669–680. [CrossRef] [PubMed]
45. Toft-Nielsen, M.; Madsbad, S.; Holst, J.J. Exaggerated secretion of glucagon-like peptide-1 (GLP-1) could cause reactive hypoglycaemia. *Diabetologia* **1998**, *41*, 1180–1186. [CrossRef] [PubMed]
46. Eloy, R.; Garaud, J.C.; Moody, A.; Jaeck, D.; Grenier, J.F. Jejunal factor stimulating insulin release in the isolated perfused canine pancreas and jejunum. *Horm. Metab. Res.* **1975**, *7*, 461–467. [CrossRef]
47. Mehagnoul-Schipper, D.J.; Lenders, J.W.; Willemsen, J.J.; Hopman, W.P. Sympathoadrenal activation and the dumping syndrome after gastric surgery. *Clin. Auton. Res.* **2000**, *10*, 301–308. [CrossRef]

48. Holdsworth, C.D.; Turner, D.; McIntyre, N. Pathophysiology of post-gastrectomy hypoglycaemia. *Br. Med. J.* **1969**, *4*, 257–259. [CrossRef]
49. Hejazi, R.A.; Patil, H.; McCallum, R.W. Dumping syndrome: Establishing criteria for diagnosis and identifying new etiologies. *Dig. Dis. Sci.* **2010**, *55*, 117–123. [CrossRef]
50. Berg, P.; McCallum, R.; Hall, M.; Sarosiek, I. Dumping Syndrome: Updated Perspectives on Etiologies and Diagnosis. *Pract. Gastroenterol.* **2014**, *38*, 30–38.
51. Arts, J.; Caenepeel, P.; Bisschops, R.; Dewulf, D.; Holvoet, L.; Piessevaux, H.; Bourgeois, S.; Sifrim, D.; Janssens, J.; Tack, J. Efficacy of the long-acting repeatable formulation of the somatostatin analogue octreotide in postoperative dumping. *Clin. Gastroenterol. Hepatol.* **2009**, *7*, 432–437. [CrossRef] [PubMed]
52. Marsk, R.; Jonas, E.; Rasmussen, F.; Näslund, E. Nationwide cohort study of post-gastric bypass hypoglycaemia including 5,040 patients undergoing surgery for obesity in 1986–2006 in Sweden. *Diabetologia* **2010**, *53*, 2307–2311. [CrossRef] [PubMed]
53. Tack, J.; Bisschops, R.; Sarnelli, G. Pathophysiology and treatment of functional dyspepsia. *Gastroenterology* **2004**, *127*, 1239–1255. [CrossRef] [PubMed]
54. Bredenoord, A.J.; Chial, H.J.; Camilleri, M.; Mullan, B.P.; Murray, J.A. Gastric accommodation and emptying in evaluation of patients with upper gastrointestinal symptoms. *Clin. Gastroenterol. Hepatol.* **2003**, *1*, 264–272. [CrossRef]
55. Abell, T.L.; Camilleri, M.; Donohoe, K.; Hasler, W.L.; Lin, H.C.; Maurer, A.H.; McCallum, R.W.; Nowak, T.; Nusynowitz, M.L.; Parman, H.P.; et al. Consensus recommendations for gastric emptying scintigraphy: A joint report of the American Neurogastroenterology and Motility Society and the Society of Nuclear Medicine. *Am. J. Gastroenterol.* **2008**, *103*, 753–763. [CrossRef] [PubMed]
56. Tougas, G.; Eaker, E.Y.; Abell, T.L.; Abrahamsson, H.; Boivin, M.; Chen, J.; Hocking, M.P.; Quigley, E.M.; Koch, K.L.; Tokayer, A.Z.; et al. Assessment of gastric emptying using a low fat meal: Establishment of international control values. *Am. J. Gastroenterol.* **2000**, *95*, 1456–1462. [CrossRef] [PubMed]
57. Keller, J.; Bassotti, G.; Clarke, J.; Dinning, P.; Fox, M.; Grover, M.; Hellström, P.M.; Ke, M.; Layer, P.; Malagelada, C.; et al. Expert consensus document: Advances in the diagnosis and classification of gastric and intestinal motility disorders. *Nat. Rev. Gastroenterol. Hepatol.* **2018**, *15*, 291–308. [CrossRef]
58. Camilleri, M. Clinical practice. Diabetic gastroparesis. *N. Engl. J. Med.* **2007**, *356*, 820–829. [CrossRef]
59. de Zwart, I.M.; de Roos, A. MRI for the evaluation of gastric physiology. *Eur. Radiol.* **2010**, *20*, 2609–2616. [CrossRef]
60. Bradshaw, L.A.; Cheng, L.K.; Chung, E.; Obioha, C.B.; Erickson, J.C.; Gorman, B.L.; Somarajan, S.; Richars, W.O. Diabetic gastroparesis alters the biomagnetic signature of the gastric slow wave. *Neurogastroenterol. Motil.* **2016**, *28*, 837–848. [CrossRef]
61. Mine, S.; Sano, T.; Tsutsumi, K.; Murakami, Y.; Ehara, K.; Saka, M.; Hara, K.; Fukagawa, T.; Udagawa, H.; Katai, H. Large-scale investigation into dumping syndrome after gastrectomy for gastric cancer. *J. Am. Coll. Surg.* **2010**, *211*, 628–636. [CrossRef] [PubMed]
62. Ritz, P.; Hanaire, H. Post-bypass hypoglycaemia: A review of current findings. *Diabetes Metab.* **2011**, *37*, 274–281. [CrossRef] [PubMed]
63. van der Kleij, F.G.; Vecht, J.; Lamers, C.B.; Masclee, A.A. Diagnostic value of dumping provocation in patients after gastric surgery. *Scand. J. Gastroenterol.* **1996**, *31*, 1162–1166. [CrossRef] [PubMed]
64. Khoo, C.M.; Muehlbauer, M.J.; Stevens, R.D.; Pamuklar, Z.; Chen, J.; Newgard, C.B.; Torquati, A. Postprandial metabolite profiles reveal differential nutrient handling after bariatric surgery compared with matched caloric restriction. *Ann. Surg.* **2014**, *259*, 687–693. [CrossRef] [PubMed]
65. Emous, M.; Ubels, F.L.; van Beek, A.P. Diagnostic tools for post-gastric bypass hypoglycaemia. *Obes. Rev.* **2015**, *16*, 843–856. [CrossRef] [PubMed]
66. Waseem, S.; Moshiree, B.; Draganov, P.V. Gastroparesis: Current diagnostic challenges and management considerations. *World J. Gastroenterol.* **2009**, *15*, 25–37. [CrossRef]
67. Ogorek, C.P.; Davidson, L.; Fisher, R.S.; Krevsky, B. Idiopathic gastroparesis is associated with a multiplicity of severe dietary deficiencies. *Am. J. Gastroenterol.* **1991**, *86*, 423–428.
68. Parkman, H.P.; Yates, K.P.; Hasler, W.L.; Nguyan, L.; Pasricha, P.J.; Snape, W.J.; Farrugia, G.; Calles, J.; Koch, K.L.; Abell, T.L.; et al. Dietary intake and nutritional deficiencies in patients with diabetic or idiopathic gastroparesis. *Gastroenterology* **2011**, *141*, 486–498. [CrossRef]

69. Bytzer, P.; Talley, N.J.; Hammer, J.; Young, L.J.; Jones, M.P.; Horowitz, M. GI symptoms in diabetes mellitus are associated with both poor glycemic control and diabetic complications. *Am. J. Gastroenterol.* **2002**, *97*, 604–611. [CrossRef]
70. Quigley, E.M. Pharmacotherapy of gastroparesis. *Expert Opin. Pharmacother.* **2000**, *1*, 881–887. [CrossRef]
71. Patterson, D.; Abell, T.; Rothstein, R.; Koch, K.; Barnett, J. A double-blind multicenter comparison of domperidone and metoclopramide in the treatment of diabetic patients with symptoms of gastroparesis. *Am. J. Gastroenterol.* **1999**, *94*, 1230–1234. [PubMed]
72. McCallum, R.W.; Ricci, D.A.; Rakatansky, H.; Behar, J.; Rhodes, J.B.; Salen, G.; Deren, J.; Ippoliti, A.; Olsen, H.W.; Falchuk, K.; et al. A multicenter placebo-controlled clinical trial of oral metoclopramide in diabetic gastroparesis. *Diabetes Care* **1983**, *6*, 463–467. [CrossRef] [PubMed]
73. Janssen, P.; Harris, M.S.; Jones, M.; Masaoka, T.; Farre, R.; Törnblom, H.; Van Oudenhove, L.; Simren, M.; Tack, J. The relation between symptom improvement and gastric emptying in the treatment of diabetic and idiopathic gastroparesis. *Am. J. Gastroenterol.* **2013**, *108*, 1382–1391. [CrossRef] [PubMed]
74. Stanghellini, V.; Tack, J. Gastroparesis: Separate entity or just a part of dyspepsia? *Gut* **2014**, *63*, 1972–1978. [CrossRef] [PubMed]
75. Rao, A.S.; Camilleri, M. Review article: Metoclopramide and tardive dyskinesia. *Aliment. Pharmacol. Ther.* **2010**, *31*, 11–19. [CrossRef] [PubMed]
76. Richards, R.D.; Davenport, K.; McCallum, R.W. The treatment of idiopathic and diabetic gastroparesis with acute intravenous and chronic oral erythromycin. *Am. J. Gastroenterol.* **1993**, *88*, 203–207. [PubMed]
77. Pasricha, P.J.; Yates, K.P.; Sarosiek, I.; McCallum, R.W.; Abell, T.L.; Koch, K.L.; Nguyen, L.A.B.; Snape, W.J.; Hasler, W.L.; Clarke, J.O.; et al. Aprepitant Has Mixed Effects on Nausea and Reduces Other Symptoms in Patients With Gastroparesis and Related Disorders. *Gastroenterology* **2018**, *154*, 65–76. [CrossRef] [PubMed]
78. Braden, B.; Caspary, W.; Börner, N.; Vinson, B.; Schneider, A.R. Clinical effects of STW 5 (Iberogast) are not based on acceleration of gastric emptying in patients with functional dyspepsia and gastroparesis. *Neurogastroenterol. Motil.* **2009**, *21*, 632–638. [CrossRef] [PubMed]
79. Friedenberg, F.; Gollamudi, S.; Parkman, H.P. The use of botulinum toxin for the treatment of gastrointestinal motility disorders. *Dig. Dis. Sci.* **2004**, *49*, 165–175. [CrossRef] [PubMed]
80. Ezzeddine, D.; Jit, R.; Katz, N.; Gopalswamy, N.; Bhutani, M.S. Pyloric injection of botulinum toxin for treatment of diabetic gastroparesis. *Gastrointest. Endosc.* **2002**, *55*, 920–923. [CrossRef] [PubMed]
81. Lacy, B.E.; Zayat, E.N.; Crowell, M.D.; Schuster, M.M. Botulinum toxin for the treatment of gastroparesis: A preliminary report. *Am. J. Gastroenterol.* **2002**, *97*, 1548–1552. [CrossRef] [PubMed]
82. Miller, L.S.; Szych, G.A.; Kantor, S.B.; Bromer, M.Q.; Knight, L.C.; Maurer, A.H.; Fisher, R.S.; Parkman, H.P. Treatment of idiopathic gastroparesis with injection of botulinum toxin into the pyloric sphincter muscle. *Am. J. Gastroenterol.* **2002**, *97*, 1653–1660. [CrossRef] [PubMed]
83. Arts, J.; Holvoet, L.; Caenepeel, P.; Bisschops, R.; Sifrim, D.; Verbeke, K.; Janssens, J.; Tack, J. Clinical trial: A randomized-controlled crossover study of intrapyloric injection of botulinum toxin in gastroparesis. *Aliment. Pharmacol. Ther.* **2007**, *26*, 1251–1258. [CrossRef] [PubMed]
84. Friedenberg, F.K.; Palit, A.; Parkman, H.P.; Hanlon, A.; Nelson, D.B. Botulinum toxin A for the treatment of delayed gastric emptying. *Am. J. Gastroenterol.* **2008**, *103*, 416–423. [CrossRef] [PubMed]
85. Angeli, T.R.; Du, P.; Midgley, D.; Paskaranandavadivel, N.; Sathar, S.; Lahr, C.; Abell, T.L.; Cheng, L.K.; O'Grady, G. Acute Slow Wave Responses to High-Frequency Gastric Electrical Stimulation in Patients With Gastroparesis Defined by High-Resolution Mapping. *Neuromodulation* **2016**, *19*, 864–871. [CrossRef] [PubMed]
86. Abell, T.; McCallum, R.; Hocking, M.; Koch, K.; Abrahamsson, H.; Leblanc, I.; Lindberg, G.; Konturek, J.; Nowak, T.; Quigley, E.M.; et al. Gastric electrical stimulation for medically refractory gastroparesis. *Gastroenterology* **2003**, *125*, 421–428. [CrossRef]
87. Chu, H.; Lin, Z.; Zhong, L.; McCallum, R.W.; Hou, X. Treatment of high-frequency gastric electrical stimulation for gastroparesis. *J. Gastroenterol. Hepatol.* **2012**, *27*, 1017–1026. [CrossRef]
88. Khashab, M.A.; Ngamruengphong, S.; Carr-Locke, D.; Bapaye, A.; Benias, P.C.; Serouya, S.; Dorwat, S.; Chaves, D.M.; Artifon, E.; de Moura, E.G.; et al. Gastric per-oral endoscopic myotomy for refractory gastroparesis: Results from the first multicenter study on endoscopic pyloromyotomy (with video). *Gastrointest. Endosc.* **2017**, *85*, 123–128. [CrossRef]

89. Khashab, M.A.; Stein, E.; Clarke, J.O.; Saxena, P.; Kumbhari, V.; Chander Roland, B.; Kalloo, A.N.; Stavropoulos, S.; Pasricha, P.; Inoue, H. Gastric peroral endoscopic myotomy for refractory gastroparesis: First human endoscopic pyloromyotomy (with video). *Gastrointest. Endosc.* **2013**, *78*, 764–768. [CrossRef]
90. Dacha, S.; Mekaroonkamol, P.; Li, L.; Shahnavaz, N.; Sakaria, S.; Keilin, S.; Willingham, F.; Christie, J.; Cai, Q. Outcomes and quality-of-life assessment after gastric per-oral endoscopic pyloromyotomy (with video). *Gastrointest. Endosc.* **2017**, *86*, 282–289. [CrossRef]
91. Gonzalez, J.M.; Benezech, A.; Vitton, V.; Barthet, M. G-POEM with antro-pyloromyotomy for the treatment of refractory gastroparesis: Mid-term follow-up and factors predicting outcome. *Aliment. Pharmacol. Ther.* **2017**, *46*, 364–370. [CrossRef] [PubMed]
92. Gonzalez, J.M.; Lestelle, V.; Benezech, A.; Cohen, J.; Vitton, V.; Grimaud, J.C.; Barthet, M. Gastric per-oral endoscopic myotomy with antropyloromyotomy in the treatment of refractory gastroparesis: Clinical experience with follow-up and scintigraphic evaluation (with video). *Gastrointest. Endosc.* **2017**, *85*, 132–139. [CrossRef] [PubMed]
93. Rodriguez, J.H.; Haskins, I.N.; Strong, A.T.; Plescia, R.L.; Allemang, M.T.; Butler, R.S.; Cline, M.S.; El-Hayek, K.; Ponsky, J.L.; Kroh, M.D. Per oral endoscopic pyloromyotomy for refractory gastroparesis: Initial results from a single institution. *Surg. Endosc.* **2017**, *31*, 5381–5388. [CrossRef] [PubMed]
94. Gourcerol, G.; Tissier, F.; Melchior, C.; Touchais, J.Y.; Huet, E.; Prevost, G.; Leroi, A.M.; Ducrotte, P. Impaired fasting pyloric compliance in gastroparesis and the therapeutic response to pyloric dilatation. *Aliment. Pharmacol. Ther.* **2015**, *41*, 360–367. [CrossRef]
95. Hibbard, M.L.; Dunst, C.M.; Swanström, L.L. Laparoscopic and endoscopic pyloroplasty for gastroparesis results in sustained symptom improvement. *J. Gastrointest. Surg.* **2011**, *15*, 1513–1519. [CrossRef]
96. Felsher, J.; Chand, B.; Ponsky, J. Decompressive percutaneous endoscopic gastrostomy in nonmalignant disease. *Am. J. Surg.* **2004**, *187*, 254–256. [CrossRef]
97. Pittman, A.C.; Robinson, F.W. Dietary management of the "dumping" syndrome. Long-term follow-up. *J. Am. Diet. Assoc.* **1962**, *40*, 108–110.
98. Robinson, F.W.; Pittman, A.C. Dietary management of postgastrectomy dumping syndrome. *Surg. Gynecol. Obstet.* **1957**, *104*, 529–534.
99. Khoshoo, V.; Reifen, R.M.; Gold, B.D.; Sherman, P.M.; Pencharz, P.B. Nutritional manipulation in the management of dumping syndrome. *Arch. Dis. Child.* **1991**, *66*, 1447–1448. [CrossRef]
100. Kellogg, T.A.; Bantle, J.P.; Leslie, D.B.; Redmond, J.B.; Slusarek, B.; Swan, T.; Buchwald, H.; Ikramuddin, S. Postgastric bypass hyperinsulinemic hypoglycemia syndrome: Characterization and response to a modified diet. *Surg. Obes. Relat. Dis.* **2008**, *4*, 492–499. [CrossRef]
101. Ukleja, A. Dumping syndrome: Pathophysiology and treatment. *Nutr. Clin. Pract.* **2005**, *20*, 517–525. [CrossRef] [PubMed]
102. Jenkins, D.J.; Gassull, M.A.; Leeds, A.R.; Metz, G.; Dilawari, J.B.; Slavin, B.; Blendis, L.M. Effect of dietary fiber on complications of gastric surgery: Prevention of postprandial hypoglycemia by pectin. *Gastroenterology* **1977**, *73*, 215–217. [CrossRef]
103. Harju, E.; Larmi, T.K. Efficacy of guar gum in preventing the dumping syndrome. *JPEN J. Parenter. Enter. Nutr.* **1983**, *7*, 470–472. [CrossRef] [PubMed]
104. Kneepkens, C.M.; Fernandes, J.; Vonk, R.J. Dumping syndrome in children. Diagnosis and effect of glucomannan on glucose tolerance and absorption. *Acta Paediatr. Scand.* **1988**, *77*, 279–286. [CrossRef] [PubMed]
105. Ng, D.D.; Ferry, R.J.; Kelly, A.; Weinzimer, S.A.; Stanley, C.A.; Katz, L.E. Acarbose treatment of postprandial hypoglycemia in children after Nissen fundoplication. *J. Pediatr.* **2001**, *139*, 877–879. [CrossRef] [PubMed]
106. Ritz, P.; Vaurs, C.; Bertrand, M.; Anduze, Y.; Guillaume, E.; Hanaire, H. Usefulness of acarbose and dietary modifications to limit glycemic variability following Roux-en-Y gastric bypass as assessed by continuous glucose monitoring. *Diabetes Technol. Ther.* **2012**, *14*, 736–740. [CrossRef] [PubMed]
107. Speth, P.A.; Jansen, J.B.; Lamers, C.B. Effect of acarbose, pectin, a combination of acarbose with pectin, and placebo on postprandial reactive hypoglycaemia after gastric surgery. *Gut* **1983**, *24*, 798–802. [CrossRef] [PubMed]
108. McLoughlin, J.C.; Buchanan, K.D.; Alam, M.J. A glycoside-hydrolase inhibitor in treatment of dumping syndrome. *Lancet* **1979**, *2*, 603–605. [CrossRef]

109. Hasegawa, T.; Yoneda, M.; Nakamura, K.; Ohnishi, K.; Harada, H.; Kyouda, T.; Yoshida, Y.; Makino, I. Long-term effect of alpha-glucosidase inhibitor on late dumping syndrome. *J. Gastroenterol. Hepatol.* **1998**, *13*, 1201–1206. [CrossRef] [PubMed]
110. Didden, P.; Penning, C.; Masclee, A.A. Octreotide therapy in dumping syndrome: Analysis of long-term results. *Aliment. Pharmacol. Ther.* **2006**, *24*, 1367–1375. [CrossRef] [PubMed]
111. Penning, C.; Vecht, J.; Masclee, A.A. Efficacy of depot long-acting release octreotide therapy in severe dumping syndrome. *Aliment. Pharmacol. Ther.* **2005**, *22*, 963–969. [CrossRef] [PubMed]
112. Deloose, E.; Bisschops, R.; Holvoet, L.; Arts, J.; De Wulf, D.; Caenepeel, P.; Lannoo, M.; Vanuytsel, T.; Andrews, C.; Tack, J. A pilot study of the effects of the somatostatin analog pasireotide in postoperative dumping syndrome. *Neurogastroenterol. Motil.* **2014**, *26*, 803–809. [CrossRef] [PubMed]
113. Vilarrasa, N.; Goday, A.; Rubio, M.A.; Caixas, A.; Pellitero, S.; Ciudin, A.; Calanas, A.; Botella, J.I.; Breton, I.; Morales, M.J.; et al. Hyperinsulinemic Hypoglycemia after Bariatric Surgery: Diagnosis and Management Experience from a Spanish Multicenter Registry. *Obes. Facts* **2016**, *9*, 41–51. [CrossRef] [PubMed]

13

# Management of Dehydration in Patients Suffering Swallowing Difficulties

**Emilie Reber [1,*], Filomena Gomes [2], Ilka A. Dähn [3], Maria F. Vasiloglou [4] and Zeno Stanga [1]**

1 Department for Diabetes, Endocrinology, Nutritional Medicine and Metabolism, Bern University Hospital, and University of Bern, Freiburgstrasse 15, 3010 Bern, Switzerland; zeno.stanga@insel.ch

2 The New York Academy of Sciences, 250 Greenwich Sweet, 40th floor, New York, NY 10007, USA; filomenisabel@hotmail.com

3 Cereneo Schweiz AG, Center for Neurology and Rehabilitation, Seestrasse 18, 6354 Vitznau, Switzerland; ilka.daehn@cereneo.ch

4 AI in Health and Nutrition Laboratory, ARTORG Center for Biomedical Engineering Research, University of Bern, Murtenstrasse 50, 3008 Bern, Switzerland; maria.vasiloglou@artorg.unibe.ch

* Correspondence: emilie.reber@insel.ch

**Abstract:** Swallowing difficulties, also called dysphagia, can have various causes and may occur at many points in the swallowing process. The treatment and rehabilitation of dysphagia represent a major interdisciplinary and multiprofessional challenge. In dysphagic patients, dehydration is frequent and often accelerated as a result of limited fluid intake. This condition results from loss of water from the intracellular space, disturbing the normal levels of electrolytes and fluid interfering with metabolic processes and body functions. Dehydration is associated with increased morbidity and mortality rates. Dysphagic patients at risk of dehydration thus require close monitoring of their hydration state, and existing imbalances should be addressed quickly. This review gives an overview on dehydration, as well as its pathophysiology, risk factors, and clinical signs/symptoms in general. Available management strategies of dehydration are presented for oral, enteral, and parenteral fluid replacement.

**Keywords:** dehydration; dysphagia; fluid intake; water

---

## 1. Introduction

Dysphagia is a dysfunction of the digestive system, consisting of a difficulty in swallowing. It affects the proper transit of the bolus in the upper digestive tract, preventing a safe oral feeding process. The main complications of dysphagia are aspiration (i.e., the passage of solid and liquid food into the respiratory tract, which can be "silent" in the absence of the protective cough reflex), aspiration pneumonia (pneumonia caused by food in the lungs), malnutrition, and dehydration. Because symptoms are very unspecific, dysphagia is frequently undetected, and either untreated or undertreated. Nevertheless, prevalence of dysphagia is high, especially among older patients with neurological disorders due to multifactorial changes of swallowing physiology, affecting at least 50% of the acute stroke population and 60% of those who suffer a severe traumatic brain injury [1,2]. In a recent systematic review with six high quality studies, the average prevalence of dysphagia in the community dwelling elderly population was 15% [3]. The same authors defined the risk factors for dysphagia as a history of clinical disease, physical frailty, and reduced ability to accomplish activities of daily living [3]. Dysphagia and the subsequent reduction of the coordination of pharyngeal muscles increase the risk of dehydration, malnutrition, pneumonia, and mortality [2]. Consequently, dysphagia may lead to dehydration—a shortage of body water due to either insufficient drinking or excess losses, or a combination of both [4]. Water and electrolyte balance is crucial for body homeostasis and is one of the most protected mechanisms in the body. Organisms can survive months without eating, but not many days without drinking, as fluid and electrolytes play major regulatory roles in many mechanisms, for example, transport systems, signal transduction, and body temperature [5].

This review highlights and discusses dehydration, as well as its pathophysiology, risk factors, and clinical signs/symptoms, focusing on dysphagic patients in particular. Possible management strategies of dehydration are presented for oral, enteral and parenteral fluid replacement.

## 2. Dysphagia

Swallowing is an essential and highly complex process of movements. This physiological process requires an exact coordination of nerval and muscular structures as well as an intact sensitivity of the mouth and throat area. The deglutition can be divided into five phases (preoral, two oral phases, pharyngeal, and oesophageal), whereby the phases run smoothly into each other and work together as muscle chains. Normally, the act of swallowing proceeds unnoticed and highly automated [6,7]. The muscle strength and the temporal orientation of the movement sequence are regulated in relation to the food/drink in the mouth (consistency and quantity). The system can be severely disturbed by diseases such as strokes, degenerative diseases, traumas, or tumours. A swallowing disorder (dysphagia) can occur in different forms. A healthy person swallows about 1,000 to 2,000 times a day [8]. The adaptation of food/drink, for example, balanced soft food or thickened liquids, may be needed to enable the patient to eat orally without an additional risk of aspiration.

Motor and cognitive performance decreases with increasing age [9,10]. Changes in the age-related swallowing disorder (presbyphagia) are the reduction of the sense of taste and smell, a reduced chewing function due to lack of oral hygiene/prosthesis, and the loss of strength to swallow food and liquids effectively and safely [10]. More than 40% of muscle mass is lost in old age [11]. Cancer patients are also severely impaired in their food intake owing to severe surgery, subsequent chemotherapy, and/or radiation. All these factors make the patients highly dependent [9,12], which leads to further health problems such as dehydration, malnutrition, anorexia, sarcopenia, and pneumonia. Older people and patients with dementia are more susceptible to stroke, pneumonia, and dehydration, which are among the most common causes of death in this population [9].

Dysphagia is associated with malnutrition, dehydration, pneumonia, reduced functional outcome, and mortality [13]. Therefore, similarly to nutritional management, populations at risk should regularly be screened for dysphagia and, when needed, further assessed by a clinical specialist (e.g., a speech-language pathologist). Patients suspected to have dysphagia after a screening test undergo assessment to determine the degree of severity of dysphagia and further treatment. Individual screening tests are performed by speech-language pathologists or trained nursing staff. They serve to identify symptoms and differentiate dysphagic patients from non-dysphagic patients. This procedure is non-invasive and can be performed quickly (in 10–15 min) while the patient is sitting in an upright position. There are several criteria that indicate that the screening test should be ceased in order to minimize the risk of aspiration (i.e., the involuntary passage of food or liquid through the vocal folds, to the lungs). Nonetheless, this test shows a sensitivity and specificity between 50% and 80% and fails to detect a significant number of aspirations [14,15].

The clinical swallowing examination is performed by speech-language pathologists. The patient sits upright at 90°. The inspection of the facial-oral structures, the oral skills, and sensitivity, as well as the oral motor arbitrary movements; the oral reflexes in the pharynx area (gag reflex, palata reflex, and so on); and the existing protective mechanisms, such as coughing and deliberate coughing, are included [16]. According to Daniels et al., liquid is gradually swallowed, thus single sips ≤20 mL of water up to 100 ml are examined (timed test) [17]. Soft and solid consistencies are also examined. Pathomechanisms like leaking anterior, nasal penetration, signs of aspiration, and residuals in the oral cavity are observed and described. Finally, an inspection of the oral cavity and a longer phonation sample are performed to clarify a sizzling voice and possibly the suspicion of penetration with aspiration [16]. In addition, instrumental examinations such as, for example, fiber optic endoscopic evaluation of swallowing (FEES; a transnasal procedure) and the video fluoroscopic swallowing study (a radiographic procedure), can be carried out.

FEES is a reportable procedure that may be completed in an outpatient clinic setting or at the bedside by passing an endoscope transnasally. It requires minimal positioning of the patient, and is thus commonly used [18]. In contrast, the video-fluoroscopy swallowing study, the gold standard for diagnosis of dysphagia, is a radiographic procedure that provides a direct, dynamic view of oral, pharyngeal, and upper oesophageal function. It, however, requires the use of a radiology suite (which can be very costly) and includes radiation exposure of the patient, who must be able to follow verbal commands (i.e., requires adequate cognitive functioning) [18]. All results will be brought together and the individual therapy plan will be defined. Regular repetitive examinations are needed to adapt swallowing treatment and the nutrition and hydration care plan.

Dysphagia therapy may be split into two categories: compensatory and rehabilitative therapies. Compensative strategies aim to maintain patient's safety when eating, while rehabilitative strategies aim to speed up the recovery process (e.g., swallowing training). Patients may be treated first with compensatory therapy and later with rehabilitation treatments. Functional oriented swallowing therapy, defined and applied by a trained speech-language pathologist, aims to create muscular conditions for largely normal swallowing and, therefore, to recover the physiological swallowing function, maintaining or improving quality of life by reducing morbidity and mortality associated with chest infections (pneumonia) and reduced nutritional status. There are also several supportive technical stimulation treatment methods available such as thermal tactile stimulation, transcranial magnetic stimulation, or transcranial direct current stimulation [19].

On the basis of the severity of dysphagia complaints and the level of alertness, the adequate food support with modified texture diets and thickened fluids will be proposed. The change of food consistency is mandatory in dysphagia, in order to reduce the need of oral manipulation, to make the swallowing process slower and safer, and to increase food and fluid intake [20]. Nevertheless, such diets lean towards less acceptance by patients, less nutritionally dense meals, less food choices, and less appealing meals than normal, leading to insufficient nutritional and fluid intake [21,22]. That is why it makes sense to make use of food fortification as well as supplemental enteral feed and fluids in these patients. Thickening agents, which are used to thicken a variety of fluids (e.g., water, tea, coffee, fruit juice), are supposed to induce a "coating feeling" in the mouth, suppressing flavour without reducing the sensation of thirst [23]. Hence, swallowing safety may be improved, but fluid intake does not substantially improve [1]. Liquid thickening is recommended in patients with dysphagia aspirating on liquids, as a way to slow the flow of the swallowed liquids, which should allow more time for airway closure and eventually reduce the risk of aspiration [24,25]. However, thickening fluids significantly decreases of the acceptance of the beverages, and thus is a practice that needs to be closely monitored. Whelan et al. showed in their study of 24 acute stroke patients with dysphagia that the intake of thickened fluids per day amounted to only 30% of the recommended 1500 mL/day [22]. The other 70% of the hydration needs had to be met through supplementary (parenteral and enteral) fluids. The group of patients who received pre-thickened fluids consumed almost double the amount of fluids than the group of patients receiving powder-thickened fluids, suggesting that the commercially available pre-thickened ready-to-drink beverages have better acceptability and can be used as a strategy to increase fluid intake among dysphagic patients (although the costs may he higher) [22].

Different food consistencies have been defined and numerous guidelines exist in many countries describing the various types of texture-modified diets and thickened fluids. These recommendations, aiming to improve patient's safety and nutritional status while avoiding aspiration pneumonia, are, however, based on best practice and are not evidence-based [26,27]. Modification of food texture and liquid thickness is a mainstay of dysphagia management. As there are only a few high-quality studies, the evidence is weak [28]. A couple of years ago, the "International Dysphagia Diet Standardisation Initiative" (IDDSI) published new global standardized definitions describing texture-modified foods and thickened liquids [29]. This terminology allows the use of a common language on multiprofessional teams (therapists, nurses, chiefs, patients, and relatives), which will support scientists working in this field, thus generating comparable research data worldwide. When applying the IDDSI definitions in each clinical setting, the food and drinks should always be tested under serving conditions. Drinks and liquidized foods are evaluated by a gravity flow test with a 10 ml syringe. This classifies beverages based on their flow rate, representing the process of drinking through a straw [29].

It is important to note that thickened liquids and adapted food consistencies are only a start to increase the quality of life of the dysphagic patients, as they work as a motivation tool and prepare them to eventually swallow food and fluid with normal consistency. Given the disadvantages of the use of thickened fluids and adapted food consistencies (which may lead to insufficient nutritional and fluid intake), it is important to control the progression of the dysphagia in order to adapt the food/drink consistency and protect the patient from being restricted to a certain consistency for too long [30].

## 3. Dehydration

Adequate water supply is indispensable to maintain cellular homeostasis and several physiological functions. Historically, total body water loss is differentiated into two types: dehydration and volume depletion [31]. Dehydration occurs when the body water losses, mostly from the intracellular volume (ICV), are higher than the intake. Low-intake dehydration is a shortage of pure water, leading to loss of both intracellular and extracellular fluid, and to raised osmolality in both compartments. Volume depletion is the result of excess losses of fluid and salts (especially sodium and sometimes other components), primarily related to a loss of extracellular volume (ECV), and clinically affecting the interstitial compartment; the fluid is lost primarily, not intracellular fluid, and serum osmolality will be normal or low. From the physiological view point, it makes sense that many physicians tend to use the term of dehydration for any loss of total body water in daily clinical practice [32].

There are numerous definitions for dehydration hampering the diagnosis. The best diagnostic approach for this complex condition thus includes history, clinical observations, laboratory tests, and physical assessment [33]. From a clinical point of view, dehydration may be defined as the rapid decrease of >3% of body weight [34]. Pathophysiologically, however, dehydration is a loss of water, resulting in a relative deficit of body water referring to sodium [35]. Consequently, increased sodium values cause the plasma osmolality to rise, reducing the ICV. This is often referred to as hypovolemic hypernatremia or hypertonic dehydration. Even if commonly used, "isotonic dehydration" and "hypotonic dehydration" differ from a pathophysiologic point of view, rather characterizing a volume depletion (loss of sodium from the ECV) than dehydration [35]. This distinction is especially relevant for the therapeutic approach [33].

If the fluid intake is too low, fluid in and around body cells concentrates, raising plasma and serum osmolality [36]. This consecutively triggers protection mechanisms (e.g., thirst and increased urine concentration by the kidney). In the elderly, with kidney function being mostly low, renal parameters do not truthfully indicate dehydration [36]. The U.S. Panel on Dietary Reference Intakes for Electrolytes and Water hence considers the plasma or serum osmolality as the main factor of hydration status, thus setting the reference standard for dehydration in older adults [37]. This is based on physiological and biochemical considerations and is accepted by experts [36]. Extracellular water loss due to diarrhoea, vomiting, or renal sodium loss (volume depletion) is, however, linked to normal or decreased plasma osmolality. While severe dehydration is not exactly defined, there are indicators of a distinctive lack of water: serum osmolality ≥300 mOsm/kg, serum sodium concentration ≥150 mmol/L, or blood urea nitrogen (BUN) to creatinine ratio ≥20. In the case of hypernatremia, free water shortage may be estimated with the following formula [35]:

$$\text{free water shortage (L)} = 0.6 \times \text{body weight (kg)} \times ((\text{plasma sodium (mmol/L)}/140) - 1)$$

### 3.1. *Adequate Intake*

The recommendations for adequate fluid intake show great variation (from 1.0 L/day in the Nordic countries to 2.2 L/day in the USA in women, 1.0–3.0 L/day in men) [36]. The European Food Safety Authority recommends an adequate intake of 2.0 L/day for women and 2.5 L/day for men of all ages [38]. Because 80% of the fluids come from beverages, adequate intake is 1.6 L/day in women and 2.0 L/day in men. Fluid requirements need to be adapted individually, for example, increased with higher activity level, fever, diarrhoea, and vomiting, or decreased in the case of heart and renal failure.

### 3.2. *Prevalence*

As dehydration is not properly defined, it is problematic to accurately assess its prevalence. Dehydration is, however, especially common in the elderly (up to 60%), depending on the definition used [39]. Bennett et al. showed that laboratory parameters indicated dehydration in 48% of elderly people admitted to an emergency department, while proper assessment of dehydration was documented only in 26% [40]. Dehydration is one of the ten most frequent diagnoses for hospital admission in older adults [41], and has been reported to be the most common fluid and electrolyte imbalance in older adults [42]. A study showed that 6.7% of inpatients aged ≥65 years were diagnosed with dehydration, with it being the principal diagnosis in 1.4% [43]. Among those suffering from swallowing difficulties, the prevalence of dehydration ranges from 44% [44] to 75% depending on the patient population, setting, and criteria used to define dehydration [45]. Nevertheless, Thomas et al. revealed that physicians misdiagnose dehydration in at least 30% of older adult inpatients [46].

### 3.3. *Impact and Risk Factors*

Elderly people tend to have diminished feeling of thirst owing to the decrease of sensitivity to the antidiuretic hormone (ADH) [47]. Numerous studies showed that adequate hydration status is normally maintained in healthy older people. Nevertheless, mental and/or physical illnesses, trauma, or operation, among others, may increase the risk of dehydration [48]. A six-month study among nursing home residents found 31% to be dehydrated during that period, and thereof, two-thirds had prior episodes of dehydration [49]. Risk factors for dehydration in dysphagic nursing home residents were, among others, severe impairment of the functional and/or cognitive function, speech disorders [45], and insufficient support at mealtime [50]. Inadequate nursing staff training, multiple medication, and being of female gender have also further been shown to increase the risk of dehydration [51]. Elderly people affected by acute infections and or chronic diseases (cardiovascular disease, diabetes, cancers), especially polymorbid patients, are at high risk of dehydration [40,41,43,51]. Dysphagia was shown to be directly linked with dehydration [4]. Evidence has shown that the clinical outcome of elderly people is worse in the presence of dysphagia [36]. High serum osmolality (>300 mOsm/kg) has been linked to an increased disability and mortality risk [36].

There are many physiological age-related alterations increasing the risk of dehydration (Figure 1) [36]. Growing age seems to dampen the two main physiological answers to reduced fluid intake: thirst and primary urine concentration (through the kidney) [36]. Moreover, fluid reserves are decreased, as body water decreases with age. In addition, common drug therapies in older people may further aggravate fluid loss, such as diuretics and laxatives therapies [36]. However, the severity of cognitive and functional impairment appears to be more relevant than only older age [36]. A study with patients suffering from dysphagia and receiving thickened fluids assessed water supply, including that from food and drinks (thickened beverages), as well as from artificial nutrition (enteral and parenteral nutrition). This study showed that estimated fluid requirements were not met for any of the patients without the use of enteral or parenteral fluids [4]. Another surprising finding of this study is that food, not thickened beverages, provided the greatest contribution to oral fluid intake, which probably reflects the general low level of acceptance of and compliance with thickened fluids. It is very important for the medical and nursing staff to be aware not only of the risk of dehydration in patients with dysphagia, but also of its clinical signs and symptoms. In collaboration with speech-language pathologists and dietitians, an individual nutrition and hydration care plan must be placed in a timely manner, as dehydration may cause severe complications and increase medical costs, morbidity, and the mortality rate [43].

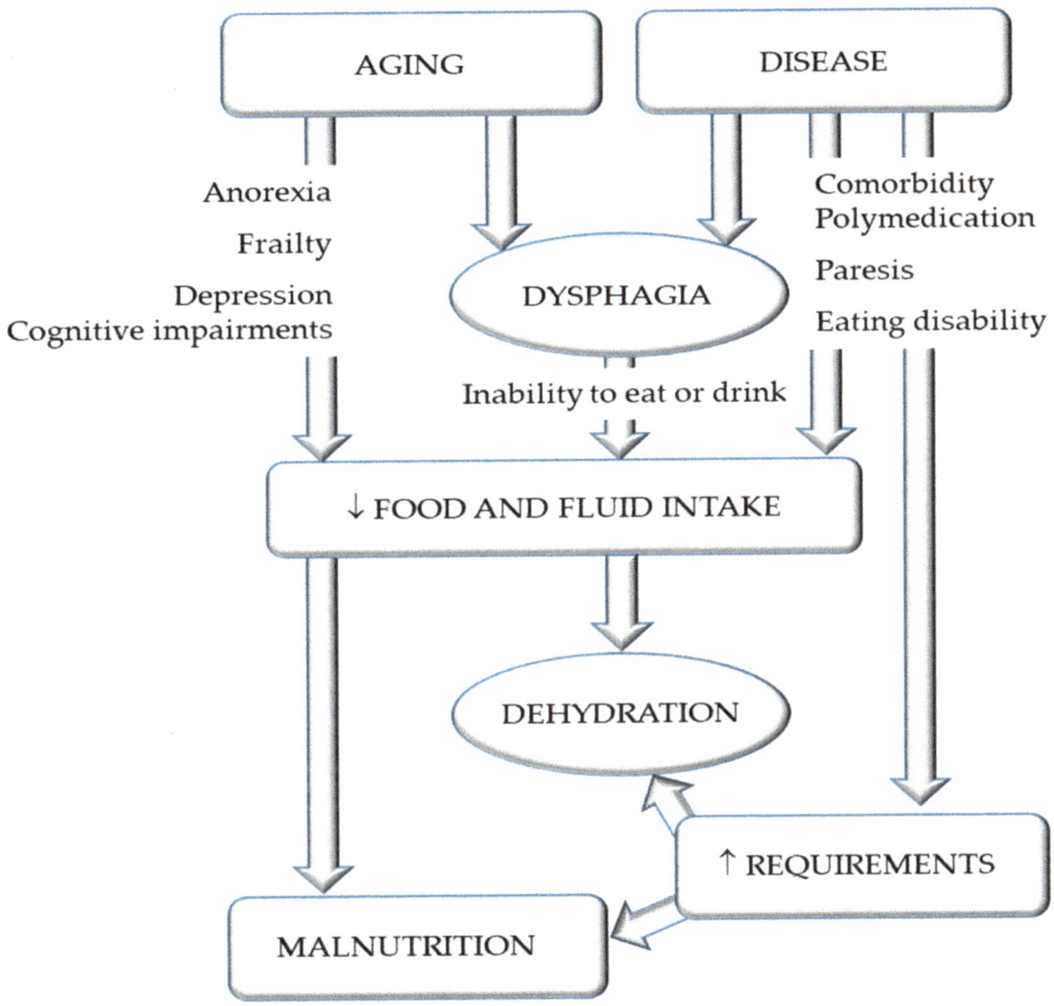


**Figure 1.** Risk factors for dehydration in dysphagia, modified after the work of [8].

## 4. Pathophysiological Considerations

### *4.1. Body Compartments*

Water distribution into the different body compartments in healthy individuals is shown in Figure 2. Body water fulfils many physiological functions: it regulates body temperature and absorbs shocks, it is a solvent for chemical reactions, it serves as transport medium, and it contributes to the removal of waste products. Water accounts for about 60% of body weight. This proportion may vary according to gender and age. Body water is generally somewhat less in women than in men owing to differences in body composition. The body water is divided intracellular (two-thirds of body water) and extracellular (one-third of body water) space. The water within the extracellular space is further divided into intravascular (1/12 of body water) and extravascular (3/4 of body water) fluid by the capillary wall. The extravascular compartment may be further divided into interstitial/transcellular fluids.

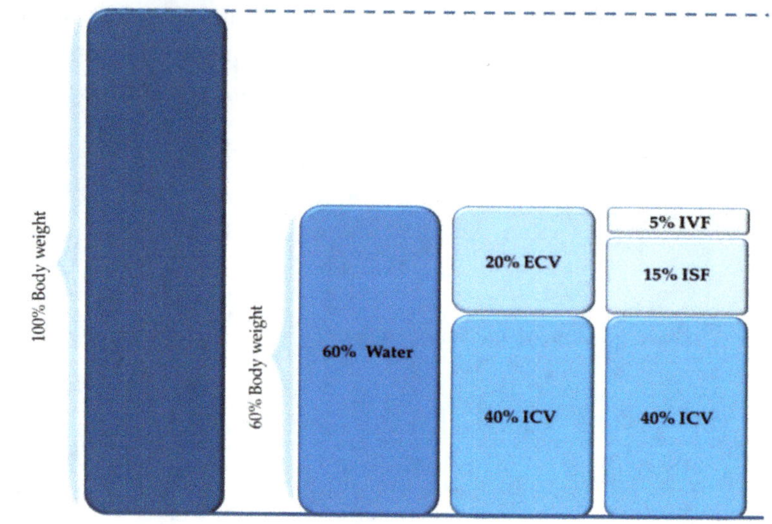


**Figure 2.** The repartition of body water within the different compartments as percentage of body weight [35]. ICV: Intracellular volume; ECV: Extracellular volume; ISF: Interstitial fluid; IVF: Intravascular fluids.

*4.2. External Fluid Balance*

Fluid balance is a complex interplay of numerous organs (e.g., skin, respiratory tract, kidneys, and gastrointestinal tract). The typical daily fluid turnover amounts to approximately 2600 mL (30–40 mL/kg body weight). Liquids represent about 1500 mL of daily input; 800 mL comes from liquids within solid food and a further 300 mL comes from oxidation water (Figure 3). The main water output (1500 mL) passes through the kidneys. The insensible perspiration composed of water losses from respiration and transpiration accounts for a substantial loss (Figure 3), while faeces alone represent a loss of 100–150 mL per day. The regulation of the sodium balance is essential for the maintenance of normal blood volume. The regulation of the water balance, however, relies on the maintenance of osmolarity. Volume maintenance has priority at any time on osmolality. The regulation of water balance also strongly relies on the capability of the kidney to excrete urine with an osmolality different from plasma, as kidneys are very efficacious in retaining sodium, but only hardly evacuate its surplus.

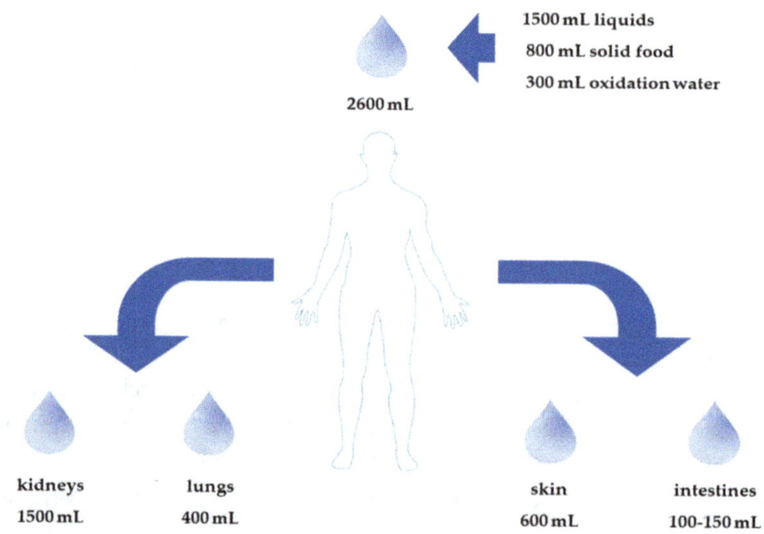


**Figure 3.** Fluid balance [35]. This figure shows the sites involved in fluid loss.

### 4.3. Internal Fluid Balance

The distribution of water within the body compartments undergoes strict control. Semipermeable cell membranes separating the intracellular and extracellular space enable the passage of water and selected molecules. The quantity of solutes per kilogram of solution is referred to as osmolality and usually fluctuates around 275 to 290 mOsm/kg. It may be directly measured or calculated with the following equation:

$$2 \times (\text{serum sodium (mmol/L)}) + \text{BUN (mg/dL)}/2.8 + \text{plasma glucose (mg/dL)}/18.$$

Tonicity is defined by the solutes determining the transcellular distribution of water, referred to as effective osmoles. Inactive osmole (e.g., urea) can freely pass the membrane and their rise in serum does not trigger water movement toward extracellular space. Nevertheless, inactive osmoles contribute to osmolality. Plasma osmolality is mostly determined by sodium (extracellular) and potassium (intracellular). Potassium in the extracellular fluid reaches 2% of the total body potassium. Anions such as chloride and bicarbonate and proteins grant the electroneutrality (Table 1). The first determining factor for the distribution of body water is the osmotic forces. Osmotic changes will immediately trigger the movement of water from lower to higher osmolarity, which has to be similar on both sides of the cell membrane.

**Table 1.** Electrolyte concentrations in the human body [5,52].

| Electrolyte | Plasma (mmol/L) | Extracellular Volume (mmol/L) | Intracellular Volume (mmol/L) |
|---|---|---|---|
| Sodium | 135–145 | 142–155 | 10–18 |
| Potassium | 3.5–5.3 | 4.0–5.5 | 120–145 |
| Calcium | 2.2–2.6 | 2.2–2.5 | 1.5 |
| Chloride | 95–105 | 98–108 | 2–6 |
| Magnesium | 0.8–1.2 | 0.7–1.2 | 15–25 |
| Phosphate | 0.81–1.45 | 0.7–1.3 | 8–20 |
| Bicarbonate | 22–30 | 22–30 | 10 |

## 5. Disorders of Fluid Balance

### 5.1. Isotonic and Hypotonic Dehydration

The term "isotonic dehydration" may be confusing to a certain degree as it in fact more refers to volume depletion than to dehydration. Isotonic dehydration occurs when the loss of water and solutes is balanced, reducing the volume of extracellular fluid, leading to reduced perfusion of the tissues, while osmolality and thus the intracellular fluid volume are kept normal (Figure 4). The reasons for this are manifold: fasting, haemorrhage, burns, gastrointestinal symptoms (vomiting, diarrhoea), drugs (sedative, diuretics), and so on. Renal perfusion is decrease owing to volume depletion and the renin–angiotensin–aldosterone system is thus activated, resulting in greater reabsorption of sodium and water. Secretion of ADH moreover causes water retention, aiming to correct volume depletion.

When sodium losses are greater than water losses, causing serum osmolality >270 mOsm/kg and sodium concentration >135 mmol/L in serum, "hypotonic dehydration" occurs. When fluids and sodium losses are partly replaced using hypotonic fluids, the extracellular space is reduced, owing to the low serum osmolality (Figure 4).

Both forms must be treated by means of isotonic fluids.

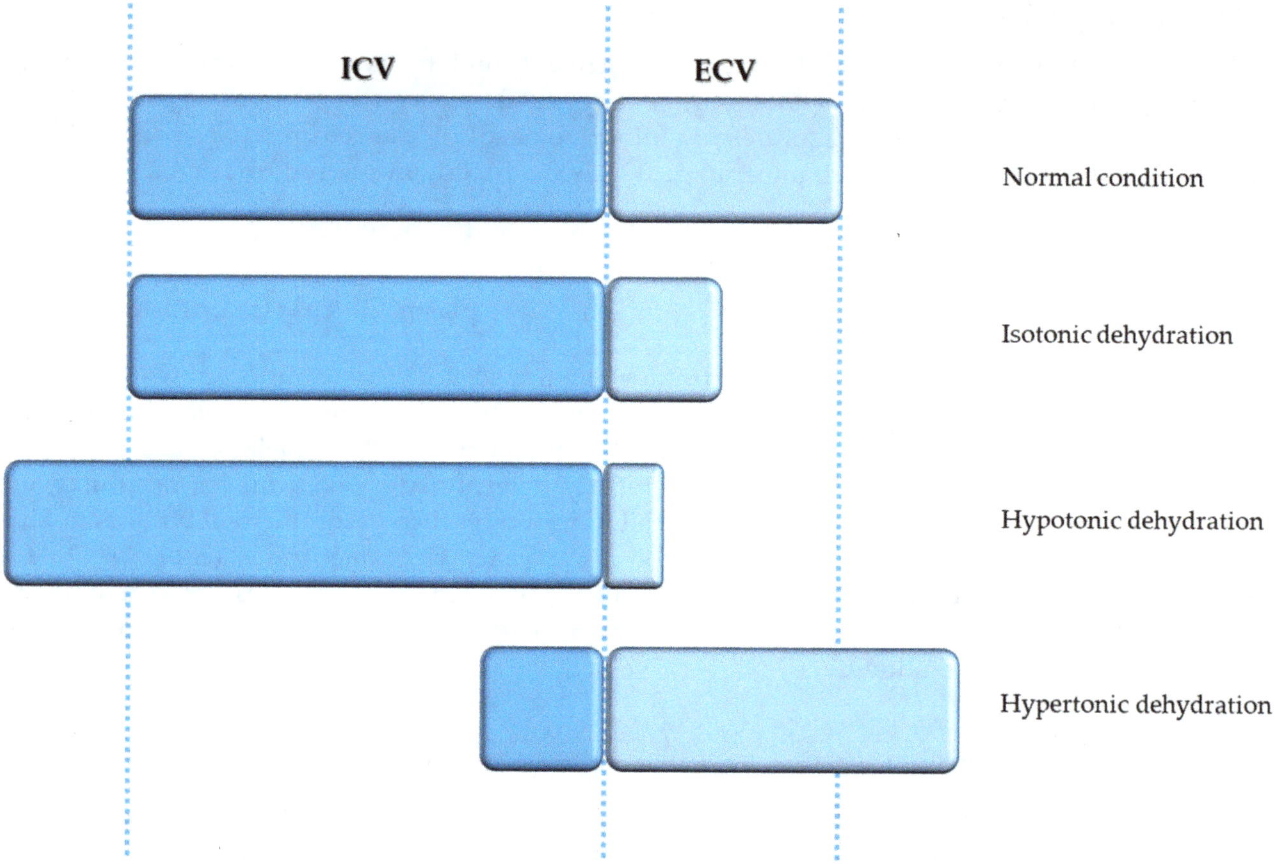


**Figure 4.** Water balance disturbances.

*5.2. Hypertonic Dehydration*

"Hypertonic dehydration" represents the pathophysiologic type of dehydration, where BUN to creatinine ratio is ≥20 and serum sodium concentrations exceed ≥150 mmol/L. Loss of water is higher than loss of sodium. The succeeding rise of sodium concentration in serum induces a rise in osmolality, which consecutively causes water to move towards the extracellular compartment, causing acute hypernatremia (Figure 4). Theses water movements also affect the brain, possibly causing a diminution in brain volume, and eventually causing rupture of veins and subsequent intracerebral or subarachnoid haemorrhage. Brain cells initially accumulate sodium and potassium, and later osmolytes (mainly myoinositol, glutamine, and glutamate), to compensate for water loss and restore volume [53,54]. As in dysphagia, hypertonic dehydration happens because of decreased water intake or as a result of either excessive (extra) renal water losses. Many factors may cause renal water losses such as renal or central diabetes insipidus, polyuric phase of acute renal failure, loop or osmotic diuretics, post obstructive disease, and so on. Extra renal water losses are the result of transcutaneous losses (e.g., sweat, fever, burns) or losses over the respiratory tract (e.g., hyperventilation). The consecutive rise in osmolality activates ADH release, and thus thirst (Figure 5). ADH secretion may be triggered by non osmolar volume-depending receptors or by supraoptic and paraventricular nuclei of the thalamus. The latest causes a reduced free water excretion. Above the threshold for ADH secretion in humans, which is 280–285 mOsm/kg, ADH secretion rises in a linear manner with rising osmolality (Figure 6). The threshold value for thirst, the major protective physiological mechanism of the body to compensate for hypernatremia, is higher than the ADH threshold [55].

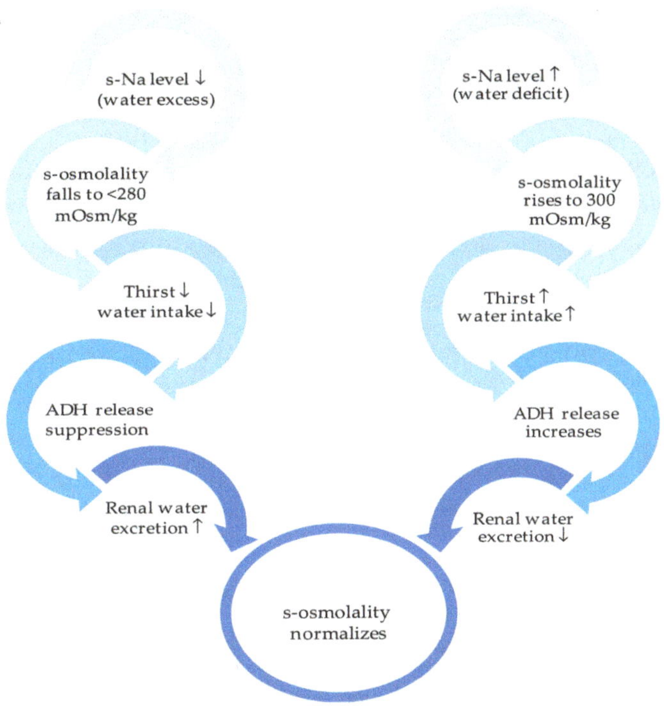


**Figure 5.** Regulation mechanisms of sodium and water. s-Na: Serum sodium; s-osmolarity: Serum osmolarity; ADH: Antidiuretic hormone.

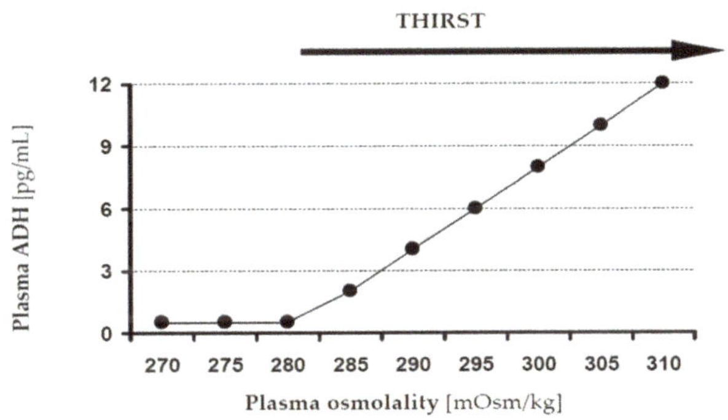


**Figure 6.** ADH release and thirst [56]. ADH: Antidiuretic hormone.

Hypotonic fluids represent the best treatment option for hypertonic dehydration.

## 6. Clinical and Biochemical Diagnostic Features

The sensitivity and specificity of dehydration signs largely depend on the volume of blood loss, where the clearest signs are heart rates changes (30 beats per minute) or severe postural dizziness leading to a lack of ability to stand [57]. Medication (e.g., beta-blockers) and older age may further influence sensitivity and specificity of these signs. Signs consecutive to fluid and electrolyte losses (e.g., due to vomiting or diarrhoea) are less clear.

Clinical signs taken alone are not very useful. A combination of at least four signs described hereafter indicates moderate to severe volume depletion. Typical clinical signs of dehydration with high scientific value are listed in Table 2. Absence of tears, transpiration, and/or thirst are among others symptoms of dehydration [33,58,59]. Clinical features with poor sensitivity and specificity are as follows: dry mucous membrane, low skin turgor, long nail bed refill time, altered respiratory pattern, changes in heart rate, dry or furrowed tongue, dry axilla, absence of tears, sunken eyes, high palpated ocular pressure, and weight loss [33,57]. The highest diagnostic utility was given by systolic blood pressure <100 mmHg in a clinical trial [58]. Owing to the loss of subcutaneous tissue with aging skin, turgor is not reliable in the elderly population. If present, dry axilla is fairly used with an appositive likelihood ratio of 2.8 (sensitivity 50%, specificity 82%) [60]. Symptoms that have a sensitivity over 80% are furrows on the tongue, dry mucous membranes, speech incoherence, extremity weakness, and orthostasis. Sunken eyes show a specificity greater than 80% and a sensitivity of 62% [32]. Central nervous system symptoms like confusion, speech difficulty, or weakness in the extremities are manifest when dehydration results in a 1% loss of body weight and are more notable at a 5% loss [32,58,61]. The development of neurologic effects is more likely to occur in acute hypernatremia developing within 48 hours than in chronic cases. Severe dehydration may cause hypotension, including the related risk of falls, reduced cardiac output, as well as consecutive reduced blood flow through organs and tissues. It may also escalate to hypovolemic shock. The risk for chronic renal disease, morbidity, and mortality are increased in the case of chronic dehydration (mild to severe) if not treated [62–64].

**Table 2.** Single signs, symptoms, and laboratory tests to identify dehydration [33,58,59].

| Assessment of Hydration Status | Feasibility of Test | Scientific Value |
|---|---|---|
| **Signs and symptoms** | | |
| Seated systolic blood pressure ≤100 mmHg | H | H |
| Blood pressure change supine/standing ≥20 mmHg | H | H |
| Thirst sensation | H | M |
| Dark urine colour | H | M |
| **Laboratory tests** | | |
| Urine specific gravity ≥1.025 | H | H |
| Blood urea nitrogen/creatinine ratio ≥20 | M | H |
| Blood osmolality calculated ≥300 mmol/kg | M | H |
| Haematocrit/haemoglobin ratio | M | M |
| Mean corpuscular volume | M | M |
| Serum sodium concentration >150 mmol/L | M | M |
| **Additional measurements** (mainly for scientific purposes) | | |
| Total body water (isotope dilution) | L | M |
| Total body water (bioelectrical impedance analysis) | H | M |
| Fluid volumes and ionic content (neutron activation analysis) | L | M |
| Blood osmolality (measured) | M | H |
| Urine osmolality | H | H |
| Salivary osmolality | H | H |
| Tear osmolality | M | M |
| Intraocular pressure (measured) | M | L |

H = high; M = medium; L = low.

Although the patient's history and physical examination may indicate the appearance of dehydration (symptoms and signs), it is obvious that medical staff should not only rely on these clinical data, but also have to integrate biochemical parameters to enable the diagnosis (Table 2) [33,58,59]. Plasma osmolarity ≥300 mOsm/kg, plasma sodium, urine specific gravity, tear, and saliva osmolality have all been shown to be suitable to diagnose dehydration [58,65,66]. For an optimal diagnostic strategy, you need at least calculate or measure BUN, glucose, creatinine, sodium, bicarbonate, and osmolality [32].

## 7. Management of Dehydration

### 7.1. General Recommendations

The identification of acute situations potentially leading to dehydration, as well as the monitoring of vital parameters, clinical signs and symptoms, and laboratory parameters (Table 2), are of utmost importance. Fluid balance (including intake and output) should additionally be monitored. Skin integrity (including mucous membranes) and drug treatments (mainly diuretics) may impact the water and electrolyte balance, as well as diseases or conditions affecting renal perfusion (e.g., heart failure, chronic kidney disease) [33,67,68]. The evidence suggests that multicomponent interventions (including increased staff awareness, assistance with drinking, support using the toilet, and a greater variety of drinks on offer) may be effective [69]. Fluid therapy may be used for resuscitation, replacement, or maintenance of the fluid balance depending on the stage of illness. The National Institute for Health and Care Excellence (NICE) provides a set of interrelated algorithms for assessment, fluid resuscitation, routine intravenous maintenance, and replacement and redistribution of fluid and electrolytes [70]. Resuscitation may be needed in the case of considerable blood loss (e.g., surgery, injury) or plasma loss (e.g., burns, acute pancreatitis). Fluids are then immediately needed to maintain circulation and organ vital function [70]. Fluid maintenance may be initiated once the vital signs and urine output are normalized.

The maintenance of fluid and electrolyte balance is the key to prevent and treat dehydration. Maintenance aims to restore insensible losses and provide sufficient water and electrolytes to maintain the normal status of body fluid compartments and sufficient water to enable the kidneys to excrete waste products. Maintenance fluid prescriptions should target the daily requirements and replace ongoing abnormal losses. Requirements of patients receiving artificial nutrition are mostly covered though the artificial nutrition itself. Special attention is needed regarding overhydration, particularly in patients suffering congestive heart failure. The best route/method/fluid for administration depends on the severity/nature/acuteness of dehydration. Oral administration should be the preferred option, although parenteral administration of fluids may be mandatory in some cases. Such prescriptions must be changed to oral administration as soon as possible, as fluids prescriptions are often maintained too long, causing infects and oedema, especially in the postoperative phase. Subcutaneous infusions should be considered to manage chronic problems, particularly in the elderly [5]. A calculation of fluids requirements has been proposed by Chidester et al. [71], suggesting the prescription of 100 mL per kilogram body weight for first 10 kg, 50 mL per kilogram for next 10 kg, and 15 mL for the remaining kilograms of body weight. When body temperature is higher than 37 °C, 100–150 mL should additionally be given.

### 7.2. Oral/Enteral Replacement

Fluid and electrolyte requirements should be met via oral or enteral routes as far as possible when fluid resuscitation is not needed [70]. The first measure to replace fluid loss should be offering thickened liquids or food with high fluids content, whereas sodium-containing food and liquids must be avoided. As previously mentioned, the evidence level for such interventions is, however, weak [72]. Enteral liquid administration (via feeding tube) may be appropriate in the case of severe dysphagia or if maintaining fluid balance is not possible. Moderate dehydration (loss of 1.5–2% body weight) may easily be corrected with the administration of oral or enteral fluids, but already alters moods and causes decreased physical and cognitive performance [62,63,73,74]. Treatment for low-intake dehydration involves administration of hypotonic fluids [36], which will help correct the fluid deficit while diluting the raised osmolality. Oral rehydration therapy (aiming the replacement of electrolytes lost in volume depletion by diarrhoea or vomiting) and sports drinks are not indicated. Hydration status should be reassessed regularly until corrected, and then regularly monitored.

### *7.3. Parenteral Replacement*

The parenteral administration of (low sodium-containing) fluids is the method of choice in the case of severe dehydration (high amounts of fluid needed) or when intravenous access is anyway given for administration of medication or nutrition [36,70]. Intravenous hydration must, however, always be regarded to as a medical treatment and not as basic care. The risk and benefit balance must be cautiously considered. Figure 7 illustrates the distribution of different fluids within body compartments after infusion. Deficits in free water must be substituted quickly if hypernatremia lasts for shorter than 48 hours. To avoid oedemas, caused by fluids shifts, high-rate administration of intravenous hypotonic solutions must be prevented. As its cells accumulate osmolytes to maintain normal cell volume, the brain is especially endangered. Brain oedema may develop as a result of hasty administration of hypotonic solutions. Fluids must hence be administered progressively, over 12 to 48 h. Hyponatraemia lasting for more than 48 h have to be corrected slowly. Not more than half of the replacement should occur in the first 24 hours of treatment, during which one should look out extremely cautiously for brain oedema, the symptoms of which may be headache or seizures. The residual replacement may occur within the next 48 to 72 h. In the case of hypernatremia, fluid replacement is considered adequate when the urine sodium concentration is over 25 mmol/L.

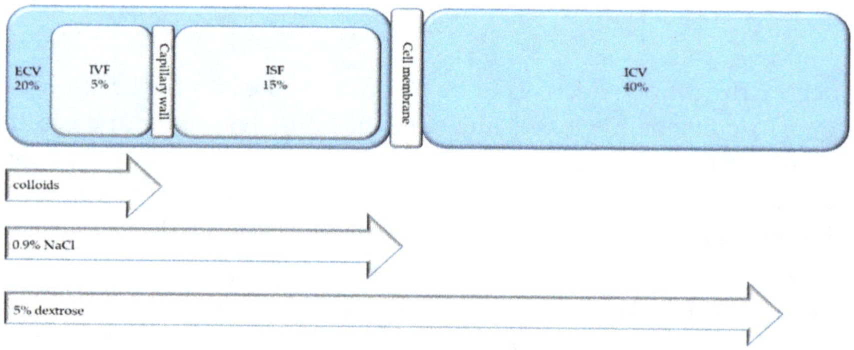


**Figure 7.** Infused fluids across the body compartments. ECV: Extracellular volume, ICV: Intracellular volume, IVF: Intravascular fluids, ISF: Interstitial fluids, NaCl: Sodium chloride.

## 8. Hypodermoclysis

Evidence has shown that adequate volumes of subcutaneous infusions are an effective treatment for dehydration, showing comparable rates of adverse effects to parenteral administration [36,75]. Many clinical trials have shown the safety and effectiveness of fluid infusion into the subcutaneous space using a fine cannula, called hypodermoclysis (HDC), making it a possible alternative to parenteral administration. HDC is particularly useful for the rehydration of patients with mild to moderate dehydration, who are cannot keep their fluid balance via the oral route [76–78]. Preferred sites for HDC are, for example, the anterior chest wall, lateral abdominal wall, inner tight, and back above or below shoulder blade. Recommendations for fluid infusion rates differ; that is, using gravity, up to 1,500 mL may be infused over 24 h at one site (rate of 20–80 mL/h), while rates of 82–148 mL/h have been recommended as well [32,79–81]. The authors' clinical experience indicates the safety of infusion of 500 mL per hour. A study using radioactive labelled injection showed that absorption into the blood occurs within one hour [82]. Infusion solutions are chosen regarding the clinical condition of the patient (balanced solutions, saline solutions, dextrose solutions, or their combination). A study among dement nursing home residents suffering dehydration showed more agitation (80%) in subjects receiving parenteral fluids compared with those receiving subcutaneous fluids (37%), regardless of the volume of administered fluid or the improvement of dehydration [83].

Subcutaneous infusions with hyaluronidase (useful enzyme to break down hyaluronic acid, thus opening the interstitial space) usually permit a more rapid infusion rate, lower rate of moderate oedema, and more comfort for the patient. Even though there are no systematic studies available, administering up to 20 mmol/L potassium chloride appears unproblematic. Local adverse effects (e.g., oedema, erythema, and cellulitis) and systemic adverse effects (e.g., heart failure or hyponatremia) occur rarely and at similar rates compared with parenteral administration [78]. The effectiveness of both methods appears to be the same. The expense for HDC is about four times less than intravenous administration and demands reduced nursing care [83,84]. HDC use may be easily used in a community setting (nursing home or home), by patients and/or their caregivers [77]. HDC is suitable to prevent dehydration or to treat mild to moderate dehydration. Intravenous fluid replacement remains mandatory, however, to treat hypovolemic shock or severe dehydration.

*Colloids and (Balanced) Crystalloids*

The volume of distribution and the metabolization of the solute are the two main factors to determine the plasma expansion capacity of a solution. Colloids are principally distributed within the intravascular space, while dextrose solutions are first metabolized and then distributed within the whole body water. Their volume expansion ability is hence limited and temporary. Resuscitation should thus be undertaken using colloids. Intravascular volume expansion is mostly done using crystalloids. If appropriated, dextrose solutions (5% or combined with saline) are used to provide free water. The expansion capacity of isotonic crystalloids, distributed within the extracellular fluids, is 20% to 25%. The remaining crystalloid volume is kept within the interstitial space. This overload of interstitial fluid has to be eliminated after the acute phase of the disease is over. Even if the use of crystalloid solutions is effective, the price to pay remains quite high. Additionally, the excessive use of sodium-containing crystalloids may cause oedema and further impair the clinical outcome. Dextrose solutions may cause potential harmful effects as well (e.g., hyponatraemia $<130$ mM). Hypochloraemic acidosis may occur as a result of the administration of saline, as they contain much higher concentrations of chloride compared with plasma. This may seriously impair the kidney function (reduced perfusion and glomerular filtration rates), the gastrointestinal function (mucosal acidosis, ileus), or other cellular dysfunction including impairment of mitochondrial function. Recent studies have shown the superiority of balanced electrolyte solutions (Hartmann's or Ringer's) on saline solutions replacing water and salt deficits, except for cases of gastric juice losses, where chloride losses are high [5]. Isotonic dextrose solutions should be used to replace deficits in free water. Colloid solutions such as albumin or hydroxyethyl starch should be used to expand volume, as they induce less salt/water overloads and oedemas than crystalloid solutions (e.g., dextrose 5%, 0.9% NaCl, and balanced crystalloids). The combination of both in varying proportions may be used in the clinical practice, depending on the patient's condition. Newly published trials show balanced crystalloids to be superior on saline solutions in critical and non-critical care [85,86]. These trials showed a lower rate of the composite outcome of death from any cause, new renal-replacement therapy, or persistent renal dysfunction with balanced crystalloids than with saline (number needed to treat 1/94).

## 9. Conclusions

Dehydration is a relevant clinical problem with severe consequences, particularly in patients suffering from dysphagia, whose fluids' intake is very restricted by the use of thickeners. At least in one-third of inpatients, dehydration is misdiagnosed and thus underestimated as well as undertreated. It is very important for the medical and nursing staff dealing with patients suffering dysphagia to be aware of dehydration, and work closely with speech-language pathologists and dietitians to place a nutrition and hydration care plan tailored to the needs and condition of each patient. Volume depletion, treated with isotonic fluids, and dehydration treated with hypotonic fluids, must be clearly taken apart. Rehydration should be treated by the oral (or enteral) route whenever possible. Parenteral rehydration must be used in severe cases. The use of HDC may be considered in the case of mild dehydration when there are contraindications for oral/enteral treatment. It represents an effective and safe treatment option, especially in patients with dysphagia.

**Author Contributions:** Conceptualization, E.R. and Z.S.; writing—original draft preparation, E.R.; writing—review and editing, F.G., I.A.D., M.F.V. and Z.S.; supervision, Z.S.

## References

1. Burgos, R.; Breton, I.; Cereda, E.; Desport, J.C.; Dziewas, R.; Genton, L.; Gomes, F.; Jesus, P.; Leischker, A.; Muscaritoli, M.; et al. ESPEN guideline clinical nutrition in neurology. *Clin. Nutr.* **2018**, *37*, 354–396. [CrossRef] [PubMed]
2. Geeganage, C.; Beavan, J.; Ellender, S.; Bath, P.M. Interventions for dysphagia and nutritional support in acute and subacute stroke. *Cochrane. Database Syst. Rev.* **2012**. [CrossRef] [PubMed]
3. Madhavan, A.; LaGorio, L.A.; Crary, M.A.; Dahl, W.J.; Carnaby, G.D. Prevalence of and Risk Factors for Dysphagia in the Community Dwelling Elderly: A Systematic Review. *J. Nutr. Health Aging* **2016**, *20*, 806–815. [CrossRef] [PubMed]
4. Vivanti, A.P.; Campbell, K.L.; Suter, M.S.; Hannan-Jones, M.T.; Hulcombe, J.A. Contribution of thickened drinks, food and enteral and parenteral fluids to fluid intake in hospitalised patients with dysphagia. *J. Hum. Nutr. Diet* **2009**, *22*, 148–155. [CrossRef] [PubMed]
5. Lobo, D.; Lewington, A.; Allison, S. Basic concepts of fluid and electrolyte therapy. *Clin. Med.* **2013**. [CrossRef]
6. Bartolome, G.; Schröter-Morasch, H. *Schluckstörungen: Diagnostik und Rehabilitation*; Elsevier, Urban & Fischer: Munich, Germany, 2013.
7. Prosiegel, M.; Weber, S. *Dysphagie: Diagnostik und Therapie: Ein Wegweiser für Kompetentes Handeln*; Springer: Berlin, Germany, 2018.
8. Wirth, R.; Dziewas, R.; Beck, A.M.; Clave, P.; Hamdy, S.; Heppner, H.J.; Langmore, S.; Leischker, A.H.; Martino, R.; Pluschinski, P.; et al. Oropharyngeal dysphagia in older persons—From pathophysiology to adequate intervention: A review and summary of an international expert meeting. *Clin. Interv. Aging* **2016**, *11*, 189–208. [CrossRef]
9. Amella, E.J. Feeding and hydration issues for older adults with dementia. *Nurs. Clin. North Am.* **2004**, *39*, 607–623. [CrossRef]
10. Kolb, C. *Nahrungsverweigerung bei Demenzkranken: PEG-Sonde-Ja oder Nein?* Mabuse-Verlag: Frankfurt am Main, Germany, 2004.
11. Schreier, M.M.; Bartholomeyczik, S. *Mangelernährung bei Alten und Pflegebedürftigen Menschen: Ursachen und Prävention aus Pflegerischer Perspektive-Review/Literaturanalyse*; Schlütersche: Hannover, Germany, 2004.
12. Baijens, L.W.; Clave, P.; Cras, P.; Ekberg, O.; Forster, A.; Kolb, G.F.; Leners, J.C.; Masiero, S.; Mateos-Nozal, J.; Ortega, O.; et al. European society for swallowing disorders—European union geriatric medicine society white paper: Oropharyngeal dysphagia as a geriatric syndrome. *Clin. Interv. Aging* **2016**, *11*, 1403–1428. [CrossRef]
13. Tagliaferri, S.; Lauretani, F.; Pela, G.; Meschi, T.; Maggio, M. The risk of dysphagia is associated with malnutrition and poor functional outcomes in a large population of outpatient older individuals. *Clin. Nutr.* **2018**. [CrossRef]
14. Logemann, J.A.; Veis, S.; Colangelo, L. A screening procedure for oropharyngeal dysphagia. *Dysphagia* **1999**, *14*, 44–51. [CrossRef]
15. Sonies, B.C. Swallowing disorders and rehabilitation techniques. *J. Pediatr. Gastroenterol. Nutr.* **1997**, *25*, S32–S33. [CrossRef] [PubMed]
16. Ickenstein, G.; Hofmayer, A.; Lindner-Pfleghar, B.; Pluschinski, P.; Riecker, A.; Schelling, A.; Prosiegel, M. Standardisierung des Untersuchungsablaufs bei neurogener oropharyngealer Dysphagie (NOD). *Neurol. Rehabil.* **2009**, *15*, 290–300.
17. Wu, M.-C.; Chang, Y.-C.; Wang, T.-G.; Lin, L.-C. Evaluating swallowing dysfunction using a 100-mL water swallowing test. *Dysphagia* **2004**, *19*, 43–47. [CrossRef] [PubMed]
18. Marcotte, P. Critical Review: Effectiveness of FEES in Comparison to VFSS at Identifying Aspiration. Available online: https://www.uwo.ca/fhs/lwm/teaching/EBP/2006_07/Marcotte.pdf (accessed on 7 November 2007).

19. Yamamura, K.; Kurose, M.; Okamoto, K. Guide to Enhancing Swallowing Initiation: Insights from Findings in Healthy Subjects and Dysphagic Patients. *Curr. Phys. Med. Rehabil. Rep.* **2018**, *6*, 178–185. [CrossRef] [PubMed]
20. Dennis, M.; Lewis, S.; Cranswick, G.; Forbes, J. FOOD: A multicentre randomised trial evaluating feeding policies in patients admitted to hospital with a recent stroke. *Health Technol. Assess.* **2006**, *10*, 1–120. [CrossRef]
21. Foley, N.; Finestone, H.; Woodbury, M.G.; Teasell, R.; Greene Finestone, L. Energy and protein intakes of acute stroke patients. *J. Nutr. Health Aging* **2006**, *10*, 171–175.
22. Whelan, K. Inadequate fluid intakes in dysphagic acute stroke. *Clin. Nutr.* **2001**, *20*, 423–428. [CrossRef]
23. Cichero, J.A. Thickening agents used for dysphagia management: Effect on bioavailability of water, medication and feelings of satiety. *Nutr. J.* **2013**. [CrossRef]
24. Clave, P.; de Kraa, M.; Arreola, V.; Girvent, M.; Farre, R.; Palomera, E.; Serra-Prat, M. The effect of bolus viscosity on swallowing function in neurogenic dysphagia. *Aliment. Pharmacol. Ther.* **2006**, *24*, 1385–1394. [CrossRef]
25. Steele, C.M.; Alsanei, W.A.; Ayanikalath, S.; Barbon, C.E.; Chen, J.; Cichero, J.A.; Coutts, K.; Dantas, R.O.; Duivestein, J.; Giosa, L.; et al. The influence of food texture and liquid consistency modification on swallowing physiology and function: A systematic review. *Dysphagia* **2015**, *30*, 2–26. [CrossRef]
26. Cichero, J.A.; Lam, P.; Steele, C.M.; Hanson, B.; Chen, J.; Dantas, R.O.; Duivestein, J.; Kayashita, J.; Lecko, C.; Murray, J.; et al. Development of international terminology and definitions for texture-modified foods and thickened fluids used in dysphagia management: The IDDSI framework. *Dysphagia* **2017**, *32*, 293–314. [CrossRef] [PubMed]
27. Marcason, W. What is the international dysphagia diet standardisation initiative? *J. Acad. Nutr. Diet* **2017**. [CrossRef] [PubMed]
28. Cichero, J.A.; Steele, C.; Duivestein, J.; Clave, P.; Chen, J.; Kayashita, J.; Dantas, R.; Lecko, C.; Speyer, R.; Lam, P.; et al. The need for international terminology and definitions for texture-modified foods and thickened liquids used in dysphagia management: Foundations of a global initiative. *Curr. Phys. Med. Rehabil. Rep.* **2013**, *1*, 280–291. [CrossRef] [PubMed]
29. International Dysphagia Diet Standardisation Committee. Complete International Dysphagia Diet Standardisation Initiative (IDDSI) Framework: Detailed Definitions. Available online: https://iddsi.org/Documents/IDDSIFramework-CompleteFramework.pdf (accessed on 29 July 2019).
30. Lippert, W.C.; Chadha, R.; Sweigart, J.R. Things We Do for No Reason: The Use of Thickened Liquids in Treating Hospitalized Adult Patients with Dysphagia. *J. Hosp. Med.* **2019**, *14*, 315–317. [CrossRef] [PubMed]
31. Mange, K.; Matsuura, D.; Cizman, B.; Soto, H.; Ziyadeh, F.N.; Goldfarb, S.; Neilson, E.G. Language guiding therapy: The case of dehydration versus volume depletion. *Ann. Intern. Med.* **1997**, *127*, 848–853. [CrossRef]
32. Thomas, D.R.; Cote, T.R.; Lawhorne, L.; Levenson, S.A.; Rubenstein, L.Z.; Smith, D.A.; Stefanacci, R.G.; Tangalos, E.G.; Morley, J.E. Understanding clinical dehydration and its treatment. *J. Am. Med. Dir. Assoc.* **2008**, *9*, 292–301. [CrossRef]
33. Armstrong, L.E.; Kavouras, S.A.; Walsh, N.P.; Roberts, W.O. Diagnosing dehydration? Blend evidence with clinical observations. *Curr. Opin. Clin. Nutr. Metab. Care.* **2016**, *19*, 434–438. [CrossRef]
34. Weinberg, A.D.; Minaker, K.L. Dehydration. Evaluation and management in older adults. Council on Scientific Affairs, American Medical Association. *JAMA* **1995**, *274*, 1552–1556. [CrossRef]
35. Stanga, Z.; Aubry, E. Dehydration in Dysphagia. In *Dysphagia: Diagnosis and Treatment*; Ekberg, O., Ed.; Springer International Publishing: Cham, Switzerland, 2019; pp. 859–871.
36. Volkert, D.; Beck, A.M.; Cederholm, T.; Cruz-Jentoft, A.; Goisser, S.; Hooper, L.; Kiesswetter, E.; Maggio, M.; Raynaud-Simon, A.; Sieber, C.C.; et al. ESPEN guideline on clinical nutrition and hydration in geriatrics. *Clin. Nutr.* **2019**, *38*, 10–47. [CrossRef]
37. Institute of Medicine; Food and Nutrition Board; Panel on Dietary Reference Intakes for Electrolytes and Water; Standing Committee on the Scientific Evaluation of Dietary Reference Intakes. *DRI, Dietary Reference Intakes for Water, Potassium, Sodium, Chloride, and Sulfate*; The National Academy Press: Washington, DC, USA, 2005.
38. EFSA Panel on Dietetic Products; Nutrition; Allergies (NDA). Scientific opinion on dietary reference values for water. *EFSA J.* **2010**. [CrossRef]

39. Stookey, J.D.; Pieper, C.F.; Cohen, H.J. Is the prevalence of dehydration among community-dwelling older adults really low? Informing current debate over the fluid recommendation for adults aged 70+years. *Public Health Nutr.* **2005**, *8*, 1275–1285. [CrossRef] [PubMed]
40. Bennett, J.A.; Thomas, V.; Riegel, B. Unrecognized chronic dehydration in older adults: Examining prevalence rate and risk factors. *J. Gerontol. Nurs.* **2004**, *30*, 22–28. [CrossRef] [PubMed]
41. Xiao, H.; Barber, J.; Campbell, E.S. Economic burden of dehydration among hospitalized elderly patients. *Am. J. Health Syst. Pharm.* **2004**, *61*, 2534–2540. [CrossRef] [PubMed]
42. Martin, J.H.; Larsen, P.D. Dehydration in the elderly surgical patient. *AORN J.* **1994**, *60*, 666–671. [CrossRef]
43. Warren, J.L.; Bacon, W.E.; Harris, T.; McBean, A.M.; Foley, D.J.; Phillips, C. The burden and outcomes associated with dehydration among US elderly, 1991. *Am. J. Public Health* **1994**, *84*, 1265–1269. [CrossRef]
44. Murray, J.; Doeltgen, S.; Miller, M.; Scholten, I. A Descriptive Study of the Fluid Intake, Hydration, and Health Status of Rehabilitation Inpatients without Dysphagia Following Stroke. *J. Nutr. Gerontol. Geriatr.* **2015**, *34*, 292–304. [CrossRef]
45. Leibovitz, A.; Baumoehl, Y.; Lubart, E.; Yaina, A.; Platinovitz, N.; Segal, R. Dehydration among long-term care elderly patients with oropharyngeal dysphagia. *Gerontology* **2007**, *53*, 179–183. [CrossRef]
46. Thomas, D.R.; Tariq, S.H.; Makhdomm, S.; Haddad, R.; Moinuddin, A. Physician misdiagnosis of dehydration in older adults. *J. Am. Med. Dir. Assoc.* **2003**, *4*, 251–254. [CrossRef]
47. Phillips, P.A.; Johnston, C.I.; Gray, L. Disturbed fluid and electrolyte homoeostasis following dehydration in elderly people. *Age Ageing* **1993**, *22*, S26–S33. [CrossRef]
48. Luckey, A.E.; Parsa, C.J. Fluid and electrolytes in the aged. *Arch. Surg.* **2003**, *138*, 1055–1060. [CrossRef]
49. Mentes, J. Oral hydration in older adults: Greater awareness is needed in preventing, recognizing, and treating dehydration. *Am. J. Nurs.* **2006**, *106*, 40–49. [CrossRef] [PubMed]
50. Kayser-Jones, J.; Schell, E.S.; Porter, C.; Barbaccia, J.C.; Shaw, H. Factors contributing to dehydration in nursing homes: Inadequate staffing and lack of professional supervision. *J. Am. Geriatr. Soc.* **1999**, *47*, 1187–1194. [CrossRef] [PubMed]
51. Lavizzo-Mourey, R.; Johnson, J.; Stolley, P. Risk factors for dehydration among elderly nursing home residents. *J. Am. Geriatr. Soc.* **1988**, *36*, 213–218. [CrossRef] [PubMed]
52. Lubos, S.; Simon, A.; Zeno, S. Water and electrolytes in health and disease. In *Basics in Clinical Nutrition*, 5th ed.; Luboš, S., Ed.; Galen: Belfast, Ireland, 2019.
53. Heilig, C.W.; Stromski, M.E.; Blumenfeld, J.D.; Lee, J.P.; Gullans, S.R. Characterization of the major brain osmolytes that accumulate in salt-loaded rats. *Am. J. Physiol.* **1989**, *257*, F1108–F1116. [CrossRef]
54. Lien, Y.H.; Shapiro, J.I.; Chan, L. Effects of hypernatremia on organic brain osmoles. *J. Clin. Invest.* **1990**, *85*, 1427–1435. [CrossRef]
55. Robertson, G.L. Physiology of ADH secretion. *Kidney Int. Suppl.* **1987**, *21*, S20–S26.
56. Robertson, G.L.; Aycinena, P.; Zerbe, R.L. Neurogenic disorders of osmoregulation. *Am. J. Med.* **1982**, *72*, 339–353. [CrossRef]
57. McGee, S.; Abernethy, W.B., 3rd; Simel, D.L. The rational clinical examination. Is this patient hypovolemic? *JAMA* **1999**, *281*, 1022–1029. [CrossRef]
58. Fortes, M.B.; Owen, J.A.; Raymond-Barker, P.; Bishop, C.; Elghenzai, S.; Oliver, S.J.; Walsh, N.P. Is this elderly patient dehydrated? Diagnostic accuracy of hydration assessment using physical signs, urine, and saliva markers. *J. Am. Med. Dir. Assoc.* **2015**, *16*, 221–228. [CrossRef]
59. Hooper, L.; Abdelhamid, A.; Attreed, N.J.; Campbell, W.W.; Channell, A.M.; Chassagne, P.; Culp, K.R.; Fletcher, S.J.; Fortes, M.B.; Fuller, N.; et al. Clinical symptoms, signs and tests for identification of impending and current water-loss dehydration in older people. *Cochrane. Database Syst. Rev.* **2015**. [CrossRef]
60. Eaton, D.; Bannister, P.; Mulley, G.P.; Connolly, M.J. Axillary sweating in clinical assessment of dehydration in ill elderly patients. *BMJ* **1994**. [CrossRef] [PubMed]
61. Lieberman, H.R. Hydration and cognition: A critical review and recommendations for future research. *J. Am. Coll. Nutr.* **2007**, *26*, 555–561. [CrossRef] [PubMed]
62. Armstrong, L.E. Challenges of linking chronic dehydration and fluid consumption to health outcomes. *Nutr. Rev.* **2012**, *70*, S121–S127. [CrossRef] [PubMed]

63. Armstrong, L.E.; Ganio, M.S.; Casa, D.J.; Lee, E.C.; McDermott, B.P.; Klau, J.F.; Jimenez, L.; Le Bellego, L.; Chevillotte, E.; Lieberman, H.R. Mild dehydration affects mood in healthy young women. *J. Nutr.* **2012**, *142*, 382–388. [CrossRef]
64. Cowen, L.E.; Hodak, S.P.; Verbalis, J.G. Age-associated abnormalities of water homeostasis. *Endocrinol. Metab. Clin. North Am.* **2013**, *42*, 349–370. [CrossRef] [PubMed]
65. Cheuvront, S.N.; Kenefick, R.W.; Charkoudian, N.; Sawka, M.N. Physiologic basis for understanding quantitative dehydration assessment. *Am. J. Clin. Nutr.* **2013**, *97*, 455–462. [CrossRef] [PubMed]
66. Sollanek, K.J.; Kenefick, R.W.; Walsh, N.P.; Fortes, M.B.; Esmaeelpour, M.; Cheuvront, S.N. Assessment of thermal dehydration using the human eye: What is the potential? *J. Therm. Biol.* **2012**, *37*, 111–117. [CrossRef]
67. Clark, W.F.; Sontrop, J.M.; Huang, S.H.; Moist, L.; Bouby, N.; Bankir, L. Hydration and Chronic Kidney Disease Progression: A Critical Review of the Evidence. *Am. J. Nephrol.* **2016**, *43*, 281–292. [CrossRef]
68. Sontrop, J.M.; Dixon, S.N.; Garg, A.X.; Buendia-Jimenez, I.; Dohein, O.; Huang, S.H.; Clark, W.F. Association between water intake, chronic kidney disease, and cardiovascular disease: A cross-sectional analysis of NHANES data. *Am. J. Nephrol.* **2013**, *37*, 434–442. [CrossRef]
69. Bunn, D.; Jimoh, F.; Wilsher, S.H.; Hooper, L. Increasing fluid intake and reducing dehydration risk in older people living in long-term care: A systematic review. *J. Am. Med. Dir. Assoc.* **2015**, *16*, 101–113. [CrossRef]
70. National Clinical Guideline Centre (UK). Intravenous Fluid Therapy: Intravenous Fluid Therapy in Adults in Hospital. Available online: https://www.nice.org.uk/guidance/cg174 (accessed on 10 December 2013).
71. Chidester, J.C.; Spangler, A.A. Fluid intake in the institutionalized elderly. *J. Am. Diet Assoc.* **1997**, *97*, 23–28. [CrossRef]
72. Beck, A.M.; Kjaersgaard, A.; Hansen, T.; Poulsen, I. Systematic review and evidence based recommendations on texture modified foods and thickened liquids for adults (above 17 years) with oropharyngeal dysphagia—An updated clinical guideline. *Clin. Nutr.* **2018**, *37*, 1980–1991. [CrossRef] [PubMed]
73. Bardis, C.N.; Kavouras, S.A.; Kosti, L.; Markousi, M.; Sidossis, L.S. Mild hypohydration decreases cycling performance in the heat. *Med. Sci. Sports Exerc.* **2013**, *45*, 1782–1789. [CrossRef] [PubMed]
74. Watson, P.; Whale, A.; Mears, S.A.; Reyner, L.A.; Maughan, R.J. Mild hypohydration increases the frequency of driver errors during a prolonged, monotonous driving task. *Physiol. Behav.* **2015**, *147*, 313–318. [CrossRef] [PubMed]
75. Turner, T.; Cassano, A.M. Subcutaneous dextrose for rehydration of elderly patients–An evidence-based review. *BMC Geriatr.* **2004**. [CrossRef] [PubMed]
76. Dasgupta, M.; Binns, M.A.; Rochon, P.A. Subcutaneous fluid infusion in a long-term care setting. *J. Am. Geriatr. Soc.* **2000**, *48*, 795–799. [CrossRef]
77. Remington, R.; Hultman, T. Hypodermoclysis to treat dehydration: A review of the evidence. *J. Am. Geriatr. Soc.* **2007**, *55*, 2051–2055. [CrossRef]
78. Slesak, G.; Schnurle, J.W.; Kinzel, E.; Jakob, J.; Dietz, P.K. Comparison of subcutaneous and intravenous rehydration in geriatric patients: A randomized trial. *J. Am. Geriatr. Soc.* **2003**, *51*, 155–160. [CrossRef]
79. Jain, S.; Mansfield, B.; Wilcox, M.H. Subcutaneous fluid administration–Better than the intravenous approach? *J. Hosp. Infect.* **1999**, *41*, 269–272. [CrossRef]
80. Sasson, M.; Shvartzman, P. Hypodermoclysis: An alternative infusion technique. *Am. Fam. Physician.* **2001**, *64*, 1575–1578.
81. Walsh, G. Hypodermoclysis: An alternate method for rehydration in long-term care. *J. Infus. Nurs.* **2005**, *28*, 123–129. [CrossRef] [PubMed]
82. Lipschitz, S.; Campbell, A.J.; Roberts, M.S.; Wanwimolruk, S.; McQueen, E.G.; McQueen, M.; Firth, L.A. Subcutaneous fluid administration in elderly subjects: Validation of an under-used technique. *J. Am. Geriatr. Soc.* **1991**, *39*, 6–9. [CrossRef] [PubMed]
83. O'Keeffe, S.T.; Lavan, J.N. Subcutaneous fluids in elderly hospital patients with cognitive impairment. *Gerontology* **1996**, *42*, 36–39. [CrossRef] [PubMed]
84. Pershad, J. A systematic data review of the cost of rehydration therapy. *Appl. Health Econ. Health Policy* **2010**, *8*, 203–214. [CrossRef]
85. Self, W.H.; Semler, M.W.; Wanderer, J.P.; Wang, L.; Byrne, D.W.; Collins, S.P.; Slovis, C.M.; Lindsell, C.J.; Ehrenfeld, J.M.; Siew, E.D.; et al. Balanced Crystalloids versus Saline in Noncritically Ill Adults. *N. Engl. J. Med.* **2018**, *378*, 819–828. [CrossRef]

# 14

# Indirect Calorimetry in Clinical Practice

**Marta Delsoglio [1], Najate Achamrah [2], Mette M. Berger [3] and Claude Pichard [1,*]**

1 Clinical Nutrition, Geneva University Hospital (HUG), 1205 Geneva, Switzerland
2 Nutrition Department, Rouen University Hospital Center, 76000 Rouen, France
3 Service of Intensive Care Medicine & Burns, University of Lausanne Hospitals (CHUV), 1005 Lausanne, Switzerland
* Correspondence: Claude.Pichard@unige.ch

**Abstract:** Indirect calorimetry (IC) is considered as the gold standard to determine energy expenditure, by measuring pulmonary gas exchanges. It is a non-invasive technique that allows clinicians to personalize the prescription of nutrition support to the metabolic needs and promote a better clinical outcome. Recent technical developments allow accurate and easy IC measurements in spontaneously breathing patients as well as in those on mechanical ventilation. The implementation of IC in clinical routine should be promoted in order to optimize the cost–benefit balance of nutrition therapy. This review aims at summarizing the latest innovations of IC as well as the clinical indications, benefits, and limitations.

**Keywords:** indirect calorimetry; indirect calorimeter; resting energy expenditure; nutrition therapy

---

## 1. Introduction

The accurate determination of patients' energy needs is required to optimize nutritional support and to reduce the deleterious effects of under- and over-feeding [1]. However nutritional requirements may be difficult to predict, especially in patients with acute or chronic conditions where many factors (e.g., stress, brain activity, endocrine profile, inflammation status, feeding state, drugs, etc.) affect their resting energy expenditure (REE). REE represents the energy expended by the body during a 24 h non-active period to maintain involuntary functions such as substrate turnover, respiration, cardiac output, and body temperature regulation [2]. In healthy sedentary adult subjects REE constitutes two-thirds of the total energy expenditure (TEE) which includes energy needed for nonobligatory expenses such as physical activity and diet-induced thermogenesis. This assumption is probably not entirely correct in sick patients where continuous nutrition, treatments and diseased-related stress increase, or decrease REE: extreme variations among individuals can be observed within the same day [3].

Indirect calorimetry (IC) is considered as the gold standard to measure REE, by measuring oxygen consumption ($VO_2$) and carbon dioxide production ($VCO_2$). Apart from REE, other parameters can be derived from IC, such as substrate (carbohydrates, fat, and protein) utilization. Indeed, the ratio between $VCO_2$ and $VO_2$ ($\frac{VCO_2}{VO_2}$) defines the respiratory quotient (RQ) that corresponds to the substrate use. The complete oxidation of glucose generates a RQ value of 1.0, while a RQ of 0.7 is indicative of a mixed substrate oxidation [2].

Recent technical developments of indirect calorimeters allow accurate, non-invasive, and easy IC measurements in spontaneously breathing patients as well as in those on mechanical ventilation. Recent trials have shown IC allows clinicians to personalize the prescription of nutrition support to the metabolic needs and to monitor the metabolic response to nutrition therapy promoting a better clinical outcome in acutely ill patients [4–8]. These results have increased the interest for IC as a tool for improving the routine nutritional evaluation and prescription.

This review aims to summarize the latest innovations of IC as well as the clinical indications, benefits, and limitations of the technique.

## 2. Indications

Equations predicting REE are relatively reliable in healthy subjects. Contrariwise, in case of disease or trauma, REE is influenced by many factors with synergic or antagonist impact (Table 1) [1,2,9]. In these conditions, predictive equations are largely inaccurate [10]. As a consequence, IC is mainly indicated in three different scenarios: (a) clinical conditions significantly modifying REE; (b) failure of a nutrition support based on predicted energy needs to maintain or restore body weight; (c) acute critical illness associated with large and dynamic changes of metabolic stress level [11]. The latter indication requires special caution, as the IC results will reflect the patient's instability: repeated IC studies are required to observe the evolution of the metabolic response to hemodynamic instability, fever, surgery, weaning from mechanical ventilation, etc. A single IC is rarely sufficient, thereby repeated measurements every second or third day are needed in patients with rapid changes of their clinical status [12–14].

**Table 1.** Factors influencing resting energy expenditure. Adapted from [1,2,9].

| Effects on REE | Factors | |
|---|---|---|
| ↑ | • Burns<br>• Hyperventilation<br>• Hyperthermia<br>• Hyperthyroidism, pheochromocytoma<br>• Inflammation (interleukins, interferons, tumor necrosis factors etc.)<br>• Metabolic acidosis | • Morbid obesity<br>• Overfeeding<br>• Physical agitation<br>• Sepsis<br>• Stress (epinephrine, cortisol, glucagon etc.) |
| ↓ | • Coma/deep sleep<br>• General anesthesia<br>• Heavy sedation<br>• Hypothermia<br>• Hypothyroidism<br>• Hypoventilation | • Gluconeogenesis<br>• Metabolic alkalosis<br>• Paralysis<br>• Sarcopenia, cachexia<br>• Starvation/underfeeding/ketosis |

Performing IC in clinical routine is recommended not only to set an optimal nutrition therapy, but also to monitor the results of the nutritional interventions, in order to avoid complications of inappropriate nutrition, i.e., of under- or over-feeding.

## 3. Practicalities

IC allows measuring REE in both mechanically ventilated and spontaneously breathing patients (Figure 1). In mechanically ventilated patients, the respiratory gas sampling is acquired by the circuit connecting the endotracheal tube to the ventilator and measured by 'breath-by-breath' or mixing chamber analyses. In spontaneously breathing subjects, a ventilated canopy hood or a fitted face-mask is used to collect inspired and expired gas. In canopy system the patient's head is surrounded by a clear rigid hood and a pump pulls air through the canopy at a constant rate. In both ventilator and canopy mode, respiratory gases are analyzed by the indirect calorimeter and used to calculate REE through Weir's equation [1]. As will be detailed below, acutely and chronically ill patients at high risk of malnutrition are the ones who benefit most from IC.

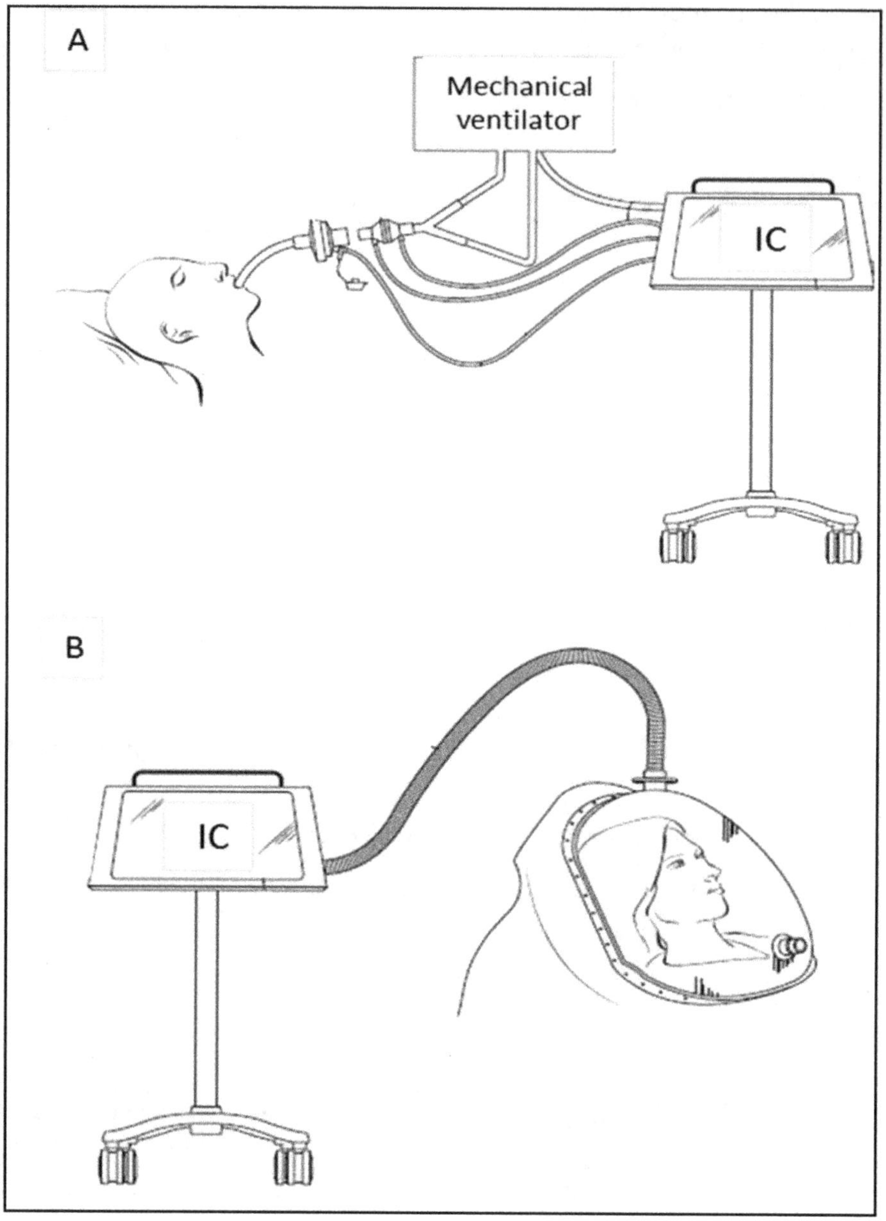


**Figure 1.** Indirect calorimetry on mechanically ventilated patient (**A**) and on spontaneous breathing patient in canopy mode (**B**). In mechanical ventilation the gas sampling is acquired by the circuit connecting the endotracheal tube to the ventilator and measured by 'breath-by-breath' or mixing chamber analyses. In spontaneous breathing mode, the subject is placed under a clear canopy with a plastic drape to avoid air leakage. Breath exchanges are collected by the calorimeter for gas analysis and enable calculation of REE using Weir's equation (REE (kcal/day) = $[(VO_2 \times 3.941) + (VCO_2 \times 1.11)] \times 1440$).

### 3.1. *Acute Diseases*

Metabolic responses to shock and injury were first described by Sir Cuthbertson [15]. According to his investigations, there is a short ebb phase starting immediately after a traumatic shock and followed by a flow phase of longer duration after 3 to 10 days (Figure 2) [16]. The ebb phase is characterized by a decrease in metabolic rate, oxygen consumption, body temperature, and enzymatic activity. The flow phase, on the contrary, is marked by an increased catabolism, with a high oxygen consumption and an elevated REE rate.

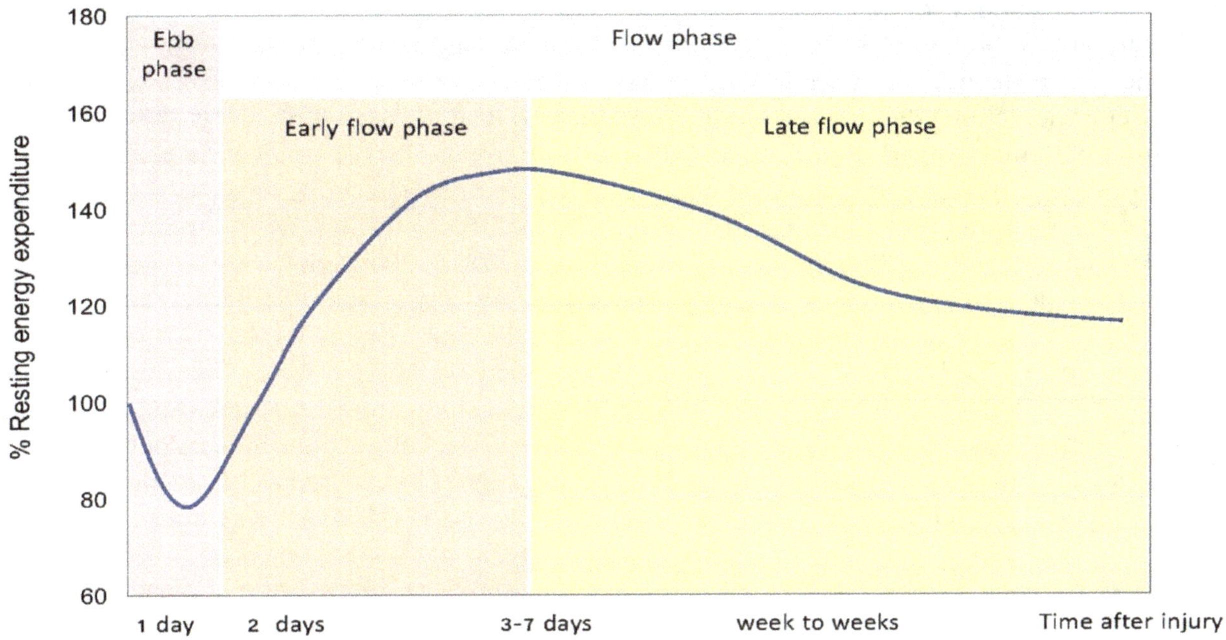


**Figure 2.** Metabolic response to injury proposed by Cuthbertson et al. A short ebb phase characterized by hypometabolism occurs immediately after the injury and is characterized by a decrease in metabolic rate, oxygen consumption, body temperature, and enzymatic activity. The ebb phase is followed by a longer hypermetabolic flow phase marked by an increased catabolism, with a high oxygen consumption and an elevated REE rate. Reused with permission from [16].

Recent studies have supported this pattern of longitudinal changes in REE in acutely ill patients [17–19]. The degree of increase from normal REE may reflect the severity of the metabolic response to the injury. However, the interaction between natural course of disease, individual inflammatory and immune system response, and medical treatments make it difficult for the clinician to evaluate caloric needs. For these reasons, IC is the only available tool enabling the individual assessment of the patients' energy needs, and to ensure precise nutritional interventions in acute conditions such as post-surgery period, pancreatitis, kidney injury, and sepsis.

The post-operative period of uncomplicated surgery has been associated with a modest 7% increase in energy metabolism as the effect of the surgical operation itself, that cannot be predicted by static equations [20]. Non-septic patients with acute pancreatitis presented a hypermetabolic state with a REE increase of 120 ± 11% compared to predicted [21]. Energy metabolism in patients with renal failure has been studied as well. Acute kidney injury (AKI) has not been shown to affect REE, but concomitant conditions, such as sepsis, mostly play role in the hypermetabolism found in these patients [22,23]. The presence of hypermetabolism has also been associated with lower age and higher vasoactive drug dose [24] and no predictive formula was able to correctly calculate energy needs in AKI patients compared to IC [25]. Sepsis is characterized by a hyperdynamic cardiovascular response against infection and has been reported to increase REE differently among patients with uncomplicated sepsis, sepsis syndrome, and septic shock (mean REE +55 ± 14%, +24 ± 12%, and +2 ± 24%) [26]. A higher REE in severe sepsis adult patients has also been associated with higher mortality [27], however further studies should investigate the effect of specific individual factors on metabolic evolution during sepsis and patient outcome.

### Critical Illness

Critical illness is frequently associated with a hypermetabolic state related to the activation of catabolic hormones and resulting in elevated REE compared to healthy subjects. However, iatrogenic factors such as beta-blockers, analgesics, and sedatives may attenuate the response and even induce a hypometabolic state. Prolonged bed rest, atrophy of the metabolically active lean body mass, and mechanical ventilation have also been reported to decrease REE [1]. In patients with multiple organ failure, the loss of lean body mass is very rapid and resulted in 22% loss in 10 days [28] and no predictive equation showed good agreement compared to REE measured by IC [29].

Trauma patients showed hypermetabolism even when heavily sedated or medically paralyzed, however those with head injury on neuromuscular blockade or in a barbiturate coma showed reduced REE compared to similar patients without these agents [30]. Brain trauma was found to increase REE with high variability among different studies, ranging from 87% to 200% compared to predicted during the first 30 days post-injury; surprisingly, in patients admitted with a brain death diagnosis, the value ranged from 75% to 200% compared to predicted during the first 7 days [31].

Similarly, post-burn hypermetabolism was shown to increase REE as high as 100% above normal as consequence of a strong catabolic response mediated by endogenous catecholamines and inflammatory cytokines. Nevertheless, this hypermetabolic state is a direct effect of burn trauma, its persistence leads to severe septic complications, multiple organ failure, and higher mortality [16]. Nutritional follow up in burn patients shows a highly dynamic and variable REE up to 160 days after injury (Figure 3) [32].

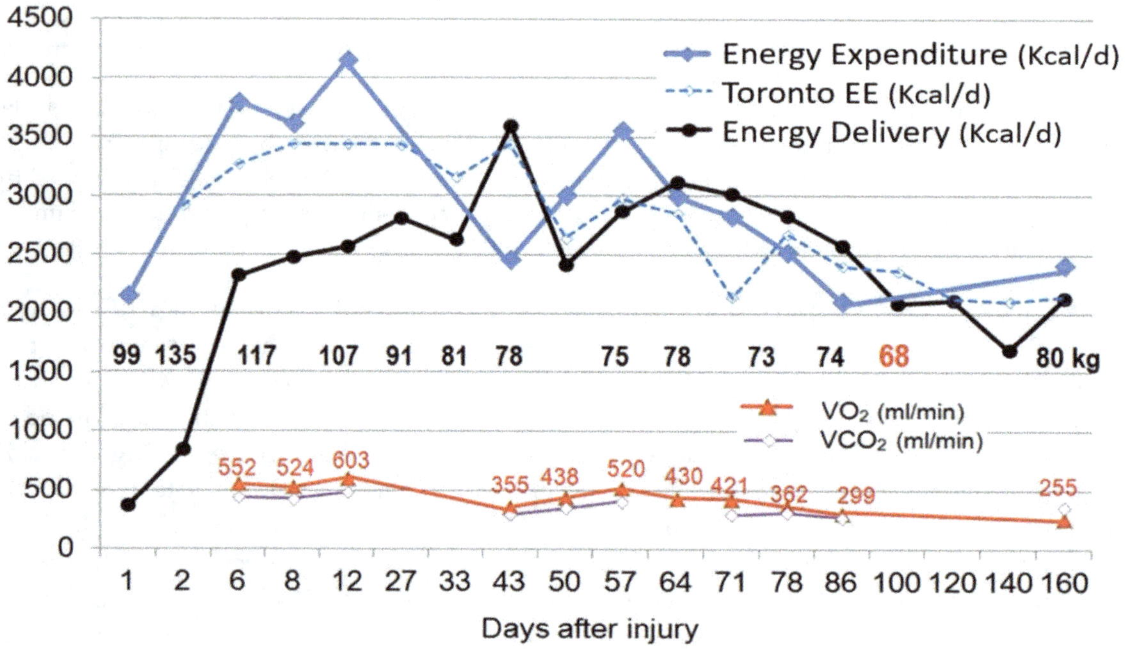


**Figure 3.** Evolution of measured REE by IC (blue), Toronto predictive equation (dashed blue), delivered energy (black), $VO_2$ (red △), and $VCO_2$ (purple ◆) in a young man weighing 99 kg upon admission with major burns covering 85% body surface over 160 days. The REE variations were important over time particularly during the early phase (weight gain due to fluid resuscitation was 36 kg by day 3), and paralleled the loss of body weight, i.e., of lean body mass (−31 kg after 3 months, with slow recovery). The REE value on day 1 corresponds to the Harris & Benedict prediction of basal EE. The figure also shows the reasonable precision of the Toronto equation, and how difficult it is to feed to measured IC value during the first 14 days. Adapted from [32].

The accurate determination of energy needs and the prevention of energy imbalance are essential in critically ill patients to avoid the harmful consequences of inadequate feeding. Underfeeding has been shown to increase hospital length of stay, infections, organ failure, to prolong mechanical ventilation, and to increase mortality, while overfeeding has been associated with hyperglycemia, hypertriglyceridemia, hepatic steatosis, azotemia, hypercapnia, and increased mortality [33]. In long staying patients with dynamic clinical conditions, IC should be repeated to monitor their nutritional requirements and avoid energy imbalance [34,35]. Optimal energy delivery targeting REE measured by IC seems to be significantly associated with reduced mortality, stressing the importance of this technique to assess caloric needs in ICU patients (Figure 4) [17].

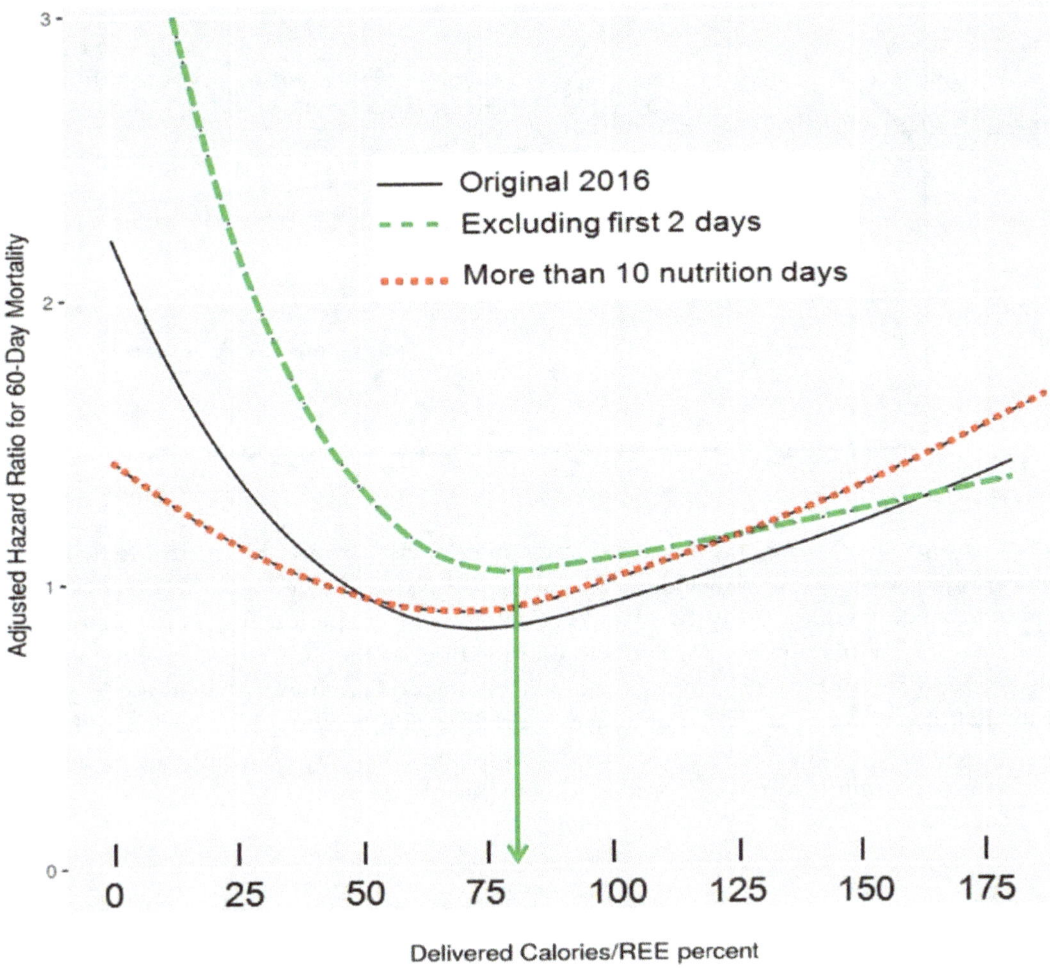


**Figure 4.** Association of delivered calories/resting energy expenditure (REE) percent by indirect calorimetry (IC) with 60-day mortality in different models: the authors recalculated their original 2016 data to integrate the fact that energy delivery increased progressively during the initial 2–3 days, reducing the mean value in stays <5 days. The lowest ICU mortality was observed when percent of delivered calories by REE obtained by IC was 80% (excluding first two feeding days) and 75% (with >10 evaluable nutrition days) ($p < 0.05$). On the contrary, increments of the ratio above that point—specifically >110%—were associated with increasing mortality ($p < 0.05$). Reproduced with permission (http://creativecommons.org/licenses/by/4.0/) [17].

The question which remains debated is the timing from which the measured REE should be prescribed as energy goal. Considering the importance of the early endogenous energy production, which is not suppressed by nutrition in the critically ill [36], feeding to measured value may result in overfeeding (Figure 5) [1]. Moreover, during the early phase of disease, catecholamines and the multiple treatments needed in these patients generate high instability and directly impact on measured REE. Tappy et al. showed that, in young starved trauma patients, the endogenous glucose production (EGP) was about 310 g/day (Figure 6), while the measured REE in these patients was 1830 kcal: feeding to the mean measured REE would clearly result in early overfeeding [37]. The figure also shows that endogenous glucose production continues in the sickest patients for many days even during feeding [8] (Figure 6). Therefore, the crude REE value provided by IC requires a careful interpretation to adequately prescribe exogenous energy supply.

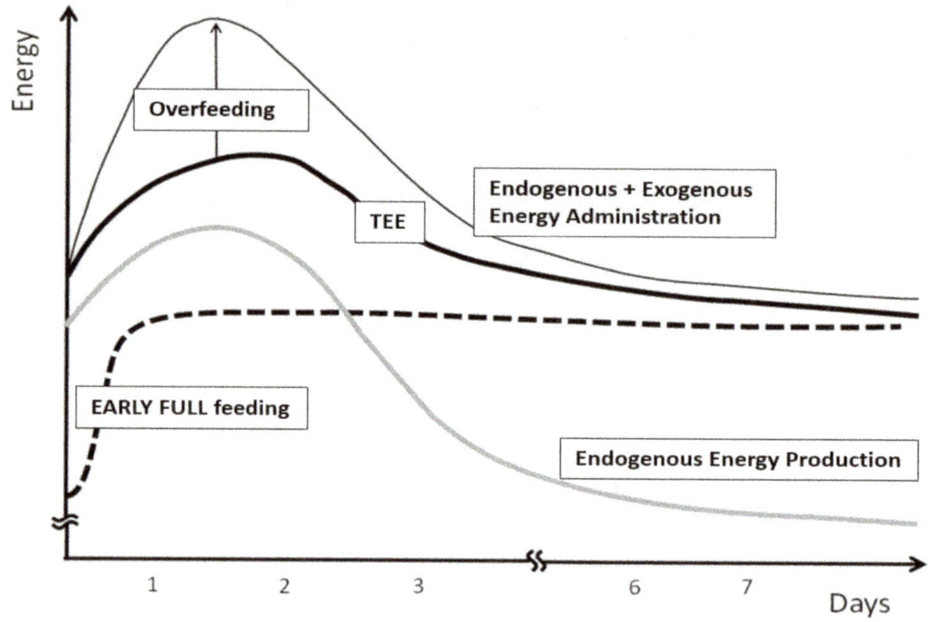


**Figure 5.** Conceptual representation of the relative overfeeding commonly resulting from early full feeding during the first days of critical illness. During this phase, the endogenous glucose production (EGP) is increased, covering up to two-thirds of total energy expenditure (TEE—solid black bold line). Full feeding in this phase will results in overfeeding, as the EGP is not attenuated by energy administration (different form healthy): exogenous feeding adds to the EGP resulting in an excessive energy availability, superior to TEE. (Solid black bold line: TEE; grey bold line: adapted endogenous energy production; dotted bold line: early energy administration; thin line: combined endogenous and exogenous energy administration). Reproduced with permission from [1].

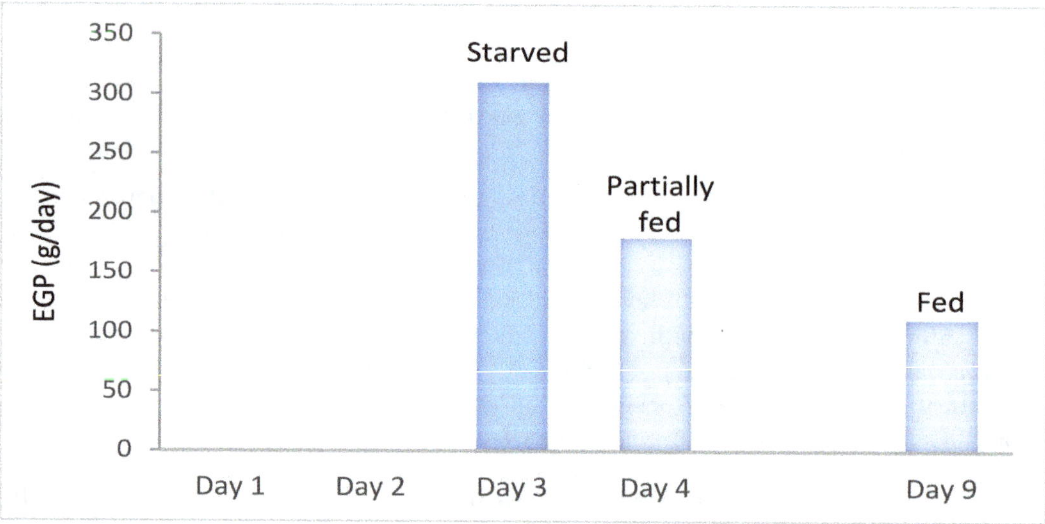


**Figure 6.** Evolution of the endogenous glucose production (EGP) over time in critically ill patients. EGP was shown to be 310 g/day in 40 years old starved trauma patients at day 3 of ICU admission (blue) [37] and then decreased to 180 and 111 g/day in older fed patients at day 4 and 9 respectively (light blue) [8]. EGP has to be considered as source of energy in order to avoid overfeeding by extrinsic energy during the first days of ICU stay. Data combined from [8,37].

There is also a debate regarding the optimal timing to cover the energy value determined by IC and the capacity of the critically ill intestine to accommodate and absorb the delivered feeding. Gastrointestinal intolerance is frequent in ICU patients and may preclude the achievement of the predefined calorie target due to the incapability of absorbing supplied nutrition [38]. The best feeding route for each patient has to be assessed in order to limit the risk of stressing the intestine and cumulative caloric deficit [39].

*3.2. Chronic Diseases*

Energy requirements may be even more difficult to predict in patients with chronic conditions due to the large individual variations in REE. Both hyper- and hypo-metabolism have been shown in chronic pathologies due to alterations in metabolism, lean body mass, organ function, and presence of inflammation. The most common pathologies with important REE alterations are described below and summarized in Table 2.

**Table 2.** Common chronic pathologies with effects on resting energy expenditure

| Condition | | Effect on REE |
|---|---|---|
| Anorexia nervosa | ↓ | Low energy intake and reduced lean body mass |
| Cancer | ↑<br>↓ | Cancer growth and inflammation<br>Progressive reduction of lean body mass |
| Chronic kidney diseases | ↑<br>↓ | Metabolic acidosis and inflammation<br>Acute and chronic renal failure |
| Chronic obstructive pulmonary disease | ↑ | Increased respiratory efforts |
| Diabetes | ↑ | Increased metabolism |
| Obesity | ↑<br>↓ | Increased lean body mass<br>Sarcopenia |
| Neuromuscular degenerative diseases | ↑<br>↓ | Inflammation and endocrine disorders<br>Dysfunction of muscle tissue |

Both hyper- and hypo-metabolism, with respectively increased or decreased REE, have been observed in cancer patients. Several factors such as type, location, and size of tumor and presence of liver metastasis may contribute to this variability [16]. Similarly some studies showed increased REE in patients with chronic kidney disease, while others reported equal or even lower REE than those of matched healthy controls [40,41]. Renal replacement therapy such as hemodialysis or peritoneal dialysis also seem to affect REE, but results are contrasted [42,43]. Neurological diseases, such as Alzheimer's, Parkinson's, Huntington's, and amyotrophic lateral sclerosis significantly affect patients' REE as consequence of motor, endocrine, and metabolic abnormalities [44]. Diabetes is known to alter macronutrient metabolism, and increase the sympathetic activity leading to 5–10% augmentation of REE. On the contrary, the administration of anti-diabetic treatments is associated with a REE decrease [45]. Patients with chronic obstructive pulmonary disease feature an increased REE associated together with the progression of the disease severity, but a decreased TEE mainly due to a reduction of physical activity [46]. Both obesity and anorexia nervosa have been associated with altered REE mainly due to the different pattern of body composition compared to normal weight subjects. Obese patients showed significantly higher REE compared to non-obese patients; however, in most cases this difference disappeared after adjusting for fat-free mass [47]. Underweight and anorectic patients showed hypometabolic status with lower REE compared to predicted as a consequence of adaptation to starvation, loss of fat, and fat-free mass [48]. Conducting IC together with body composition measurement is useful to further optimize the nutrition prescription in these patients.

## 4. Benefits

The major benefit of performing IC in clinical practice is the prevention of both under- and over-feeding among patients with different conditions, thanks to the precise assessment and control of their energy needs. Inappropriate feeding has been associated with increased risk of infectious and non-infectious complications, length of hospitalization, more frequent readmission, and mortality, especially in ICU patients. Patients at risk of malnutrition were also found to be more likely to go to rehabilitation or nursing facilities rather than home after discharge [49]. In addition to negative outcomes in hospitalized patients, malnutrition also represents an economic burden for hospitals and the society [50]. In the ICU setting, supplemental parenteral nutrition (SPN) guided by IC has been shown to allow personalized and optimal nutrition in patients intolerant to full enteral nutrition. A reduction of nosocomial infections in the patients on SPN versus those on exclusive and insufficient enteral nutrition has been reported [5]. In depth analysis has further shown that the provision of SPN compared to exclusive enteral nutrition turned out to be a cost saving strategy [51,52]. Up to now, only four studies based their nutritional intervention on measured REE by IC [53]. A meta-analysis of available studies nevertheless shows that interventions guided by IC versus equations have significantly better clinical outcomes [34]. Promoting a systematic use of IC to individually optimize nutrition support among in- and out-patients, should result in meaningful clinical benefits and cost advantages. A large-scale study providing the benefits related to the use of IC to guide the prescription of nutrition support is needed.

## 5. Limitations

IC is the gold standard for measuring REE and for guiding nutrition support; however, several factors may limit the accuracy and/or the feasibility of the measurement (Table 3). During mechanical ventilation, air leakages in the respiratory circuit (particularly elevated in case of tracheostomy), high positive end expiratory pressure (PEEP > 10), fraction of inspired oxygen ($FiO_2$) > 80%, and presence of other gases than $O_2$, $CO_2$, and $N_2$ lead to unreliable results [1]. Thoracic drains are also a frequent cause of leakage in cardiothoracic units. Factors causing instability—such as agitation, fever, sedatives, and vasoactive adjustments during IC—limit the agreement between measured and real REE [54]. Likewise, organ support therapies such as continuous renal replacement therapy (CRRT) affect the respiratory pattern due to $CO_2$ removal, therefore measured REE does not reflect patient's real needs [54]. Similarly, to calculate real REE on extracorporeal membrane oxygenation (ECMO) patients requires gas exchange analysis by IC at both ventilator and ECMO sides [55,56].

**Table 3.** Factors limiting the reliability and feasibility of IC measurement.

| Factors Limiting IC Measurement |
| --- |
| • Agitation, fever, sedatives, and vasoactive adjustments during measurement |
| • Air leakages in respiratory circuit |
| • Dialysis or continuous renal replacement therapy |
| • ECMO |
| • Mechanical ventilation with PEEP > 10<br>• Mechanical ventilation with $FiO_2$ > 80%<br>• Noninvasive ventilation<br>• Other gases than $O_2$, $CO_2$, and $N_2$: helium |
| • Supplemental oxygen in spontaneous breathing patients |

Moreover, not all subjects are good candidates to IC (i.e., spontaneous breathing patients who are claustrophobic, nauseous, vomiting, or do not tolerate a face mask or being under a canopy cannot undergo IC measurement). Patients who require supplemental oxygen or undergoing noninvasive ventilation are also difficult to test due to limitations of software and techniques. Other restraints for performing IC in clinical routine are related to the equipment and maintenance cost, poor health insurance reimbursement, lack of trained manpower, difficulties interpreting the results, and lack of time to carry out the measurements [13].

## 6. Current Developments

Many indirect calorimeters are commercially available, but most of them are bulky, expensive and poorly accurate compared to a reference device [57–60]. Some indirect calorimeters use the 'breath-by-breath' technology and generate rapid readings by measuring short intervals of gas samples, but this method is error-prone due to the response time of gas analyzers and software. Others are equipped with a mixing chamber and offer more stable measurements, because the gas is physically 'averaged' before being analyzed. However, the presence of the mixing chamber (3–5 L) results in a large dimension device, which requires prolonged measurements (>20 min) to allow gas concentrations stability. This limits the possibility of doing short-time reliable measurements [57–60].

In recent years, hand-held calorimeters such as the MedGem™ and BodyGem™ (Microlife, Dunedin, FL, USA) have also been developed. While traditional indirect calorimeters measure $VO_2$ and $VCO_2$, the hand-held devices measure only $VO_2$, while RQ is assumed to be 0.85. Advantages of these devices are portability, low degree of technical expertise required, and low cost. However, they cannot be used in ventilated patients, do not measure $VCO_2$, and are not validated in hospitalized patients [61].

Indeed, several comparison studies have been conducted both in adults and children comparing standard metabolic carts to determine whether the MedGem™ device is accurate and reliable. The hand-held calorimeter showed discrepant results compared to Deltatrac® in anorexia nervosa patients and healthy controls [62], overestimating REE by 8–11% [63] and agreeing only about 45% of the time in ambulatory adults [64]. MedGem® showed agreement only 21% of the time with Vmax measures in outpatients with cirrhosis [65] and tended to overestimate REE in obese individuals [66]. Similarly, it was found inaccurate in children and adolescents with and without obesity, overestimating REE by 7–10% [67,68] compared to other indirect calorimeters such as Parvomedics® and Deltatrac®, and underestimating by 8% [69] compared to Vmax®.

An international multicentric study (ICALIC), supported by two academic societies (ESPEN and ESICM), has recently led to the evaluation of a new generation calorimeter (Q-NRG®) developed to overcome the issue of inaccuracy, high cost, and lack of time [1]. It is equipped with a micro mixing chamber (2 mL) and features the technical characteristics required for measuring REE in both mechanically ventilated and spontaneous breathing subjects. In vitro evaluation showed gas analyzers' accuracy within 2% difference against a mass spectrometer (MS) for the measurements of predefined gas mixtures and within 5% in a mechanically ventilated setting at oxygen enrichment up to 70% for measurements of simulated $VO_2$ and $VCO_2$ [70]. Q-NRG® also showed very good accuracy and intra- and inter-unit precision in canopy mode both in vitro and in vivo compared to MS in healthy volunteers [71]. Studies to evaluate the ergonomics of the Q-NRG® in the ICU and hospitalized patients are ongoing within the frame of ICALIC study: they compare the currently used calorimeters. In addition to accuracy and precision, the innovation and performances of this new calorimeter are reactivity, portability, battery-powered, affordability, monthly gas calibration, and warm-up free operations. Current innovations also led to the development of original devices to facilitate the personal monitoring of REE. An example is the Breezing® device, a pocket-sized indirect calorimeter that measures oxygen consumption and carbon dioxide production rate in breath with a colorimetric technology. This device showed good agreement with the results from the Douglas Bag method for $VO_2$, $VCO_2$, EE, and RQ in healthy subjects but no tests were performed in clinical setting [72].

## 7. Alternative Methods to IC

So far, predictive equations remain the most common REE estimation method. They allow a rapid calculation of REE using anthropometric data (height, weight, sex, etc.) and have been validated among different group of hospitalized patients, but none is optimal (Table 4). Most of these equations have been developed in healthy subjects, resulting in large errors in case of critical illness and chronic diseases, despite the use of the correction factors [73]. Other methods for assessing REE have been explored and compared to IC in order to find a valid alternative.

Fick's principle uses cardiac output data, hemoglobin concentration, and arterial and mixed venous oxygen concentrations obtained from a pulmonary artery catheter to calculate REE. Comparison with IC in critically ill patients showed poor correlation with high variability between absolute values and variations of $VO_2$ measured, unacceptable for clinical use [74,75]. The error found may be mostly related to five factors: the accuracy of the blood gas analyzer used to calculate arterial and venous oxygen content, the mixed of venous and bronchial arterial blood sample, the hemoglobin levels, the cardiac output variation over the respiratory cycle and the assumption of a fixed RQ to calculate REE [74,76].

The calculation of EE based on $CO_2$ measurement collected from mechanical ventilators ($EEVCO_2$) has also been proposed. This technique considers a fixed value of RQ to calculate the oxygen consumption ($VO_2$) and REE through the Weir formula. Mainly due to the variability of RQ in critically ill patients, the accuracy of $EEVCO_2$ compared to the Deltatrac® metabolic monitor is poor [77–80].

The doubly labeled water method implies the oral administration of water with both hydrogen and oxygen atoms labeled with non-radioactive isotopes ($^2H/^1H$ and $^{18}O/^{16}O$) and uses their elimination rates in body liquids to calculate $CO_2$ production. By assuming a fixed RQ this method allows calculating TEE in any subjects and any environment, and can been used in complementation to IC to calculate Physical Activity Level [81,82]. However, this technique is expensive and requires long time to get the results, limiting its use in daily clinical practice [3].

Motion sensors devices initially developed for fitness settings may be useful in clinical practice to monitor activity induced energy expenditure (AEE), in particular for patients undergoing physiotherapy during rehabilitation programs, as well as for the management of daily activity and the dietary programs in patients with obesity and/or diabetes. These devices are wearable on the arm, wrist, or waist; user-friendly; relatively low-cost; and non-invasive. Energy expenditure is derived from acceleration data and individual parameters (sex, age, weight, heart rate) using manufacturer's confidential algorithms. However, the energy expenditure derived from these devices generally over- or underestimates the energy expenditure measured by IC by at least 10% [83]. Further studies are needed to validate their accuracy in clinical practice.

Measurements of body composition by bioelectrical impedance analysis (BIA) or dual energy X-ray absorptiometry (DXA) can be used to estimate REE. To this purpose predictive formula including FFM and FM values have been developed. This approach has been shown quite inaccurate in clinical populations compared to IC [73,84,85] and cannot be adopted in critically ill patients due to their abnormalities in hydration state and serum electrolyte concentrations that cause errors in the BIA-derived estimates of FFM and FM [86].

**Table 4.** Some predictive equations commonly used in clinical practice and tested among different hospitalized patients against IC.

| Equations | Parameters Used for Calculation | Accuracy Rate * |
|---|---|---|
| **General Hospitalized Population** | | |
| 25 kcal/kg | 25 × WT | 43% [10]<br>23% [87] |
| Harris & Benedict (1919) | M: 13.75 × WT + 5.00 × HT − 6.75 × age + 66.47<br>F: 9.56 × WT + 1.85 × HT − 0.67 × age + 655.09 | 43% [10]<br>38% [87] |
| Ireton-Jones (1992) | 1925 − 10 × age + 5 × WT + (281 if male) + (292 if trauma) + (851 if burn) | 28% [10] |
| Mifflin-St Jeor (1990) | M: 10 × WT + 6.25 × HT − 5 × age + 5<br>F: 10 × WT + 6.25 × HT − 5 × age − 161 | 35% [10]<br>32% [87] |
| Schofield (1985) | 8.4 × WT + 4.7 × HT + 200 | 42% [87] |
| **Anorexic Patients (BMI < 16)** | | |
| Bernstein et al. (1983) | M: 11.02 × WT + 10.23 × HT − 5.8 × age − 1032<br>F: 7.48 × WT − 0.42 × HT − 3 × age + 844 | 40% [73] |
| Harris & Benedict (1919) | M: 13.75 × WT + 5.00 × HT − 6.75 × age + 66.47<br>F: 9.56 × WT + 1.85 × HT − 0.67 × age + 655.09 | 39% [73] |
| Huang et al. (2004) | 10.16 × WT + 3.93 × HT − 1.44 × age + 273.82 × sex + 60.65 | 43% [73] |
| Lazzer et al. (2007) | M: 0.05 × WT + 4.65 × HT − 0.02 × age − 3.60<br>F: 0.04 × WT + 3.62 × HT − 2.68 | 39% [73] |
| Mifflin-St Jeor (1990) | M: 10 × WT + 6.25 × HT − 5 × age + 5<br>F: 10 × WT + 6.25 × HT − 5 × age − 161 | 40% [73] |
| Müller et al. (2004) | 0.05 × WT + 1.01 × sex + 0.015 × age + 3.21 | 37% [73] |
| Owen (1987) | M: WT × 10.2 + 879<br>F: WT × 7.18 + 795 | 41% [73] |
| **Obese Patients (BMI > 30)** | | |
| Bernstein et al. (1983) | M: 11.02 × WT + 10.23 × HT − 5.8 × age − 1032<br>F: 7.48 × WT − 0.42 × HT − 3 × age + 844 | 16% [88]<br>21% [89] |
| Harris & Benedict (1919) | M: 13.75 × WT + 5.00 × HT − 6.75 × age + 66.47<br>F: 9.56 × WT + 1.85 × HT − 0.67 × age + 655.09 | 64% [88] |
| Huang et al. (2004) | 10.16 × WT + 3.93 × HT − 1.44 × age + 273.82 × sex + 60.65 | 66% [88]<br>53% [89]<br>54% [90] |
| Lazzer et al. (2007) | M: 0.05 × WT + 4.65 × HT − 0.02 × age − 3.60<br>F: 0.04 × WT + 3.62 × HT − 2.68 | 58% [88]<br>46% [90] |
| Mifflin-St Jeor (1990) | M: 10 × WT + 6.25 × HT − 5 × age + 5<br>F: 10 × WT + 6.25 × HT − 5 × age − 161 | 52% [89]<br>56% [90] |
| Müller et al. (2004) | 0.05 × WT + 1.10 × sex + 0.016 × age + 2.92 | 60% [88]<br>58% [89]<br>47% [90] |
| Owen (1987) | M: WT × 10.2 + 879<br>F: WT × 7.18 + 795 | 38% [73]<br>40% [89] |

**Table 4.** *Cont.*

| Equations | Parameters Used for Calculation | Accuracy Rate * |
|---|---|---|
| **Critically Ill Patients** | | |
| 25 Kcal/Kg | 25 × WT | 12% [91] |
| Harris-Benedict (1919) | M: 13.75 × WT + 5.00 × HT − 6.75 × age + 66.47<br>F: 9.56 × WT + 1.85 × HT − 0.67 × age + 655.09 | 31% [91]<br>32% [92] |
| Ireton-Jones (1997) | 1925 − 10 × age + 5 × WT + (281 if M) + (292 if trauma) + (851 if burn) | 37% [93] |
| Mifflin-St Jeor (1990) | M: 10 × WT + 6.25 × HT − 5 × age + 5<br>F: 10 × WT + 6.25 × HT − 5 × age − 161 | 18% [91]<br>35% [10] |
| Owen (1987) | M: WT × 10.2 + 879<br>F: WT × 7.18 + 795 | 12% [91] |
| Penn State (2003) | 0.85 × HB + 175 × Tmax + 33 × Ve − 6433 | 43% [10] |
| Swinamer (1990) | 945 × BSA − 6.4 × age + 108 T + 24.2 × RR + 81.7 × VT − 4349 | 55% [93]<br>45% [10] |

* % of patients where the predicted value (by equation) is within 10% of measured value (by IC). BSA, body surface area ($m^2$); HB, Harris–Benedict value; HT, height (cm); RR, respiratory rate (breath/min); sex: males (M) = 1, female (F); T, temperature (°C); Tmax, maximum temperature (°C) in previous 24 h; TV, tidal volume (L); Ve, expired minute ventilation at the time of collection (L/min); WT, weight (kg).

The agreement of predictive equations compared to IC results in critically ill patients was shown not to exceed 55%, especially in overweight or obese sarcopenic patients, and after prolonged physical immobilization [33,35,94]. Poor agreement is mainly due to the influence of body temperature, nutrition support, presence of sepsis, level of sedation, and therapies on REE [13]. The magnitude and the duration of the variations depend mostly on the severity of the disease with a considerable individual variability that cannot be assessed by equations [95]. Moreover, most of the equations base their calculations on anthropometric parameters, such as the body weight, which is often unknown and largely influenced by fluid retention or dehydration, leading to unreliable results [96].

Predictive equations tend to over (↑) or under (↓)—estimate REE in patients with chronic diseases such as:

- chronic obstructive pulmonary disease (↓) [97]
- chronic kidney disease (↑) [98]
- amyotrophic lateral sclerosis (↓) [85]
- fibro-calculous pancreatic diabetes and diabetes type 2 (↓) [99]
- cancer (↑) [100]
- cirrhosis (↓) [101]

Similarly, predictive equations are inaccurate in patients with extreme BMI (BMI < 16 kg/$m^2$ and BMI > 40 kg/$m^2$) [102]. Errors are mainly due to an excessive or deficient fat mass, which is less metabolically active than the lean body mass, and to the body weight considered for the calculation (current, ideal, adjusted, or estimated) [73]. Therefore, it seems clear that standard factors to estimate the energy needs of individual patients are inappropriate and should be discouraged to guide nutrition support. Pragmatically, the ESPEN guideline suggests to use the simplest equation in critically ill patients—i.e., 20 kcal/kg/day during the first days—and in absence of IC to increase to 25 kcal/kg/day after 7 days [34].

## 8. Conclusions

The optimization of nutrition therapy is crucial for global patient care. In order to prevent under- and over-feeding and their related complications, it is important to accurately assess REE in individual patients and to ensure adapted nutrition support. IC is considered as the gold standard to this purpose and ideally any patients in whom energy needs are uncertain should be measured. Recent developments should facilitate the widespread use of IC in medical routine and promote better clinical outcomes. Considering the ongoing debate, the widespread use of IC might finally enable the design of prospective studies which will be able to determine the optimal dose of energy to deliver during the different stages of disease, i.e., the ratio of the energy delivered to measured REE and timing of feeding.

**Author Contributions:** M.D.: conceptualization, writing—original draft preparation, visualization; N.A.: writing—review and editing; M.M.B.: writing—review and editing, supervision; C.P.: writing—review and editing, supervision.

## References

1. Oshima, T.; Berger, M.M.; De Waele, E.; Guttormsen, A.B.; Heidegger, C.P.; Hiesmayr, M.; Singer, P.; Wernerman, J.; Pichard, C. Indirect calorimetry in nutritional therapy. A position paper by the ICALIC study group. *Clin. Nutr.* **2017**, *36*, 651–662. [CrossRef]
2. Gupta, R.D.; Ramachandran, R.; Venkatesan, P.; Anoop, S.; Joseph, M.; Thomas, N. Indirect Calorimetry: From Bench to Bedside. *Indian J. Endocrinol. Metab.* **2017**, *21*, 594–599. [CrossRef]
3. Fraipont, V.; Preiser, J.C. Energy Estimation and Measurement in Critically Ill Patients. *J. Parenter. Enter. Nutr.* **2013**, *37*, 705–713. [CrossRef]
4. Singer, P.; Anbar, R.; Cohen, J.; Shapiro, H.; Shalita-Chesner, M.; Lev, S.; Grozovski, E.; Theilla, M.; Frishman, S.; Madar, Z. The tight calorie control study (TICACOS), a prospective, randomized, controlled pilot study of nutritional support in critically ill patients. *Intensiv. Care Med.* **2011**, *37*, 601–609. [CrossRef]
5. Heidegger, C.P.; Berger, M.M.; Graf, S.; Zingg, W.; Darmon, P.; Costanza, M.C.; Thibault, R.; Pichard, C. Optimisation of energy provision with supplemental parenteral nutrition in critically ill patients: A randomised controlled clinical trial. *Lancet* **2013**, *381*, 385–393. [CrossRef]
6. Petros, S.; Horbach, M.; Seidel, F.; Weidhase, L. Hypocaloric vs Normocaloric Nutrition in Critically Ill Patients: A Prospective Randomized Pilot Trial. *J. Parenter. Enter. Nutr.* **2016**, *40*, 242–249. [CrossRef]
7. Allingstrup, M.J.; Kondrup, J.; Wiis, J.; Claudius, C.; Pedersen, U.G.; Hein-Rasmussen, R.; Bjerregaard, M.R.; Steensen, M.; Jensen, T.H.; Lange, T.; et al. Early goal-directed nutrition versus standard of care in adult intensive care patients: The single-centre, randomised, outcome assessor-blinded EAT-ICU trial. *Intensiv. Care Med.* **2017**, *43*, 1637–1647. [CrossRef]
8. Berger, M.M.; Pantet, O.; Jacquelin-Ravel, N.; Charriere, M.; Schmidt, S.; Becce, F.; Audran, R.; Spertini, F.; Tappy, L.; Pichard, C. Supplemental parenteral nutrition improves immunity with unchanged carbohydrate and protein metabolism in critically ill patients: The SPN2 randomized tracer study. *Clin. Nutr.* **2018**. [CrossRef]
9. Merritt, R. Use of indirect calorimetry in critically ill patients. In *The ASPEN Nutrition Support Practice Manual*, 2nd ed.; American Society for Parenteral and Enteral Nutrit: Silver Spring, MD, USA, 2006; pp. 277–280.
10. Boullata, J.; Williams, J.; Cottrell, F.; Hudson, L.; Compher, C. Accurate determination of energy needs in hospitalized patients. *J. Am. Diet. Assoc.* **2007**, *107*, 393–401. [CrossRef]
11. Wooley, J.A.; Sax, H.C. Indirect calorimetry: Applications to practice. *Nutr. Clin. Pract.* **2003**, *18*, 434–439. [CrossRef]

12. Berger, M.M.; Reintam-Blaser, A.; Calder, P.C.; Casaer, M.; Hiesmayr, M.J.; Mayer, K.; Montejo, J.C.; Pichard, C.; Preiser, J.C.; van Zanten, A.R.H.; et al. Monitoring nutrition in the ICU. *Clin. Nutr.* **2019**, *38*, 584–593. [CrossRef]
13. Singer, P.; Singer, J. Clinical Guide for the Use of Metabolic Carts: Indirect Calorimetry-No Longer the Orphan of Energy Estimation. *Nutr. Clin. Pract.* **2016**, *31*, 30–38. [CrossRef]
14. Weissman, C.; Kemper, M.; Hyman, A.I. Variation in the resting metabolic rate of mechanically ventilated critically ill patients. *Anesth. Analg.* **1989**, *68*, 457–461. [CrossRef]
15. Cuthbertson, D.P.; Angeles Valero Zanuy, M.A.; Leon Sanz, M.L. Post-shock metabolic response. 1942. *Nutr. Hosp.* **2001**, *16*, 176–182.
16. Rattanachaiwong, S.; Singer, P. Indirect Calorimetry as Point of Care Testing. *Clin. Nutr.* **2019**. [CrossRef]
17. Zusman, O.; Theilla, M.; Cohen, J.; Kagan, I.; Bendavid, I.; Singer, P. Resting energy expenditure, calorie and protein consumption in critically ill patients: A retrospective cohort study. *Crit. Care* **2016**, *20*, 367. [CrossRef]
18. Plank, L.D.; Hill, G.L. Sequential metabolic changes following induction of systemic inflammatory response in patients with severe sepsis or major blunt trauma. *World J. Surg.* **2000**, *24*, 630–638. [CrossRef]
19. Plank, L.D.; Connolly, A.B.; Hill, G.L. Sequential changes in the metabolic response in severely septic patients during the first 23 days after the onset of peritonitis. *Ann. Surg.* **1998**, *228*, 146–158. [CrossRef]
20. Brandi, L.S.; Oleggini, M.; Lachi, S.; Frediani, M.; Bevilacqua, S.; Mosca, F.; Ferrannini, E. Energy metabolism of surgical patients in the early postoperative period: A reappraisal. *Crit. Care Med.* **1988**, *16*, 18–22. [CrossRef]
21. Dickerson, R.N.; Vehe, K.L.; Mullen, J.L.; Feurer, I.D. Resting energy expenditure in patients with pancreatitis. *Crit. Care Med.* **1991**, *19*, 484–490. [CrossRef]
22. Schneeweiss, B.; Graninger, W.; Stockenhuber, F.; Druml, W.; Ferenci, P.; Eichinger, S.; Grimm, G.; Laggner, A.N.; Lenz, K. Energy metabolism in acute and chronic renal failure. *Am. J. Clin. Nutr.* **1990**, *52*, 596–601. [CrossRef]
23. Soncini Sanches, A.C.; de Góes, C.R.; Nogueira Berbel Bufarah, M.; Balbi, A.L.; Ponce, D. Does Acute Kidney Injury Alter Energy Metabolism of Septic Patients? *Arch. Ren. Dis. Manag.* **2016**, *2*, 19–23. [CrossRef]
24. Goes, C.R.; Balbi, A.L.; Ponce, D. Evaluation of Factors Associated with Hypermetabolism and Hypometabolism in Critically Ill AKI Patients. *Nutrients* **2018**, *10*, 505. [CrossRef]
25. Sabatino, A.; Theilla, M.; Hellerman, M.; Singer, P.; Maggiore, U.; Barbagallo, M.; Regolisti, G.; Fiaccadori, E. Energy and Protein in Critically Ill Patients with AKI: A Prospective, Multicenter Observational Study Using Indirect Calorimetry and Protein Catabolic Rate. *Nutrients* **2017**, *9*, 802. [CrossRef]
26. Kreymann, G.; Grosser, S.; Buggisch, P.; Gottschall, C.; Matthaei, S.; Greten, H. Oxygen consumption and resting metabolic rate in sepsis, sepsis syndrome, and septic shock. *Crit. Care Med.* **1993**, *21*, 1012–1019. [CrossRef]
27. Wu, C.; Wang, X.Y.; Yu, W.K.; Tian, F.; Liu, S.T.; Li, P.; Li, J.; Li, N. Hypermetabolism in the Initial Phase of Intensive Care Is Related to a Poor Outcome in Severe Sepsis Patients. *Ann. Nutr. Metab.* **2015**, *66*, 188–195. [CrossRef]
28. Puthucheary, Z.A.; Rawal, J.; McPhail, M.; Connolly, B.; Ratnayake, G.; Chan, P.; Hopkinson, N.S.; Phadke, R.; Dew, T.; Sidhu, P.S.; et al. Acute skeletal muscle wasting in critical illness. *JAMA* **2013**, *310*, 1591–1600. [CrossRef]
29. Jeon, J.; Kym, D.; Cho, Y.S.; Kim, Y.; Yoon, J.; Yim, H.; Hur, J.; Chun, W. Reliability of resting energy expenditure in major burns: Comparison between measured and predictive equations. *Clin. Nutr.* **2018**. [CrossRef]
30. McClave, S.A.; Martindale, R.G.; Kiraly, L. The use of indirect calorimetry in the intensive care unit. *Curr. Opin. Clin. Nutr. Metab. Care* **2013**, *16*, 202–208. [CrossRef]
31. Foley, N.; Marshall, S.; Pikul, J.; Salter, K.; Teasell, R. Hypermetabolism following moderate to severe traumatic acute brain injury: A systematic review. *J. Neurotrauma* **2008**, *25*, 1415–1431. [CrossRef]
32. Berger, M.M.; Pichard, C. Feeding should be individualized in the critically ill patients. *Curr. Opin. Crit. Care* **2019**, *25*, 307–313. [CrossRef]
33. Ndahimana, D.; Kim, E.K. Energy Requirements in Critically Ill Patients. *Clin. Nutr. Res.* **2018**, *7*, 81–90. [CrossRef]

34. Singer, P.; Blaser, A.R.; Berger, M.M.; Alhazzani, W.; Calder, P.C.; Casaer, M.P.; Hiesmayrh, M.; Mayeri, K.; Montejoj, J.C.; Pichard, C.; et al. ESPEN guideline on clinical nutrition in the intensive care unit. *Clin. Nutr.* **2019**, *38*, 48–79. [CrossRef]
35. Zusman, O.; Kagan, I.; Bendavid, I.; Theilla, M.; Cohen, J.; Singer, P. Predictive equations versus measured energy expenditure by indirect calorimetry: A retrospective validation. *Clin. Nutr.* **2018**. [CrossRef]
36. Wolfe, R.R. Sepsis as a modulator of adaptation to low and high carbohydrate and low and high fat intakes. *Eur. J. Clin. Nutr.* **1999**, *53*, S136–S142. [CrossRef]
37. Tappy, L.; Schwarz, J.M.; Schneiter, P.; Cayeux, C.; Revelly, J.P.; Fagerquist, C.K.; Jéquier, E.; Chioléro, R. Effects of isoenergetic glucose-based or lipid-based parenteral nutrition on glucose metabolism, de novo lipogenesis, and respiratory gas exchanges in critically ill patients. *Crit. Care Med.* **1998**, *26*, 860–867. [CrossRef]
38. Viana, M.V.; Pantet, O.; Bagnoud, G.; Martinez, A.; Favre, E.; Charriere, M.; Favre, D.; Eckert, P.; Berger, M.M. Metabolic and Nutritional Characteristics of Long-Stay Critically Ill Patients. *J. Clin. Med.* **2019**, *8*, 985. [CrossRef]
39. Reignier, J.; Boisrame-Helms, J.; Brisard, L.; Lascarrou, J.B.; Ait Hssain, A.; Anguel, N.; Argaud, L.; Asehnoune, K.; Asfar, P.; Bellec, F.; et al. Enteral versus parenteral early nutrition in ventilated adults with shock: A randomised, controlled, multicentre, open-label, parallel-group study (NUTRIREA-2). *Lancet* **2018**, *391*, 133–143. [CrossRef]
40. Avesani, C.M.; Draibe, S.A.; Kamimura, M.A.; Dalboni, M.A.; Colugnati, F.A.; Cuppari, L. Decreased resting energy expenditure in non-dialysed chronic kidney disease patients. *Nephrol. Dial. Transplant.* **2004**, *19*, 3091–3097. [CrossRef]
41. Neyra, R.; Chen, K.Y.; Sun, M.; Shyr, Y.; Hakim, R.M.; Ikizler, T.A. Increased resting energy expenditure in patients with end-stage renal disease. *J. Parenter. Enteral. Nutr.* **2003**, *27*, 36–42. [CrossRef]
42. Kamimura, M.A.; Draibe, S.A.; Avesani, C.M.; Canziani, M.E.; Colugnati, F.A.; Cuppari, L. Resting energy expenditure and its determinants in hemodialysis patients. *Eur. J. Clin. Nutr.* **2007**, *61*, 362–367. [CrossRef]
43. Ikizler, T.A.; Wingard, R.L.; Sun, M.; Harvell, J.; Parker, R.A.; Hakim, R.M. Increased energy expenditure in hemodialysis patients. *J. Am. Soc. Nephrol.* **1996**, *7*, 2646–2653.
44. Cekici, H.; Acar Tek, N. Determining energy requirement and evaluating energy expenditure in neurological diseases. *Nutr. Neurosci.* **2018**, 1–11. [CrossRef]
45. Huggett, R.J.; Scott, E.M.; Gilbey, S.G.; Stoker, J.B.; Mackintosh, A.F.; Mary, D.A. Impact of type 2 diabetes mellitus on sympathetic neural mechanisms in hypertension. *Circulation* **2003**, *108*, 3097–3101. [CrossRef]
46. Farooqi, N.; Carlsson, M.; Haglin, L.; Sandstrom, T.; Slinde, F. Energy expenditure in women and men with COPD. *Clin. Nutr. ESPEN* **2018**, *28*, 171–178. [CrossRef]
47. Carneiro, I.P.; Elliott, S.A.; Siervo, M.; Padwal, R.; Bertoli, S.; Battezzati, A.; Prado, C.M. Is Obesity Associated with Altered Energy Expenditure? *Adv. Nutr.* **2016**, *7*, 476–487. [CrossRef]
48. Cuerda, C.; Ruiz, A.; Velasco, C.; Breton, I.; Camblor, M.; Garcia-Peris, P. How accurate are predictive formulas calculating energy expenditure in adolescent patients with anorexia nervosa? *Clin. Nutr.* **2007**, *26*, 100–106. [CrossRef]
49. Yeh, D.D.; Fuentes, E.; Quraishi, S.A.; Cropano, C.; Kaafarani, H.; Lee, J.; King, D.R.; DeMoya, M.; Fagenholz, P.; Butler, K.; et al. Adequate Nutrition May Get You Home: Effect of Caloric/Protein Deficits on the Discharge Destination of Critically Ill Surgical Patients. *JPEN* **2016**, *40*, 37–44. [CrossRef]
50. Milte, R.K.; Ratcliffe, J.; Miller, M.D.; Crotty, M. Economic evaluation for protein and energy supplementation in adults: Opportunities to strengthen the evidence. *Eur. J. Clin. Nutr.* **2013**, *67*, 1243–1250. [CrossRef]
51. Correia, M.; Perman, M.I.; Pradelli, L.; Omaralsaleh, A.J.; Waitzberg, D.L. Economic burden of hospital malnutrition and the cost-benefit of supplemental parenteral nutrition in critically ill patients in Latin America. *J. Med. Econ.* **2018**, *21*, 1047–1056. [CrossRef]
52. Pradelli, L.; Graf, S.; Pichard, C.; Berger, M.M. Supplemental parenteral nutrition in intensive care patients: A cost saving strategy. *Clin. Nutr.* **2018**, *37*, 573–579. [CrossRef]
53. Berger, M.M.; Pichard, C. Parenteral nutrition in the ICU: Lessons learned over the past few years. *Nutrition* **2019**, *59*, 188–194. [CrossRef]
54. Haugen, H.A.; Chan, L.N.; Li, F. Indirect calorimetry: A practical guide for clinicians. *Nutr. Clin. Pract.* **2007**, *22*, 377–388. [CrossRef]

55. De Waele, E.; van Zwam, K.; Mattens, S.; Staessens, K.; Diltoer, M.; Honore, P.M.; Czapla, J.; Nijs, J.; La Meir, M.; Huyghens, L.; et al. Measuring resting energy expenditure during extracorporeal membrane oxygenation: Preliminary clinical experience with a proposed theoretical model. *Acta Anaesthesiol. Scand.* **2015**, *59*, 1296–1302. [CrossRef]
56. Wollersheim, T.; Frank, S.; Muller, M.C.; Skrypnikov, V.; Carbon, N.M.; Pickerodt, P.A.; Spies, C.; Mai, K.; Spranger, J.; Weber-Carstens, S. Measuring Energy Expenditure in extracorporeal lung support Patients (MEEP)-Protocol, feasibility and pilot trial. *Clin. Nutr.* **2018**, *37*, 301–307. [CrossRef]
57. Graf, S.; Karsegard, V.L.; Viatte, V.; Heidegger, C.P.; Fleury, Y.; Pichard, C.; Genton, L. Evaluation of three indirect calorimetry devices in mechanically ventilated patients: Which device compares best with the Deltatrac II(®)? A prospective observational study. *Clin. Nutr.* **2015**, *34*, 60–65. [CrossRef]
58. Graf, S.; Karsegard, V.L.; Viatte, V.; Maisonneuve, N.; Pichard, C.; Genton, L. Comparison of three indirect calorimetry devices and three methods of gas collection: A prospective observational study. *Clin. Nutr.* **2013**, *32*, 1067–1072. [CrossRef]
59. Sundstrom, M.; Tjader, I.; Rooyackers, O.; Wernerman, J. Indirect calorimetry in mechanically ventilated patients. A systematic comparison of three instruments. *Clin. Nutr.* **2013**, *32*, 118–121. [CrossRef]
60. Cooper, J.A.; Watras, A.C.; O'Brien, M.J.; Luke, A.; Dobratz, J.R.; Earthman, C.P.; Schoeller, D.A. Assessing validity and reliability of resting metabolic rate in six gas analysis systems. *J. Am. Diet. Assoc.* **2009**, *109*, 128–132. [CrossRef]
61. Hipskind, P.; Glass, C.; Charlton, D.; Nowak, D.; Dasarathy, S. Do handheld calorimeters have a role in assessment of nutrition needs in hospitalized patients? A systematic review of literature. *Nutr. Clin. Pract.* **2011**, *26*, 426–433. [CrossRef]
62. Hlynsky, J.; Birmingham, C.L.; Johnston, M.; Gritzner, S. The agreement between the MedGem indirect calorimeter and a standard indirect calorimeter in anorexia nervosa. *Eat. Weight Disord.* **2005**, *10*, e83–e87. [CrossRef]
63. Alam, D.S.; Hulshof, P.J.; Roordink, D.; Meltzer, M.; Yunus, M.; Salam, M.A.; van Raaij, J.M. Validity and reproducibility of resting metabolic rate measurements in rural Bangladeshi women: Comparison of measurements obtained by Medgem and by Deltatrac device. *Eur. J. Clin. Nutr.* **2005**, *59*, 651–657. [CrossRef]
64. Frankenfield, D.C.; Coleman, A. An evaluation of a handheld indirect calorimeter against a standard calorimeter in obese and nonobese adults. *JPEN* **2013**, *37*, 652–658. [CrossRef]
65. Schock, L.; Lam, L.; Tandon, P.; Taylor, L.; Raman, M. Indirect Calorimetry Performance Using a Handheld Device Compared to the Metabolic Cart in Outpatients with Cirrhosis. *Nutrients* **2019**, *11*, 1030. [CrossRef]
66. Anderson, E.J.; Sylvia, L.G.; Lynch, M.; Sonnenberg, L.; Lee, H.; Nathan, D.M. Comparison of energy assessment methods in overweight individuals. *J. Acad. Nutr. Diet.* **2014**, *114*, 273–278. [CrossRef]
67. White, D.A.; Staggs, V.S.; Williams, V.; Edwards, T.C.; Shook, R.; Shakhnovich, V. Handheld Indirect Calorimetry as a Clinical Tool for Measuring Resting Energy Expenditure in Children with and without Obesity. *Child. Obes.* **2019**, *15*, 280–287. [CrossRef]
68. Fields, D.A.; Kearney, J.T.; Copeland, K.C. MedGem hand-held indirect calorimeter is valid for resting energy expenditure measurement in healthy children. *Obesity (Silver Spring)* **2006**, *14*, 1755–1761. [CrossRef]
69. Woo, P.; Murthy, G.; Wong, C.; Hursh, B.; Chanoine, J.P.; Elango, R. Assessing resting energy expenditure in overweight and obese adolescents in a clinical setting: Validity of a handheld indirect calorimeter. *Pediatr Res.* **2017**, *81*, 51–56. [CrossRef]
70. Oshima, T.; Dupertuis, Y.M.; Delsoglio, M.; Graf, S.; Heidegger, C.P.; Pichard, C. In vitro validation of indirect calorimetry device developed for the ICALIC project against mass spectrometry. *Clin. Nutr. ESPEN.* **2019**, *32*, 50–55. [CrossRef]
71. Delsoglio, M.; Dupertuis, Y.M.; Oshima, T.; van der Plas, M.; Pichard, C. Evaluation of the accuracy and precision of a new generation indirect calorimeter in canopy dilution mode. *Clin. Nutr.* **2019**, in press.
72. Xiaojun, X.; Quach, A.; Bridgeman, D.; Tsow, F.; Forzani, E.; Tao, N. Personalized Indirect Calorimeter for Energy Expenditure (EE) Measurement. *Glob. J. Obes. Diabetes Metab. Syndr.* **2015**. [CrossRef]
73. Jesus, P.; Achamrah, N.; Grigioni, S.; Charles, J.; Rimbert, A.; Folope, V.; Petit, A.; Déchelotte, P.; Coëffier, M. Validity of predictive equations for resting energy expenditure according to the body mass index in a population of 1726 patients followed in a Nutrition Unit. *Clin. Nutr.* **2015**, *34*, 529–535. [CrossRef]

74. Soussi, S.; Vallee, F.; Roquet, F.; Bevilacqua, V.; Benyamina, M.; Ferry, A.; Cupaciu, A.; Chaussard, M.; De Tymowski, C.; Boccara, D.; et al. Measurement of Oxygen Consumption Variations in Critically Ill Burns Patients: Are the Fick Method and Indirect Calorimetry Interchangeable? *Shock* **2017**, *48*, 532–538. [CrossRef]
75. Inadomi, C.; Terao, Y.; Yamashita, K.; Fukusaki, M.; Takada, M.; Sumikawa, K. Comparison of oxygen consumption calculated by Fick's principle (using a central venous catheter) and measured by indirect calorimetry. *J. Anesth.* **2008**, *22*, 163–166. [CrossRef]
76. Ogawa, A.M.; Shikora, S.A.; Burke, L.M.; Heetderks-Cox, J.E.; Bergren, C.T.; Muskat, P.C. The thermodilution technique for measuring resting energy expenditure does not agree with indirect calorimetry for the critically ill patient. *J. Parenter. Enter. Nutr.* **1998**, *22*, 347–351. [CrossRef]
77. Oshima, T.; Graf, S.; Heidegger, C.P.; Genton, L.; Pugin, J.; Pichard, C. Can calculation of energy expenditure based on CO2 measurements replace indirect calorimetry? *Crit. Care* **2017**, *21*, 13. [CrossRef]
78. Stapel, S.N.; de Grooth, H.J.S.; Alimohamad, H.; Elbers, P.W.G.; Girbes, A.R.J.; Weijs, P.J.M.; Oudemans-van Straaten, H.M. Ventilator-derived carbon dioxide production to assess energy expenditure in critically ill patients: Proof of concept. *Crit. Care* **2015**, *19*, 370. [CrossRef]
79. Rousing, M.L.; Hahn-Pedersen, M.H.; Andreassen, S.; Pielmeier, U.; Preiser, J.C. Energy expenditure in critically ill patients estimated by population-based equations, indirect calorimetry and CO2-based indirect calorimetry. *Ann. Intensiv. Care* **2016**, *6*, 16. [CrossRef]
80. Kagan, I.; Zusman, O.; Bendavid, I.; Theilla, M.; Cohen, J.; Singer, P. Validation of carbon dioxide production (VCO2) as a tool to calculate resting energy expenditure (REE) in mechanically ventilated critically ill patients: A retrospective observational study. *Crit. Care* **2018**, *22*, 186. [CrossRef]
81. de Carvalho Bastone, A.; Ferriolli, E.; Pfrimer, K.; de Souza Moreira, B.; Diz, J.B.M.; Dias, J.M.D.; Dias, R.C. Energy Expenditure in Older Adults Who Are Frail: A Doubly Labeled Water Study. *J. Geriatr. Phys. Ther.* **2017**. [CrossRef]
82. Schutz, Y. Respiration chamber calorimetry and doubly labeled water: Two complementary aspects of energy expenditure? *Eur. J. Clin. Nutr.* **2018**, *72*, 1310–1313. [CrossRef]
83. Wahl, Y.; Duking, P.; Droszez, A.; Wahl, P.; Mester, J. Criterion-Validity of Commercially Available Physical Activity Tracker to Estimate Step Count, Covered Distance and Energy Expenditure during Sports Conditions. *Front. Physiol.* **2017**, *8*, 725. [CrossRef]
84. Hashizume, N.; Tanaka, Y.; Yoshida, M.; Fukahori, S.; Ishii, S.; Saikusa, N.; Masui, D.; Higashidate, N.; Sakamoto, S.; Tsuruhisa, S.; et al. Resting energy expenditure prediction using bioelectrical impedance analysis in patients with severe motor and intellectual disabilities. *Brain Dev. Jpn.* **2019**, *41*, 352–358. [CrossRef]
85. Jesus, P.; Marin, B.; Fayemendy, P.; Nicol, M.; Lautrette, G.; Sourisseau, H.; Preux, P.M.; Couratier, P.; Desport, J.C. Resting energy expenditure equations in amyotrophic lateral sclerosis, creation of an ALS-specific equation. *Clin. Nutr.* **2019**, *38*, 1657–1665. [CrossRef]
86. Barak, N.; Wall-Alonso, E.; Cheng, A.; Sitrin, M.D. Use of bioelectrical impedance analysis to predict energy expenditure of hospitalized patients receiving nutrition support. *JPEN* **2003**, *27*, 43–46. [CrossRef]
87. Kruizenga, H.M.; Hofsteenge, G.H.; Weijs, P.J. Predicting resting energy expenditure in underweight, normal weight, overweight, and obese adult hospital patients. *Nutr. Metab. (Lond.)* **2016**, *13*, 85. [CrossRef]
88. Achamrah, N.; Jesus, P.; Grigioni, S.; Rimbert, A.; Petit, A.; Dechelotte, P.; Folope, V.; Coëffier, M. Validity of Predictive Equations for Resting Energy Expenditure Developed for Obese Patients: Impact of Body Composition Method. *Nutrients* **2018**, *10*, 63. [CrossRef]
89. Orozco-Ruiz, X.; Pichardo-Ontiveros, E.; Tovar, A.R.; Torres, N.; Medina-Vera, I.; Prinelli, F.; Lafortuna, C.L.; Guevara-Cruz, M. Development and validation of new predictive equation for resting energy expenditure in adults with overweight and obesity. *Clin. Nutr.* **2018**, *37 Pt A*, 2198–2205. [CrossRef]
90. Cancello, R.; Soranna, D.; Brunani, A.; Scacchi, M.; Tagliaferri, A.; Mai, S.; Marzullo, P.; Zambon, A.; Invitti, C. Analysis of Predictive Equations for Estimating Resting Energy Expenditure in a Large Cohort of Morbidly Obese Patients. *Front. Endocrinol. (Lausanne)* **2018**, *9*, 367. [CrossRef]
91. Kross, E.K.; Sena, M.; Schmidt, K.; Stapleton, R.D. A comparison of predictive equations of energy expenditure and measured energy expenditure in critically ill patients. *J. Crit. Care* **2012**, *27*, 321.e5. [CrossRef]
92. Costa, N.A.; Marinho, A.D.; Cancado, L.R. Nutritional requirements of the critically ill patient. *Rev. Bras. Ter. Intensiv.* **2012**, *24*, 270–277. [CrossRef]

93. MacDonald, A.; Hildebrandt, L. Comparison of formulaic equations to determine energy expenditure in the critically ill patient. *Nutrition* **2003**, *19*, 233–239. [CrossRef]
94. Pichard, C.; Oshima, T.; Berger, M.M. Energy deficit is clinically relevant for critically ill patients: Yes. *Intensiv. Care Med.* **2015**, *41*, 335–338. [CrossRef]
95. Frankenfield, D.C.; Ashcraft, C.M. Estimating energy needs in nutrition support patients. *J. Parenter. Enter. Nutr.* **2011**, *35*, 563–570. [CrossRef]
96. Graf, S.; Pichard, C.; Genton, L.; Oshima, T.; Heidegger, C.P. Energy expenditure in mechanically ventilated patients: The weight of body weight! *Clin. Nutr.* **2017**, *36*, 224–228. [CrossRef]
97. Ramos, F.M.; Rossato, L.T.; Ramires, B.R.; Pimentel, G.D.; Venancio, L.S.; Orsatti, F.L.; de Oliveira, E.P. Comparison of predictive equations of resting energy expenditure in older adults with chronic obstructive pulmonary disease. *Rev. Port. Pneumol. (2006)* **2017**, *23*, 40–42. [CrossRef]
98. Kamimura, M.A.; Avesani, C.M.; Bazanelli, A.P.; Baria, F.; Draibe, S.A.; Cuppari, L. Are prediction equations reliable for estimating resting energy expenditure in chronic kidney disease patients? *Nephrol. Dial. Transplant.* **2011**, *26*, 544–550. [CrossRef]
99. Behera, K.K.; Joseph, M.; Shetty, S.K.; Chacko, A.; Sahoo, M.K.; Mahendri, N.V.; Nair, V.; Nadig, S.; Thomas, N. Resting energy expenditure in subjects with fibro-calculous pancreatic diabetes. *J. Diabetes* **2014**, *6*, 158–163. [CrossRef]
100. Khor, S.M.; Mohd, B.B. Assessing the resting energy expenditure of cancer patients in the Penang General Hospital. *Malays. J. Nutr.* **2011**, *17*, 43–53.
101. Eslamparast, T.; Vandermeer, B.; Raman, M.; Gramlich, L.; Den Heyer, V.; Belland, D.; Ma, M.; Tandon, P. Are Predictive Energy Expenditure Equations Accurate in Cirrhosis? *Nutrients* **2019**, *11*, 334. [CrossRef]
102. Frankenfield, D.C. Bias and accuracy of resting metabolic rate equations in non-obese and obese adults. *Clin. Nutr.* **2013**, *32*, 976–982. [CrossRef]

# 15

# Efficacy and Efficiency of Nutritional Support Teams

**Emilie Reber [1,*], Rachel Strahm [1], Lia Bally [1], Philipp Schuetz [2,3] and Zeno Stanga [1]**

1 Department of Diabetes, Endocrinology, Nutritional Medicine and Metabolism, Bern University Hospital, and University of Bern, Freiburgstrasse 15, 3010 Bern, Switzerland
2 Department of Medical University, Division of General Internal and Emergency Medicine, Kantonsspital Aarau, Tellstrasse 25, 5000 Aarau, Switzerland
3 Department for Clinical Research, Medical Faculty, University of Basel, 4001 Basel, Switzerland
* Correspondence: emilie.reber@insel.ch

**Abstract:** Malnutrition is frequent in patients during a hospital admission and may further worsen during the hospital stay without appropriate nutritional support. Malnutrition causes greater complication rates, morbidity, and mortality rates, which increases the length of hospital stay and prolongs rehabilitation. Early recognition of individual nutritional risk and timely initiation of a tailored nutritional therapy are crucial. Recent evidence from large-scale trials suggests that efficient nutritional management not only improves the nutritional status, but also prevents negative clinical outcomes and increases patients' quality of life. Multifaceted clinical knowledge is required to ensure optimal nutritional support, according to a patient's individual situation and to avoid potential complications. Furthermore, clear definition of responsibilities and structuring of patient, and work processes are indispensable. Interdisciplinary and multiprofessional nutritional support teams have been built up to ensure and improve the quality and safety of nutritional treatments. These teams continuously check and optimize the quality of procedures in the core areas of nutritional management by implementing nutritional screening processes using a validated tool, nutritional status assessment, an adequate nutritional care plan development, prompt and targeted nutritional treatment delivery, and provision of accurate monitoring to oversee all aspects of care, from catering to artificial nutrition. The foundation of any nutritional care plan is the identification of patients at risk. The aim of this narrative review is to provide an overview about composition, tasks, and challenges of nutritional support teams, and to discuss the current evidence regarding their efficiency and efficacy in terms of clinical outcome and cost effectiveness.

**Keywords:** nutritional support team; nutritional management; malnutrition; efficacy

---

## 1. Introduction

Malnutrition, which is defined as a state resulting from the lack of intake or uptake of nutrition leading to altered body composition, decreased mental and physical function, and impaired clinical outcome, is a lurking threat at hospitals in developing countries as well as in industrialized countries [1–5]. Up to 50% of admitted patients are malnourished or at high risk for malnutrition. Acutely ill patients frequently suffer from inflammation and subsequent anorexia, which leads to inadequate food intake and, therefore, to a catabolic state. Under these circumstances, the nutritional status further deteriorates, which may cause rapid weight loss [6].

The association between malnutrition and adverse clinical outcome is well described in the literature [7–32]. Nutritional treatment is urgently needed in malnourished patients to counteract negative metabolic and clinical consequences, to speed up recovery processes, and to enable better quality of life and patient autonomy [2,28,33–35].

The term "food chain" (Figure 1) has been adopted to emphasize that all stages in nutritional care must be adequate, from screening of patients and planning of menus to the distribution and serving of the food [36,37]. Because of the risks, and need for nutritional support, it is desirable for hospitals to appoint a multidisciplinary and multiprofessional nutrition steering group, including the clinical nutrition team, to oversee all aspects of nutritional care, from catering to artificial nutrition [36].

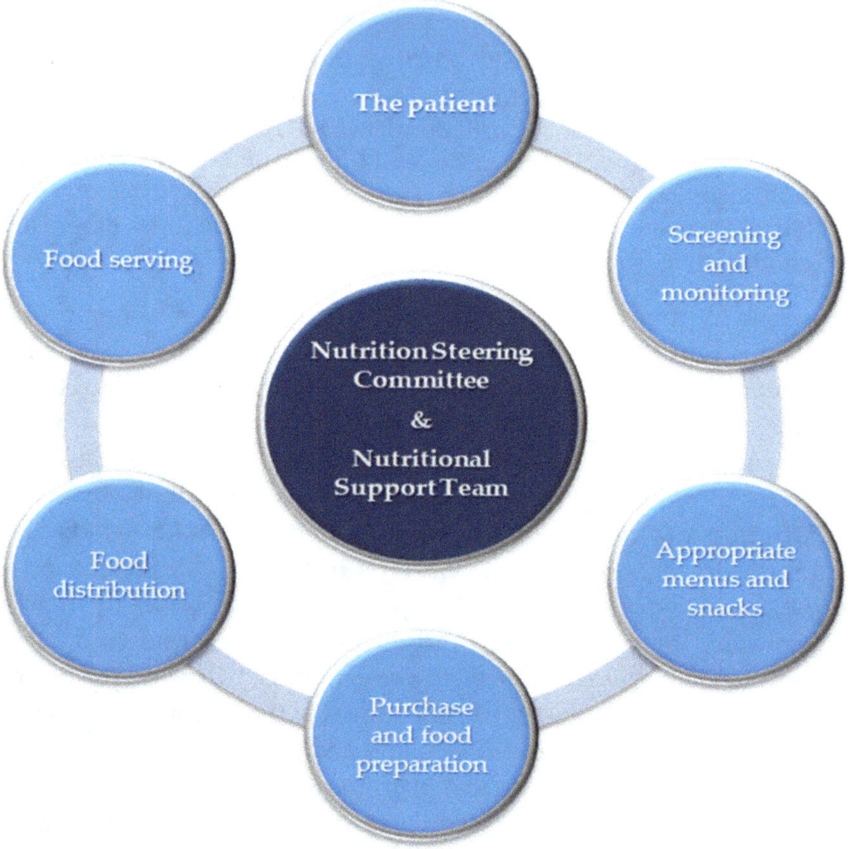
The patient
Screening and monitoring
Appropriate menus and snacks
Purchase and food preparation
Food distribution
Food serving
Nutrition Steering Committee
&
Nutritional Support Team

**Figure 1.** The food chain [36]. The food chain has been adopted to emphasize that all stages in the provision of food must be adequate, from screening of patients and planning of menus to the distribution and serving of the food.

Appropriate, high-quality hospital food is part of a multimodal therapy that includes a wide selection of meals, snacks between meals, and the option of fortified food. The majority of hospitals in industrialized countries should be able to provide such meals, which enable patients to meet their nutritional needs. The problem is that the number of hospitals have now outsourced the hospital kitchen, e.g., to catering companies, which may make it difficult to offer best quality food to patients. Meals may, for example, be frozen and unfrozen or heated twice, which causes an important loss of quality, e.g., regarding micronutrients. Remarkably, more than 40% of meals are left on the patient's plate and wasted, which means a patients' food consumption meets less than 80% of their nutritional needs, and causes additional costs for the hospital [38,39].

The high prevalence of malnutrition implies a close monitoring of food intake, on the one hand, by means of adequate meal-ordering systems and, on the other hand, by sensitizing hospital medical staff to nutritional issues. The keys to better manage nutritional support in hospitals are: (1) enhanced awareness and (2) profound knowledge of this complex matter. Attention to the organization is needed from the medical staff on the ward such as to prevent interruption of meals due to procedures or rounds, and to provide support for disabled patients who need assistance with eating. Such essential tasks have been shown to improve clinical outcomes and reduce healthcare costs in several studies [40–42].

In hospitals, competent nutritional management should rely on two structures: nutritional steering committees and multiprofessional nutritional support teams (NSTs) (Figure 2). The nutrition steering committee is the legislative body with direct access to hospital management (staff function). This committee consists of representative nurses, physicians, pharmacists, dieticians, cooks, managers, controllers, NST members, etc. [43]. It is responsible for promoting good nutrition as a policy, with explicit written nutritional standards, protocols, and guidelines. Further responsibilities are meant to guarantee choice of a wide range of meals and to support continuous improvement and monitoring of the nutritional therapy in terms of quality, safety, and medical efficacy [44]. This committee is also responsible for education, teaching, training, and research coordination. The nutrition steering committee and the NST should also collaborate closely with other hospitals and, in case of tertiary urban hospitals with the University as well as national and international nutritional societies, for clinical research and teaching purposes. NST exercises an executive function throughout the hospital (Figure 3). An optimal functioning institutionalized NST as described above is possible in an urban setting due to the high personal and financial resources allocated. In suburban or rural regions, it is also possible to build an NST but in a reduced format. Our long-lasting clinical experience shows that a single dietician with a physician with special interest in clinical nutrition can overtake the most important clinical tasks of an NST. There is a great opportunity to perform high standing qualitative nutritional care in any setting even if a dietician is available only once a week.

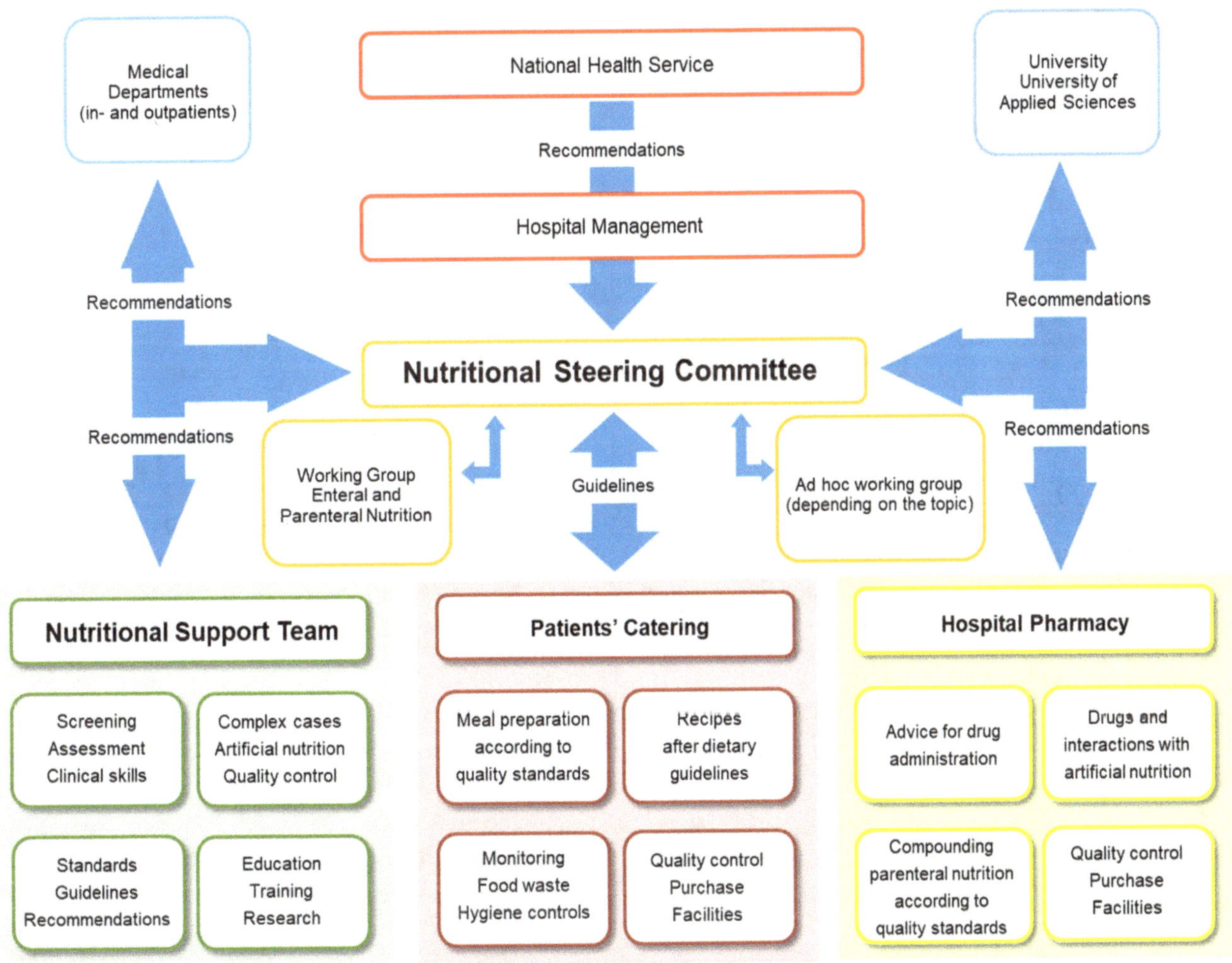


**Figure 2.** Nutritional management structure, with the Bern University Hospital, as an example.

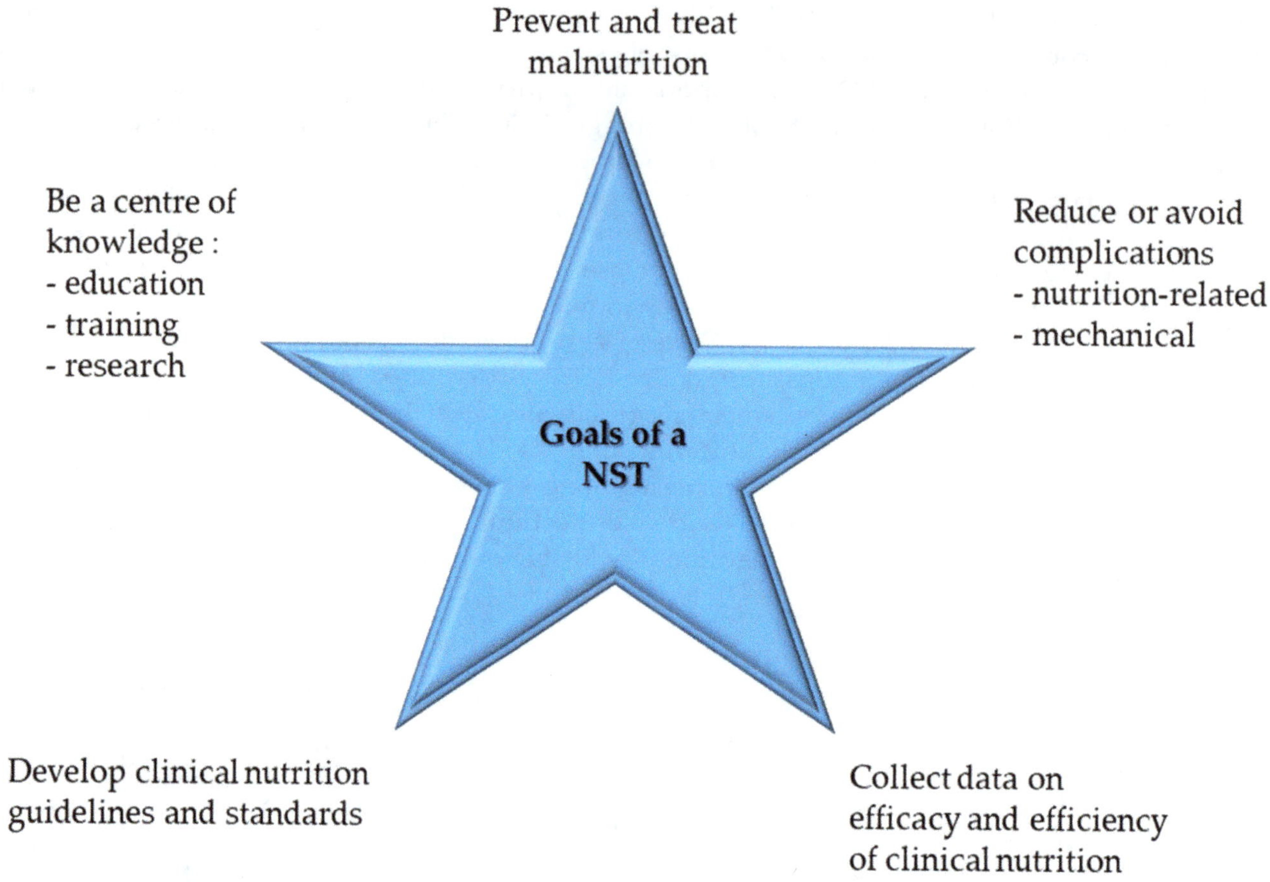


**Figure 3.** Goals of an NST, modified after [43].

Even though there has been considerable interest in NST to improve nutritional care and, thereby, patient outcomes, there is still a lack of strong scientific evidence mainly due to only a few randomized controlled studies with small heterogeneous study populations, different treatments, and non-standardized outcomes. The aim of this narrative review is to provide an overview about composition, tasks, and challenges of nutritional support teams and discuss the current evidence regarding their efficiency and efficacy in terms of clinical outcome and cost effectiveness.

## 2. Development of NSTs

While tube feeding (enteral nutrition) has been used since the Renaissance, parenteral nutrition was first successfully used in 1968 [45,46]. At that point, nutritional therapy was established in the clinical setting. Years later, case reports on negative outcomes caused by inadequate nutritional therapies were published. Several studies showed that medical staff often overlooks the clinical signs of malnutrition, which leads to longer hospital stays and higher mortality rates [17].

NSTs were developed to counteract these concerns. At the same time, international societies such as the American Society for Clinical Nutrition (ASPEN, 1976) and the European Society for Clinical Nutrition and Metabolism (ESPEN, 1979) were created. Their primary objective was to study metabolic problems associated with acute diseases and their nutritional implications, and to provide each patient with timely and appropriate nutritional care. A study in 2005 found that NST were present in 2.8% of the hospitals in Germany, 7.9% in Austria, and 2.4% in Switzerland [48]. Ten years later, a Swiss survey indicated that 62% of the country's hospitals had an NST composed of at least one physician and one dietician [49]. Currently, data from the "Nutrition Day Worldwide" shows that most hospitals (mostly urban hospitals) in Europe (approximately 66%) and in the USA (approximately 60%) have such NSTs. This shows the rising importance of clinical nutrition in the industrialized countries [50].

## 3. NST Composition and Collaboration

Simon Allison (Nottingham, UK) defines an NST as a multiprofessional team including professionals from different disciplines who are good communicators and possess knowledge of the optimal delivery of nutritional therapy [51,52]. An NST improves and ensures the therapy quality and reduces health care costs by preventing needless interventions (e.g., ensuring the appropriateness of indication, stopping unnecessary long fluid therapies, preventing unnecessary catheter removals) and optimizing current treatments (e.g., combining nutritional and drug therapies) [7,23,29]. Smooth multiprofessional and interdisciplinary cooperation as well as impeccable communication are key for the success of an NST. Such a team is traditionally composed of physicians, dieticians, and nurses specialized in clinical nutrition, and pharmacists, with the dieticians primarily assuming the lead in coordinating nutritional care during a hospital stay and, thereafter, in the outpatient clinic [17,53–56].

The composition of the team may vary according to the local needs and options in terms of human resources. Additionally, intensive collaboration with hospital departments responsible for infectious diseases and hospital hygiene is advisable, particularly in the area of parenteral nutrition. This cooperation allows the NST to share knowledge and competence in catheter handling, which is important for preventing, diagnosing, and possibly treating catheter-related bloodstream infections [17]. Other specialists may also collaborate with the NST, such as physiotherapists, occupational therapists, psychotherapists, or social workers [54,56]. Multiprofessional collaboration has to be perceived as an opportunity to integrate the personal and professional expertise of each individual.

## 4. Tasks and Challenges of NSTs

While the nutritional steering committee has a legislative role, an NST has an executive function throughout the hospital in terms of implementing standards, protocols, and guidelines in daily clinical practice. The core task of an NST is to ensure and promote high-level, evidence-based management of nutrition and to transfer this theoretical knowledge into clinical practice. The foundation of any nutritional care plan (Figure 4) is assessment of nutritional risk and early adequate provision of nutritional support to patients at risk of or suffering from malnutrition. Nutritional support is considered an essential part of the multimodal medical therapy concept, which has demonstrated good therapeutic outcomes. The individual tasks of the members of an NST are shown in Table 1.

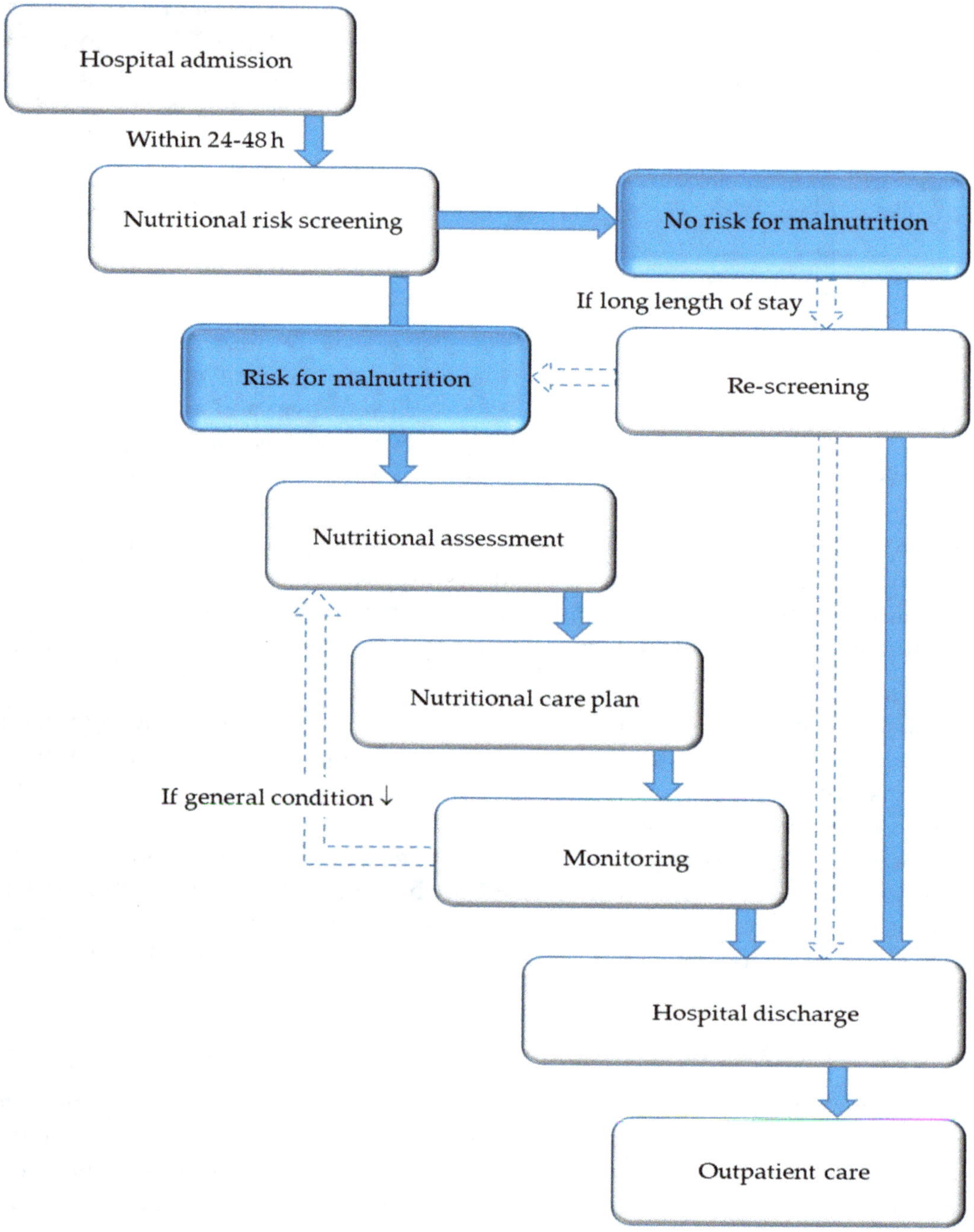


**Figure 4.** Nutritional care algorithm.

**Table 1.** Individual tasks of NST members [43].

| Professional Function | Nutritional Care Tasks |
|---|---|
| Nurse | • Gives advice on routes, methods, and systems for delivery of enteral/parenteral nutrition;<br>• Assesses adequacy of access to nutrition therapy;<br>• Advises on use of tubes, feeding pumps, and enteral/parenteral equipment;<br>• Implements and adapts protocols on methods of delivering enteral/parenteral nutrition to establish uniformity, save costs, and prevent mechanical complications;<br>• Educates on enteral/parenteral nutrition and highly complex nutritional therapy;<br>• Conducts research on complex nutritional therapy. |
| Physician | • Prescribes and manages enteral/parenteral therapy;<br>• Promotes the established nutrition therapy within the host specialty;<br>• Provides professional input for highly complex nutritional therapy;<br>• Supports ongoing research and projects on complex nutritional therapy;<br>• Informs colleagues, physicians in training, and members on the board of directors of the importance of good nutrition therapy on the ward. |
| Dietician | • Gives advice on enteral/parenteral nutrition (indications, choice of feeding solution, nutritional goals);<br>• Advises about options for enteral/parenteral nutrition and other nutrients (e.g., immuno-nutrition, vitamins, trace elements);<br>• Edits, implements, and adapts protocols on enteral/parenteral nutrition and complex nutritional therapy;<br>• Develops and interprets screening tools; initiates and performs nutritional assessment;<br>• Contributes to education and conducts research on complex nutritional solutions. |
| Pharmacist | • Provides logistical support for parenteral nutrition;<br>• Oversees and provides information about possible chemical/pharmaceutical interactions between parenteral nutrition components;<br>• Provides professional input on the composition of parenteral nutrition, on stability and compatibility of parenteral admixtures, and on drug/medication interactions with enteral/parenteral nutrition;<br>• Supports ongoing research projects on complex nutritional therapy, develops and implements parenteral nutrition protocols. |

### *4.1. Screening and Assessment*

One of the most important missions of a, NST is to educate, to teach, and to train professionals in the skills related to clinical nutrition [51,53,56]. Sharing knowledge and experience with medical staff, health care providers, and students is part of effective nutritional management [55]. Awareness for malnutrition (sensitization), education, and training are, however, lacking [57]. It is a core task of the NST to implement nutritional standards, protocols, and guidelines in daily clinical practice, by establishing proper protocols for screening, assessment, and action [53,58]. The consequences of malnutrition are frequently underestimated and malnutrition is, unfortunately, rarely documented as a distinct diagnosis in medical reports and nurses' charts despite being of central medical and economic importance in hospitals [57].

The first step of nutritional care is the identification of patients at nutritional risk using simple, quick, and validated screening tools. Nutritional screening should be performed in all inpatients (and, preferably, also outpatients) within 24–48 h after hospital admission, respectively, as well as admission on the ward/intermediate care unit/intensive care unit. Nutritional screening should be performed by trained medical staff, at best, multi-professionally from nurses and physicians in charge of the patients, but, alternatively, from nurses, dietitians, or physicians only [59,60]. The Nutritional Risk Screening 2002 (NRS 2002) (Figure 5) is a widely used and well-validated screening tool used in hospitals to determine whether the patient is at nutritional risk [61]. If confirmed, a care plan has to be developed, based on more detailed nutritional assessment to determine the degree/severity of malnutrition. Patients with special metabolic, functional, or clinical problems that cannot be cared for by standard means should be referred to nutrition experts for more detailed nutritional assessment and design of a care plan.

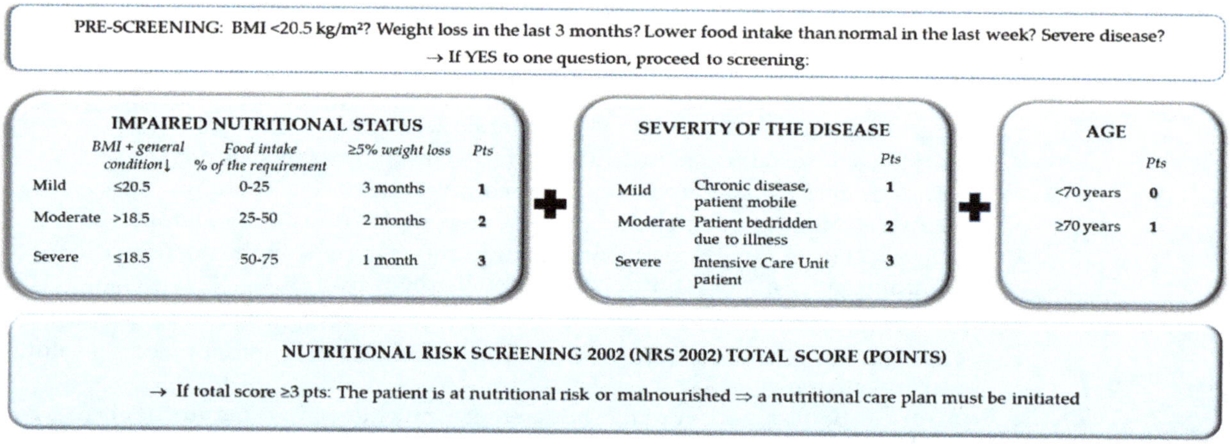


**Figure 5.** Nutritional risk screening 2002 [61].

Formal quantification of food intake may be helpful. Nutritional assessment can be carried out for at least two days using food diaries or food intake charts (e.g., semi-quantitative plate diagram) that are kept by nursing staff [62]. These can be used by dietitians to calculate energy and protein intake. Anthropometric measurements such as body weight, height, body mass index (BMI = weight ÷ (height in meters)$^2$), and, if applicable, mid-upper arm circumference or triceps skin fold tests may also be included [62,63]. In addition, according to the local circumstances and standards of care, the following additional measurements may complete the nutritional assessment: body composition (bioelectrical impedance analysis), muscle function (handgrip strength), activities of daily living (Barthel index), quality of life (mainly questionnaires such as SF-36 [64]), and calculation of energy requirements (e.g., Harris and Benedict formula, indirect calorimetry) [63]. Routine laboratory parameters (e.g., complete blood count, lipid profile, electrolytes, and liver parameters) may give information on the patient's nutritional state (proof of nutrient deficiency, information about the etiology of malnutrition, and follow-up of nutritional therapy), the disease severity and activity, and body composition changes to identify patients at nutritional risk [65]. However, none of these markers is very specific for nutritional deficiencies, and their medical interpretation is only possible in the context of the patient's clinical status and history. Thus, nutrition-related factors are hardly ever the sole cause of conspicuous laboratory findings, and there is no such thing as an optimal surrogate marker for malnutrition [65].

Laboratory values must, therefore, always be interpreted in a clinical context [66]. Nitrogen balance, albumin, prealbumin, transferrin, retinol binding protein, insulin growth factor-1, creatinine-height index, and total lymphocyte count are among the few parameters that may be used to quantify malnutrition in malnourished patients [65]. Concerning micronutrients, several potential deficiencies have been associated with malnutrition, including vitamins (i.e., vitamin B12, folic acid, fat-soluble vitamins A, D, E, K) and trace elements (especially zinc, iron, and selenium). The goal of nutritional assessment is to gain an understanding of the patient's nutritional status in order to develop a nutritional care plan containing an accurate calculation of the individual energy and protein requirements and choice of the most appropriate form of feeding (normal food, special consistency, fortified meals, snacks, oral nutritional supplements, or artificial nutrition support).

To call attention to the daily work of an NST (screening, assessment, and nutritional therapy) and, for the reimbursement of this procedure by insurance companies, it is crucial to record, document, and use the code for malnutrition in the Diagnosis Related Groups (DRG) tariff system. It is, therefore, important that the additional revenues arising from use of the DRG code for malnutrition and its therapy are reinvested to cover costs and promote NSTs.

### 4.2. Nutritional Therapy

NST offers a hospital-wide service with the aim to improve the quality of nutritional therapies targeting complex multimorbid patients, and, in general, to "fight against malnutrition." From a clinical and therapeutic standpoint, nutritional management starts with the identification of patients at nutritional risk—a status that will subsequently guide clinical decision-making—and focuses on those patients likely to benefit from nutritional therapy [67]. Using clinically important endpoints, there is now a substantial body of evidence showing that nutrition support improves outcome when it is implemented appropriately [28]. Thus, after an assessment has been completed and the severity of malnutrition has been determined, the attending medical staff—in cooperation with the NST—sets the individual nutritional plan and the strategy to achieve these goals (Figure 6). While the objective is always to fully meet the individual energy and protein requirements, one should strive for a nutritional intake of at least 75% of those needs [3,68]. Achievement of the goals set and adherence to therapy should be re-evaluated every 24–48 h. If necessary, the nutritional intervention should be adapted. Escalation of the support strategy—i.e., from oral to enteral or from enteral to parenteral nutrition—should be considered within five days [28].

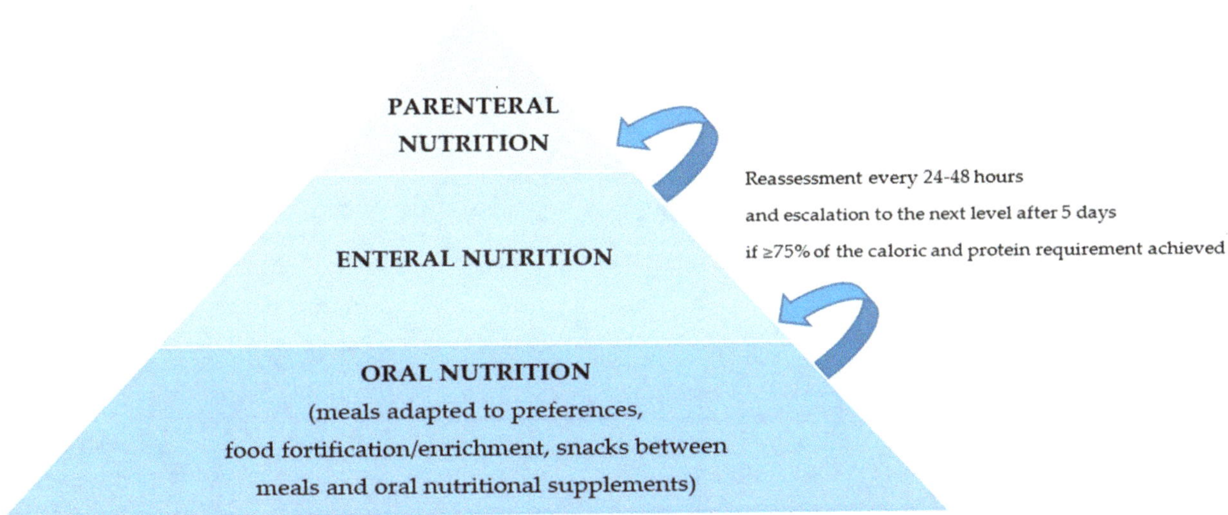


**Figure 6.** Strategy for nutritional therapy. The nutritional therapy is designed by an NST based on the patient's needs and current situation. The most physiologic route of nutrition delivery is preferable. Nutritional therapy should be regularly re-evaluated and escalated if needed.

### 4.3. Monitoring and Safety

An NST ensures the correct handling of the artificial nutrition, and reviews the appropriateness of the therapies and related prescriptions [51]. The initiation of a nutritional therapy in complex clinical situations and its proper documentation are also tasks of an NST [69]. An NST ensures the quality and safety of nutritional interventions, especially artificial nutrition, which helps to reduce potential mechanical and metabolic complications (e.g., blood glucose issues and refeeding syndrome) as well as infections [70]. The NST has a consultative role for the treating medical staff in the hospital and takes over the management of the nutritional therapy in outpatients.

### 4.4. Outpatient Management

Nutritional therapy is normally initialized during the hospital stay, and continued after discharge under close monitoring. The NST plays a key role in management of the therapy during the transition from the inpatient to the outpatient setting (Figure 7). The NST carries out regular visits on the wards, and, subsequently, plans and organizes the hospital discharge from a medical as well as a therapeutic point of view. It monitors the patients, when possible, in regular consultations in the outpatient' clinic. If artificial nutrition is needed at home, the multiprofessional NST instructs and educates patients as well as relatives and caregivers in close cooperation with the treating medical staff. After discharge, the NST remains the core contact for patients, their relatives, their general practitioners, and home care services regarding problems with nutritional therapy (intricate nutrition-related questions, complications, problems with devices, etc.). The NST also plays a central role in the outpatient setting, embedded in the complex interdisciplinary and multiprofessional therapeutic-medical network.

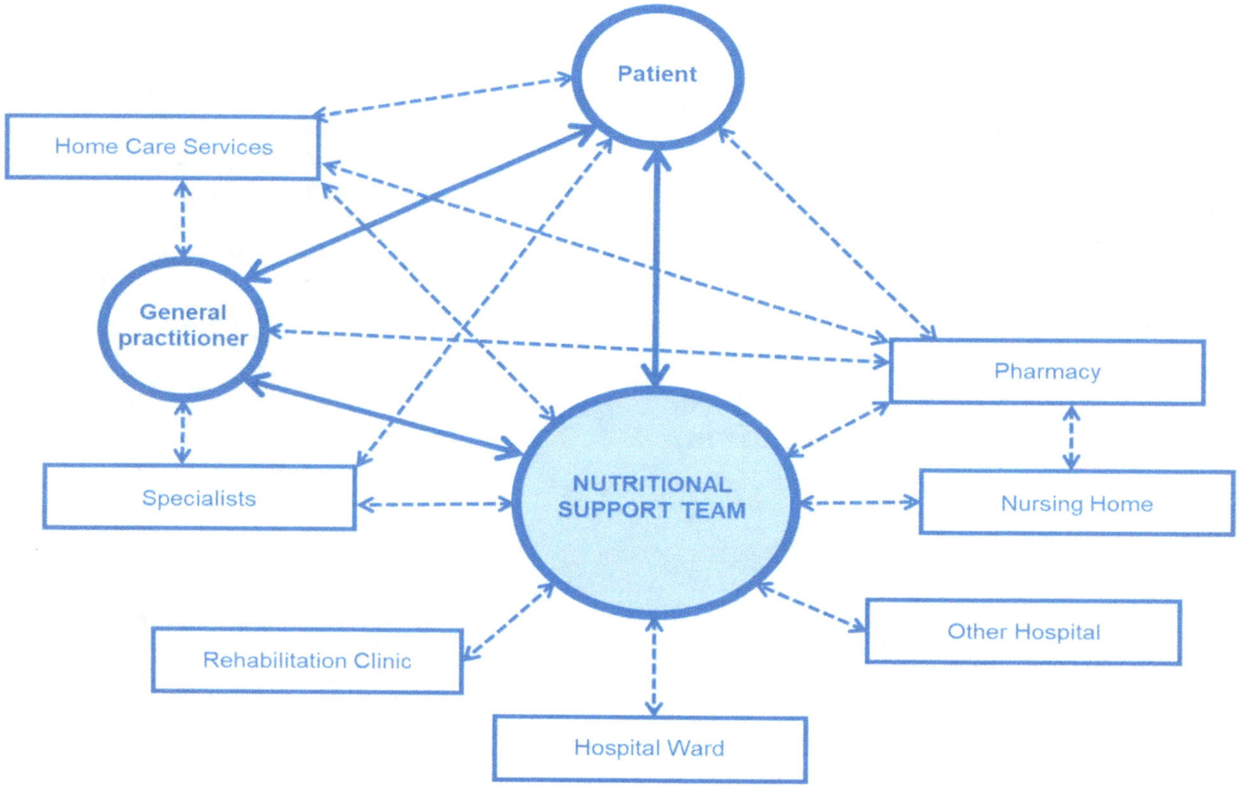


**Figure 7.** Network of an NST. NST has a central role in the management of patients with complex nutritional therapy in the inpatient and outpatient setting, during the hospital stay and beyond.

### 4.5. Standards and Processes

An NST monitors the clinical outcomes of the patients and regulates/optimizes processes of the nutritional intervention accordingly. Furthermore, NST periodically checks operating procedures as well as patient procedures, and proposes changes to optimize nutritional care. A good example is the transition from parenteral to enteral nutrition, or from enteral to oral therapy [58]. Since this is the platform of evidence-based practice, operational tasks of an NST include guaranteeing a wide range of meal choices, applying standards of care, implementing medical guidelines, developing standards for consultations, implementing evidence-based nutritional treatment, and maintaining high standards for the quality of hospital food (recipe management) in close collaboration with the catering department [36].

### *4.6. Education, Training, and Research*

An NST also oversees and coordinates education and training in the field of nutritional management, according to the local possibilities and settings. This includes the dissemination of experience, expertise, and skills to trainees, students, and residents as well as other medical and para-medical staff. Multiprofessional work, connected thinking, and effective interdisciplinary communication are mandatory [54–56,71,72]. NST can ensure optimal treatment quality only when all professions and disciplines cooperate smoothly and the patient is given a place.

A respectful and strength-based team culture is the goal. Nutritional interventions and counseling should be scientifically-based whenever possible, and should correspond to the latest knowledge (evidence-based practice). The level of evidence that informs the daily clinical practice of an NST is not always satisfactory and is often based on long-term experience and expertise.

Beyond teaching, knowledge transfer, and skill development, NST should be able to perform clinical translational research and run clinical studies. A trial hypothesis may be generated in response to the concerns and challenges of everyday practice. Exchange of ideas, networking, and cooperation with other hospitals, universities, institutes, and societies is essential in this context, depending on the hospital setting [56].

## 5. Efficacy, Efficiency, and Positive Outcomes

An NST is often involved in defining the indications for and implementing artificial nutrition [73]. Through the involvement of an NST, there are significantly more correct indications for parenteral nutrition, and, as a result, many labor-intensive interventions can be avoided [53]. In the study of Sriram et al., the number of indicated parenteral therapies increased from 71.3% to 83.4% between 2003 and 2006 due to the intervention of NST [29]. At the same time, non-indicated interventions decreased from 16.5% to 8.9%, which is a sign of higher treatment quality [29]. Boitano et al. investigated compliance with the ASPEN guidelines for parenteral nutrition, which were implemented between 2007 and 2010 [7]. Through changes in the prescription forms, implementation of NST visits on the wards, and the education of physicians, the number of non-indicated therapies could be reduced. The percentage of indicated parenteral therapies increased from 60% to 97%, and around 85% of the patients were able to meet their energy and protein needs, versus 54% before [7]. The close monitoring of nutritional therapy showed an increase in correctly documented laboratory values from 53% to 83%. Additionally, the percentage of patients with hyperglycemia, which is the most frequent complication of parenteral nutrition, could be reduced from 47% to 3% [7]. Besides the obvious increase in treatment quality, the hospital was able to save a total of $5.3 million USD. In the study of Trujillo et al., including consecutive patients treated with parenteral nutrition, 15% of the nutritional interventions were non-indicated and 23% could have been avoided, for a total cost savings of $183,309 per year [32]. Through the interventions of an NST, metabolic complications could also be significantly reduced, from 66% to 34%, which represents $510,746 USD yearly. During 1997, in a Swiss university hospital, 69% of the parenteral nutrition prescriptions were done without involvement of an NST, and 28% of these were non-indicated [23]. Of these non-indicated therapies, 58% were inadequate. In 62% of the patients, energy intake was too low. In 20% of the patients, it was too high, and an additional 17% of patients received no vitamins or trace elements. After an NST was involved, the percentage of patients receiving parenteral nutrition decreased to 35% (2765 bags in 1995 vs 1812 bags in 1998), which leads to more enteral tube feeding. Furthermore, the number of catheter-related infections decreased from 25 (1995) to 3 (1998). Through the direct involvement of an NST, a total of 245,000 Euros per year could be saved [23]. In England, savings of over 50,715 British Pounds were achieved yearly, through the NST monitoring among medical and surgical patients [20]. Through the involvement of an NST, Chris Anderson et al. demonstrated a reduction of the yearly parenteral nutrition costs from $2107 to $1784 USD (mean total per day on parenteral nutrition) [8].

Already in the 1970s and 1980s, studies showed the efficacy (drop in severe catheter-related infections) and the associated cost-effectiveness of involving an NST [9,11,13,17,18,25,26]. Later on, further studies revealed that NST optimizes nutritional therapy and decreases metabolic complications. Moreover, through its interventions, NST is able to reduce the occurrence of electrolyte imbalance, especially in patients on home parenteral nutrition [44–47,57,74]. The recent study of Park et al. showed that the early intervention of an NST in critically ill patients with gastrointestinal diseases positively influences survival [22]. A significant reduction in 90-day mortality under oral nutritional therapy was reported in the study of Deutz et al. [10]. Benefits of NST interventions (oral, enteral, or parenteral) on patients' clinical outcomes could be demonstrated in many other randomized controlled trials over the last two decades, including improved energy and protein intake, shorter length of hospital stay, fewer complications, a lower elective rehospitalization rate, less weight loss, improved muscle function, and an improvement in quality of life [12,14–16,19,21,24,27,28,30,51]. In the study of Johansen et al., NST was responsible for the nutritional management only in the intervention group [19]. The primary endpoint was a composite of nutrition-related factors, which may influence the length of the hospital stay (mobilization, signs of infection, complications). Energy and protein intake of ≥75% of the requirements could be achieved in 62% of the patients in the intervention group versus 36% in the control group [19]. The hospital length of stay of patients who developed complications was significantly shorter in the intervention group [19]. Nutritional therapy may be carried out easily at home with the support of home care services, which results in substantial cost savings [31].

More recently, the efficacy and efficiency of an NST (counseling, therapy, and patient procedures, according to a protocol) were confirmed in the multicenter randomized, controlled Effect of early nutritional support on Frailty, Functional Outcomes, and Recovery of malnourished medical inpatients Trial (EFFORT) of Schuetz et al. [28]. In this study, more than 2000 polymorbid medical inpatients at nutritional risk (NRS 2002 total score ≥3) were randomly assigned to either receive a standard hospital diet versus individualized nutritional support, according to a nutritional protocol [75]. After 30 days, the positive effect of the individualized nutritional management through an NST could be shown. A total of 79% of the intervention group reached their energy and protein requirements, with 76% even within three days (high compliance rate). In the control group, 54% of the patients reached their energy requirements, and 55% reached the protein requirements. Quality of life, functional status, and clinical outcome were also significantly improved. Improved outcome can be translated into a need to treat 25 patients to prevent one adverse clinical outcome and 37 to prevent one death [28]. Notably, there was no increase in side-effects or complications, such as refeeding syndrome, associated with nutritional support [76,77]. These results show that malnutrition is a mostly modifiable risk factor and that a global strategy aimed at meeting the needs of individual patients is of decisive importance. Cachexia may not be fully reversed with nutritional support but remains essential until refractory cachexia occurs [78,79] (Table 2).

**Table 2.** Clinical studies showing efficacy and efficiency of NST.

| Outcome | Correct Indication | Cost Savings | Decreased Complication Rates | Reduced Mortality | Improved Monitoring | Increased Dietary Intake | Positive Influence of Individualized Nutritional Support |
|---|---|---|---|---|---|---|---|
| Studies | Boitano et al. [7]<br>Piquet et al. [23]<br>Trujilo et al. [32]<br>Sriram et al. [29] | Boitano et al. [7]<br>ChrisAnderson et al. [8]<br>Curry et al. [9]<br>Faubion et al. [11]<br>Goldmann et al. [13]<br>Jacobs et al. [18]<br>Kennedy et al. [20]<br>Piquet et al. [23]<br>Ryan et al. [25]<br>Sanders et al. [26]<br>Trujilo et al. [32] | Boitano et al. [7]<br>Curry et al. [9]<br>Faubion et al. [11]<br>Gariballa et al. [12]<br>Goldmann et al. [13]<br>Ha et al. [14]<br>Hegerova et al. [15]<br>Hickson et al. [16]<br>Jacobs et al. [18]<br>Johansen et al. [19]<br>Norman et al. [21,41]<br>Piquet et al. [23]<br>Ruefenacht et al. [24]<br>Ryan et al. [25]<br>Sanders et al. [26]<br>Somanchi et al. [27]<br>Schuetz et al. [28]<br>Starke et al. [30]<br>Stratton et al. [31]<br>Trujilo et al. [32]<br>ten Dam et al. [43]<br>Dudrick et al. [45]<br>Fürst et al. [46]<br>Butterworth [47]<br>Allison [51]<br>Council of Europe [57] | Park et al. [22]<br>Schuetz et al. [28]<br>Deutz et al. [10] | Boitano et al. [7]<br>Kennedy et al. [20] | Boitano et al. [7]<br>Gariballa et al. [12]<br>Ha et al. [14]<br>Hegerova et al. [15]<br>Hickson et al. [16]<br>Johansen et al. [19]<br>Norman et al. [21,41]<br>Ruefenacht et al. [24]<br>Somanchi et al. [27]<br>Schuetz et al. [28]<br>Starke et al. [30]<br>Stratton et al. [31]<br>ten Dam et al. [43]<br>Dudrick et al. [45]<br>Fürst et al. [46]<br>Allison [51]<br>Council of Europe [57] | Johansen et al. [19]<br>Ruefenacht et al. [24]<br>Schuetz et al. [28] |

## 6. Strength of Evidence Regarding Nutritional Support Teams

Evidence-based medicine is intended to optimize the decision-making of physicians and patients by emphasizing the use of evidence from well-designed and well-conducted research including typically randomized trials and meta-analyses summarizing effects of such single trials. For many fields of clinical nutrition, including NSTs, there has been an important lack of large-scale interventional studies providing such high-quality evidence, and much of today's knowledge is based on observational research and experience of physician and dieticians. As a consequence, current clinical practice guidelines, often give weak recommendations regarding nutritional topics. However, as outlined above, there are some new and important clinical trials in the field, which provide strong evidence in favor of nutritional support and thus also in favor of NSTs [10,28]. However, there is clearly room for further improvements in our understanding on how to best use nutrition in individual patients.

## 7. Conclusions and Outlook

Malnutrition is a mostly modifiable condition with potentially deleterious consequences, if left untreated. Malnourished patients can be detected early and treated in a timely fashion through comprehensive nutritional care management. This contributes to improvements in the patient's clinical outcome, as recently shown in the EFFORT trial [28]. An interdisciplinary approach and nutritional therapies are effective in cost containment (improving quality of treatment, avoiding unnecessary interventions, and simplifying management), which is especially relevant for the modern healthcare policy. These results show that NSTs should be widely propagated and implemented in a hospital. There is growing evidence from clinical trials demonstrating the efficacy and efficiency of NSTs. The success of nutritional medicine strongly depends on their institutionalization and visibility of the field and the role of the NSTs in modern multimodal medical care. The key task of NSTs is to implement a comprehensive nutritional care system, so that every patient who could potentially benefit from nutritional support receives it rapidly, adequately, and with the highest standards of quality.

**Author Contributions:** Conceptualization, E.R. and Z.S. Writing—original draft preparation, E.R. Writing—review and editing, E.R., R.S., L.B., and P.S. Supervision, Z.S.

## References

1. Aeberhard, C.; Birrenbach, T.; Joray, M.; Muhlebach, S.; Perrig, M.; Stanga, Z. Simple training tool is insufficient for appropriate diagnosis and treatment of malnutrition: A pre-post intervention study in a tertiary center. *Nutrition* **2016**, *32*, 355–361. [CrossRef] [PubMed]
2. Felder, S.; Lechtenboehmer, C.; Bally, M.; Fehr, R.; Deiss, M.; Faessler, L.; Kutz, A.; Steiner, D.; Rast, A.C.; Laukemann, S.; et al. Association of nutritional risk and adverse medical outcomes across different medical inpatient populations. *Nutrition* **2015**, *31*, 1385–1393. [CrossRef] [PubMed]
3. McWhirter, J.P.; Pennington, C.R. Incidence and recognition of malnutrition in hospital. *BMJ* **1994**, *308*, 945–948. [CrossRef] [PubMed]
4. Pirlich, M.; Schutz, T.; Norman, K.; Gastell, S.; Lubke, H.J.; Bischoff, S.C.; Bolder, U.; Frieling, T.; Güldenzoph, H.; Hahn, K.; et al. The German hospital malnutrition study. *Clin. Nutr.* **2006**, *25*, 563–572. [CrossRef] [PubMed]
5. Sorensen, J.; Kondrup, J.; Prokopowicz, J.; Schiesser, M.; Krahenbuhl, L.; Meier, R.; Liberda, M. EuroOOPS: An international, multicentre study to implement nutritional risk screening and evaluate clinical outcome. *Clin. Nutr.* **2008**, *27*, 340–349. [CrossRef] [PubMed]
6. Rinninella, E.; Cintoni, M.; De Lorenzo, A.; Anselmi, G.; Gagliardi, L.; Addolorato, G.; Miggiano, G.A.; Gasbarrini, A.; Mele, M.C. May nutritional status worsen during hospital stay? A sub-group analysis from a cross-sectional study. *Intern. Emerg. Med.* **2019**, *14*, 51–57. [CrossRef] [PubMed]

7. Boitano, M.; Bojak, S.; McCloskey, S.; McCaul, D.S.; McDonough, M. Improving the safety and effectiveness of parenteral nutrition: Results of a quality improvement collaboration. *Nutr. Clin. Pract.* **2010**, *25*, 663–671. [CrossRef]
8. ChrisAnderson, D.; Heimburger, D.C.; Morgan, S.L.; Geels, W.J.; Henry, K.L.; Conner, W.; Hensrud, D.D.; Thompson, G.; Weinsier, R.L. Metabolic complications of total parenteral nutrition: Effects of a nutrition support service. *JPEN J. Parenter. Enteral. Nutr.* **1996**, *20*, 206–210. [CrossRef]
9. Curry, C.R.; Quie, P.G. Fungal septicemia in patients receiving parenteral hyperalimentation. *N. Engl. J. Med.* **1971**, *285*, 1221–1225. [CrossRef]
10. Deutz, N.E.; Matheson, E.M.; Matarese, L.E.; Luo, M.; Baggs, G.E.; Nelson, J.L.; Hegazi, R.A.; Tappenden, K.A.; Ziegler, T.R. NOURISH Study Group. Readmission and mortality in malnourished, older, hospitalized adults treated with a specialized oral nutritional supplement: A randomized clinical trial. *Clin. Nutr.* **2016**, *35*, 18–26. [CrossRef]
11. Faubion, W.C.; Wesley, J.R.; Khalidi, N.; Silva, J. Total parenteral nutrition catheter sepsis: Impact of the team approach. *JPEN J. Parenter. Enteral. Nutr.* **1986**, *10*, 642–645. [CrossRef]
12. Gariballa, S.; Forster, S.; Walters, S.; Powers, H. A randomized, double-blind, placebo-controlled trial of nutritional supplementation during acute illness. *Am. J. Med.* **2006**, *119*, 693–699. [CrossRef]
13. Goldmann, D.A.; Maki, D.G. Infection control in total parenteral nutrition. *JAMA* **1973**, *223*, 1360–1364. [CrossRef]
14. Ha, L.; Hauge, T.; Spenning, A.B.; Iversen, P.O. Individual, nutritional support prevents undernutrition, increases muscle strength and improves QoL among elderly at nutritional risk hospitalized for acute stroke: A randomized, controlled trial. *Clin. Nutr.* **2010**, *29*, 567–573. [CrossRef]
15. Hegerova, P.; Dedkova, Z.; Sobotka, L. Early nutritional support and physiotherapy improved long-term self-sufficiency in acutely ill older patients. *Nutrition* **2015**, *31*, 166–170. [CrossRef]
16. Hickson, M.; Bulpitt, C.; Nunes, M.; Peters, R.; Cooke, J.; Nicholl, C.; Frost, G. Does additional feeding support provided by health care assistants improve nutritional status and outcome in acutely ill older in-patients?—A randomised control trial. *Clin. Nutr.* **2004**, *23*, 69–77. [CrossRef]
17. National Institute for Health and Clinical Excellence. Nutrition Support for Adults: Oral Nutrition Support, Enteral Tube Feeding and Parenteral Nutrition (clinical guideline 32). Available online: https://www.nice.org.uk/Guidance/CG32 (accessed on 20 August 2019).
18. Jacobs, D.O.; Melnik, G.; Forlaw, L.; Gebhardt, C.; Settle, R.G.; DiSipio, M.; Rombeau, J.L. Impact of a nutritional support service on VA surgical patients. *J. Am. Coll. Nutr.* **1984**, *3*, 311–315. [CrossRef]
19. Johansen, N.; Kondrup, J.; Plum, L.M.; Bak, L.; Norregaard, P.; Bunch, E.; Bærnthsen, H.; Andersen, J.R.; Larsen, I.H.; Martinsen, A. Effect of nutritional support on clinical outcome in patients at nutritional risk. *Clin. Nutr.* **2004**, *23*, 539–550. [CrossRef]
20. Kennedy, J.F.; Nightingale, J.M. Cost savings of an adult hospital nutrition support team. *Nutrition* **2005**, *21*, 1127–1133. [CrossRef]
21. Norman, K.; Kirchner, H.; Freudenreich, M.; Ockenga, J.; Lochs, H.; Pirlich, M. Three month intervention with protein and energy rich supplements improve muscle function and quality of life in malnourished patients with non-neoplastic gastrointestinal disease–a randomized controlled trial. *Clin. Nutr.* **2008**, *27*, 48–56. [CrossRef]
22. Park, Y.E.; Park, S.J.; Park, Y.; Cheon, J.H.; Kim, T.I.; Kim, W.H. Impact and outcomes of nutritional support team intervention in patients with gastrointestinal disease in the intensive care unit. *Medicine* **2017**, *96*, e8776. [CrossRef]
23. Piquet, M.A.; Bertrand, P.C.; Roulet, M. Role of a nutrition support team in reducing the inappropriate use of parenteral nutrition. *Clin. Nutr.* **2004**, *23*, 437; author reply 8. [CrossRef]
24. Rufenacht, U.; Ruhlin, M.; Wegmann, M.; Imoberdorf, R.; Ballmer, P.E. Nutritional counseling improves quality of life and nutrient intake in hospitalized undernourished patients. *Nutrition* **2010**, *26*, 53–60. [CrossRef]
25. Ryan, J.A., Jr.; Abel, R.M.; Abbott, W.M.; Hopkins, C.C.; Chesney, T.M.; Colley, R.; Phillips, K.; Fischer, J.E. Catheter complications in total parenteral nutrition: A prospective study of 200 consecutive patients. *N. Engl. J. Med.* **1974**, *290*, 757–761. [CrossRef]
26. Sanders, R.A.; Sheldon, G.F. Septic complications of total parenteral nutrition: A five year experience. *Am. J. Surg.* **1976**, *132*, 214–220. [CrossRef]

27. Somanchi, M.; Tao, X.; Mullin, G.E. The facilitated early enteral and dietary management effectiveness trial in hospitalized patients with malnutrition. *JPEN J. Parenter. Enteral. Nutr.* **2011**, *35*, 209–216. [CrossRef]
28. Schuetz, P.; Fehr, R.; Baechli, V.; Geiser, M.; Gomes, F.; Kutz, A.; Tribolet, P.; Bregenzer, T.; Braun, N.; Hoess, C. Individualized nutritional support in medical inpatients at nutritional risk: A randomized clinical trial. *Lancet* **2019**, *393*, 2312–2321. [CrossRef]
29. Sriram, K.; Cyriac, T.; Fogg, L.F. Effect of nutritional support team restructuring on the use of parenteral nutrition. *Nutrition* **2010**, *26*, 735–739. [CrossRef]
30. Starke, J.; Schneider, H.; Alteheld, B.; Stehle, P.; Meier, R. Short-term individual nutritional care as part of routine clinical setting improves outcome and quality of life in malnourished medical patients. *Clin. Nutr.* **2011**, *30*, 194–201. [CrossRef]
31. Stratton, R.J.; Green, C.J.; Elia, M. *Disease-Related Malnutrition: An Evidence-Based Approach to Treatment*; CABI Publishing: Wallingford, UK, 2003.
32. Trujillo, E.B.; Young, L.S.; Chertow, G.M.; Randall, S.; Clemons, T.; Jacobs, D.O.; Robinson, M.K. Metabolic and monetary costs of avoidable parenteral nutrition use. *JPEN J. Parenter. Enteral. Nutr.* **1999**, *23*, 109–113. [CrossRef]
33. Casaer, M.P.; Hermans, G.; Wilmer, A.; Van den Berghe, G. Impact of early parenteral nutrition completing enteral nutrition in adult critically ill patients (EPaNIC trial): A study protocol and statistical analysis plan for a randomized controlled trial. *Trials* **2011**, *12*, 21. [CrossRef]
34. Kubrak, C.; Jensen, L. Malnutrition in acute care patients: A narrative review. *Int. J. Nurs. Stud.* **2007**, *44*, 1036–1054. [CrossRef]
35. Villet, S.; Chiolero, R.L.; Bollmann, M.D.; Revelly, J.P.; Cayeux, R.N.M.; Delarue, J.; Berger, M.M. Negative impact of hypocaloric feeding and energy balance on clinical outcome in ICU patients. *Clin. Nutr.* **2005**, *24*, 502–509. [CrossRef]
36. Iff, S.; Leuenberger, M.; Rosch, S.; Knecht, G.; Tanner, B.; Stanga, Z. Meeting the nutritional requirements of hospitalized patients: An interdisciplinary approach to hospital catering. *Clin. Nutr.* **2008**, *27*, 800–805. [CrossRef]
37. Allison, S.; Stanga, Z.G.; Odlund Olin, A. Organization of nutritional care. In *Basics in Clinical Nutrition*, 3rd ed.; Sobotka, L., Ed.; Galen: Prague, Czechia, 2011; pp. 135–139.
38. Barton, A.D.; Beigg, C.L.; Macdonald, I.A.; Allison, S.P. High food wastage and low nutritional intakes in hospital patients. *Clin. Nutr.* **2000**, *19*, 445–449. [CrossRef]
39. Dias-Ferreira, C.; Santos, T.; Oliveira, V. Hospital food waste and environmental and economic indicators—A Portuguese case study. *Waste Manag.* **2015**, *46*, 146–154. [CrossRef]
40. Elia, M.; Parsons, E.L.; Cawood, A.L.; Smith, T.R.; Stratton, R.J. Cost-effectiveness of oral nutritional supplements in older malnourished care home residents. *Clin. Nutr.* **2018**, *37*, 651–658. [CrossRef]
41. Norman, K.; Pirlich, M.; Smoliner, C.; Kilbert, A.; Schulzke, J.D.; Ockenga, J.; Lochs, H.; Reinhold, T. Cost-effectiveness of a 3-month intervention with oral nutritional supplements in disease-related malnutrition: A randomised controlled pilot study. *Eur. J. Clin. Nutr.* **2011**, *65*, 735–742. [CrossRef]
42. Zhong, Y.; Cohen, J.T.; Goates, S.; Luo, M.; Nelson, J.; Neumann, P.J. The Cost-Effectiveness of Oral Nutrition Supplementation for Malnourished Older Hospital Patients. *Appl. Health Econ. Health Policy* **2017**, *15*, 75–83. [CrossRef]
43. ten Dam, S.; Droop, A.; Arjaans, W.; de Groot, S.; van Bokhorst-de van der Schueren, M. Organisation of Nutritional Care Ethical and Legal Aspects. Module 11.1 Organisation of a nutritional support team, 2012. Available online: https://lllnutrition.com/mod/page/view.php?id=3422 (accessed on 20 August 2019).
44. Ockenga, J.; Valentini, L. Organisationsstruktur der ernährungsmedizinischen Kompetenz, Ernährungsteams und Ernährungskommissionen. In *Ernährungsmedizin*, 5th ed.; Biesalski, H.K., Bischoff, S.C., Pirlich, M., Weimann, A., Eds.; Georg Thieme Verlag KG: Stuttgart, Germany, 2017; pp. 469–476.
45. Dudrick, S.J., Wilmore, D.W.; Vars, H.M.; Rhoads, J.E. Long-term total parenteral nutrition with growth, development, and positive nitrogen balance. *Surgery* **1968**, *64*, 134–142.
46. Fürst, P.; Stehle, P. Künstliche Ernährung–gestern, heute, morgen. *Transfus. Med. Hemother.* **1990**, *17*, 237–244. [CrossRef]
47. Butterworth, C.E. The skeleton in the hospital closet. 1974. *Nutrition* **1994**, *10*, 435–441.

48. Shang, E.; Hasenberg, T.; Schlegel, B.; Sterchi, A.B.; Schindler, K.; Druml, W.; Koletzko, B.; Meier, R. An European survey of structure and organisation of nutrition support teams in Germany, Austria and Switzerland. *Clin. Nutr.* **2005**, *24*, 1005–1013. [CrossRef]
49. Aubry, E.; Mareschal, J.; Gschweitl, M.; Zvingelis, M.; Schuetz, P.; Stanga, Z. Facts zum Management der Klinischen Ernährung—Eine Online-Befragung. *Aktuel. Ernahrungsmed.* **2018**, *42*, 452–460. [CrossRef]
50. NutritionDay Worldwide 2018. Available online: https://www.nutritionday.org/en/about-nday/national-reports/index.html (accessed on 20 August 2019).
51. Allison, S.P. Nutritional support—Who needs it and who does it? *Clin. Nutr.* **1992**, *11*, 165–166. [CrossRef]
52. Allison, S. Hospital food as treatment. In *A Report by a Working Party of BAPEN*; BAPEN: Maidenhead, UK, 1999.
53. Delegge, M.; Wooley, J.A.; Guenter, P.; Wright, S.; Brill, J.; Andris, D.; Wagner, P.; Filibeck, D. ASPEN Board of Directors. The state of nutrition support teams and update on current models for providing nutrition support therapy to patients. *Nutr. Clin. Pract.* **2010**, *25*, 76–84.
54. Nightingale, J. Nutrition support teams: How they work, are set up and maintained. *Frontline Gastroenterol.* **2010**, *1*, 171–177. [CrossRef]
55. Payne-James, J. Cost-effectiveness of nutrition support teams. Are they necessary? *Nutrition* **1997**, *13*, 928–930. [CrossRef]
56. Suchner, U.; Dormann, A.; Hund-Wissner, E.; Shang, E.; Senkal, M. Anforderungen an Struktur und Funktion eines Ernährungsteams. *Anaesthesist* **2000**, *49*, 675–684. [CrossRef]
57. Council of Europe, Committee of Ministers. Resolution ResAP (2003) on Food and Nutritional Care in Hospitals. 2004. Available online: https://search.coe.int/cm/Pages/result_details.aspx?ObjectID=09000016805de855 (accessed on 20 August 2019).
58. Schneider, P.J. Nutrition support teams: An evidence-based practice. *Nutr. Clin. Pract.* **2006**, *21*, 62–67. [CrossRef]
59. Reber, E.; Gomes, F.; Bally, L.; Schuetz, P.; Stanga, Z. Nutritional Management of Medical Inpatients. *J. Clin. Med.* **2019**, *8*, 1130. [CrossRef]
60. Reber, E.; Gomes, F.; Vasiloglou, M.F.; Schuetz, P.; Stanga, Z. Nutritional Risk Screening and Assessment. *J. Clin. Med.* **2019**, *8*, 1065. [CrossRef]
61. Kondrup, J.; Rasmussen, H.H.; Hamberg, O.; Stanga, Z. Nutritional risk screening (NRS 2002): A new method based on an analysis of controlled clinical trials. *Clin. Nutr.* **2003**, *22*, 321–336. [CrossRef]
62. Soeters, P.B.; Reijven, P.L.; van Bokhorst-de van der Schueren, M.A.; Schols, J.M.; Halfens, R.J.; Meijers, J.M.; van Gemerta, W.G. A rational approach to nutritional assessment. *Clin. Nutr.* **2008**, *27*, 706–716. [CrossRef]
63. Barbosa-Silva, M.C. Subjective and objective nutritional assessment methods: What do they really assess? *Curr. Opin. Clin. Nutr. Metab. Care* **2008**, *11*, 248–254. [CrossRef]
64. Ware, J.E., Jr.; Sherbourne, C.D. The MOS 36-item short-form health survey (SF-36). I. Conceptual framework and item selection. *Med. Care* **1992**, *30*, 473–483. [CrossRef]
65. Keller, U. Nutritional Laboratory Markers in Malnutrition. *J. Clin. Med.* **2019**, *8*, 775. [CrossRef]
66. Leuenberger, M.; Nuoffer, J.-M.; Stanga, Z. Sinnvolle laborchemische Diagnostik in der Mangelernährung. *Pipette* **2007**, *2*, 15–19.
67. Allison, S.P. Malnutrition, disease, and outcome. *Nutrition* **2000**, *16*, 590–593. [CrossRef]
68. Kondrup, J.; Bak, L.; Hansen, B.S.; Ipsen, B.; Ronneby, H. Outcome from nutritional support using hospital food. *Nutrition* **1998**, *14*, 319–321. [CrossRef]
69. Valentini, L.; Jadma, K. Zehn Jahre Ernährungsteam in Österreich: Definitionen, Aufgaben und Perspektiven. *J. Ernärhrungsmed.* **2004**, *6*, 17–23.
70. Laesser, C.; Cumming, P.; Reber, E.; Stanga, Z.; Muka, T.; Bally, L. Management of Glucose Control in Noncritically Ill, Hospitalized Patients Receiving Parenteral and/or Enteral Nutrition: A Systematic Review. *JCM* **2019**, *8*, 935. [CrossRef]
71. Burch, N.E.; Stewart, J.; Smith, N. Are nutrition support teams useful? Results from the NCEPOD study into parenteral nutrition. *Gut* **2011**, *60* (Suppl. 1), A2. [CrossRef]
72. Rasmussen, N.M.L.; Belqaid, K.; Lugnet, K.; Nielsen, A.L.; Rasmussen, H.H.; Beck, A.M. Effectiveness of multidisciplinary nutritional support in older hospitalised patients: A systematic review and meta-analyses. *Clin. Nutr. ESPEN* **2018**, *27*, 44–52. [CrossRef]

73. Riley, K.; Sulo, S.; Dabbous, F.; Partridge, J.; Kozmic, S.; Landow, W.; VanDerBosch, G.; Falson, M.K.; Sriram, K. Reducing Hospitalizations and Costs: A Home Health Nutrition-Focused Quality Improvement Program. *JPEN J. Parenter. Enteral. Nutr.* **2019**. [CrossRef]
74. Valentini, L.; Volkert, D.; Schütz, T.; Ockenga, J.; Pirlich, M.; Druml, W.; Schindler, K.; Ballmer, P.E.; Bischoff, S.C.; Weimann, A.; et al. Leitlinie der Deutschen Gesellschaft für Ernährungsmedizin (DGEM). *Aktuelle Ernährungsmedizin* **2013**, *38*, 97–111. [CrossRef]
75. Bounoure, L.; Gomes, F.; Stanga, Z.; Keller, U.; Meier, R.; Ballmer, P.; Fehr, R.; Mueller, B.; Genton, L.; Bertrand, P.C.; et al. Detection and treatment of medical inpatients with or at-risk of malnutrition: Suggested procedures based on validated guidelines. *Nutrition* **2016**, *32*, 790–798. [CrossRef]
76. Friedli, N.; Stanga, Z.; Sobotka, L.; Culkin, A.; Kondrup, J.; Laviano, A.; Mueller, B.; Schuetz, P. Revisiting the refeeding syndrome: Results of a systematic review. *Nutrition* **2017**, *35*, 151–160. [CrossRef]
77. Friedli, N.; Stanga, Z.; Culkin, A.; Crook, M.; Laviano, A.; Sobotka, L.; Kressig, R.W.; Kondrup, J.; Mueller, B.; Schuetz, P. Management and prevention of refeeding syndrome in medical inpatients: An evidence-based and consensus-supported algorithm. *Nutrition* **2018**, *47*, 13–20. [CrossRef]
78. Arends, J.; Baracos, V.; Bertz, H.; Bozzetti, F.; Calder, P.C.; Deutz, N.E.P.; Erickson, N.; Laviano, A.; Lisanti, M.P.; Lobo, D.N.; et al. ESPEN expert group recommendations for action against cancer-related malnutrition. *Clin. Nutr.* **2017**, *36*, 1187–1196. [CrossRef]
79. Fearon, K.; Strasser, F.; Anker, S.D.; Bosaeus, I.; Bruera, E.; Fainsinger, R.L.; Jatoi, A.; Loprinzi, C.; MacDonald, N.; Mantovani, G.; et al. Definition and classification of cancer cachexia: An international consensus. *Lancet Oncol.* **2011**, *12*, 489–495. [CrossRef]

# Permissions

All chapters in this book were first published by MDPI; hereby published with permission under the Creative Commons Attribution License or equivalent. Every chapter published in this book has been scrutinized by our experts. Their significance has been extensively debated. The topics covered herein carry significant findings which will fuel the growth of the discipline. They may even be implemented as practical applications or may be referred to as a beginning point for another development.

The contributors of this book come from diverse backgrounds, making this book a truly international effort. This book will bring forth new frontiers with its revolutionizing research information and detailed analysis of the nascent developments around the world.

We would like to thank all the contributing authors for lending their expertise to make the book truly unique. They have played a crucial role in the development of this book. Without their invaluable contributions this book wouldn't have been possible. They have made vital efforts to compile up to date information on the varied aspects of this subject to make this book a valuable addition to the collection of many professionals and students.

This book was conceptualized with the vision of imparting up-to-date information and advanced data in this field. To ensure the same, a matchless editorial board was set up. Every individual on the board went through rigorous rounds of assessment to prove their worth. After which they invested a large part of their time researching and compiling the most relevant data for our readers.

The editorial board has been involved in producing this book since its inception. They have spent rigorous hours researching and exploring the diverse topics which have resulted in the successful publishing of this book. They have passed on their knowledge of decades through this book. To expedite this challenging task, the publisher supported the team at every step. A small team of assistant editors was also appointed to further simplify the editing procedure and attain best results for the readers.

Apart from the editorial board, the designing team has also invested a significant amount of their time in understanding the subject and creating the most relevant covers. They scrutinized every image to scout for the most suitable representation of the subject and create an appropriate cover for the book.

The publishing team has been an ardent support to the editorial, designing and production team. Their endless efforts to recruit the best for this project, has resulted in the accomplishment of this book. They are a veteran in the field of academics and their pool of knowledge is as vast as their experience in printing. Their expertise and guidance has proved useful at every step. Their uncompromising quality standards have made this book an exceptional effort. Their encouragement from time to time has been an inspiration for everyone.

The publisher and the editorial board hope that this book will prove to be a valuable piece of knowledge for researchers, students, practitioners and scholars across the globe.

# List of Contributors

**Yousang Ko, Yong Bum Park, Eun-Kyung Mo and Jin-Wook Moon**
Department of Internal Medicine, Division of Pulmonary, Allergy and Critical Care Medicine, Kangdong Sacred Heart Hospital, Hallym University College of Medicine, Seoul 05355, Korea
College of Medicine, Lung Research Institute of Hallym University, Chuncheon 24253, Korea

**Changwhan Kim**
Department of Internal Medicine, School of Medicine, Jeju National University Hospital, Jeju National University, Jeju 63241, Korea

**Alfredo Fernández-Quintela, Iñaki Milton-Laskibar, Jenifer Trepiana, Saioa Gómez-Zorita, Naroa Kajarabille and María P. Portillo**
Nutrition and Obesity Group, Department of Pharmacy and Food Science, University of the Basque Country (UPV/EHU) and Lucio Lascaray Research Institute, 01006 Vitoria, Spain
CIBEROBN Physiopathology of Obesity and Nutrition, Institute of Health Carlos III, 01006 Vitoria, Spain
Bioaraba Health Research Institute, 01009 Vitoria, Spain

**Asier Léniz**
Nutrition and Obesity Group, Department of Pharmacy and Food Science, University of the Basque Country (UPV/EHU) and Lucio Lascaray Research Institute, 01006 Vitoria, Spain
Bioaraba Health Research Institute, 01009 Vitoria, Spain
Basque Health Service (Osakidetza), Integrated Health Care Organization Araba, 01009 Álava, Spain

**Marcela González**
Nutrition and Food Science Department, Faculty of Biochemistry and Biological Sciences, National University of Litoral and National Scientific and Technical Research Council (CONICET), Santa Fe 3000, Argentina

**Irene Hoyas**
Department of Endocrinology and Nutrition, University Hospital Doce de Octubre, 28041 Madrid, Spain

**Jane Fletcher**
Nutrition Nurses, Queen Elizabeth Hospital Birmingham, University Hospitals Birmingham NHS Foundation Trust, Mindelsohn Way, Edgbaston, Birmingham B15 2WG, UK

**Kalliopi-Anna Poulia**
Department of Nutrition and Dietetics, Laiko General Hospital of Athens, 11527 Athens, Greece

**Maria F. Vasiloglou**
Diabetes Technology Research Group, ARTORG Center for Biomedical Engineering Research, University of Bern, Murtenstrasse 50, 3008 Bern, Switzerland

**Miguel Leon-Sanz**
Medical School, University Complutense, 28040 Madrid, Spain

**Andrea Kopp Lugli**
Intensive Care Unit and Intermediate Care Unit, Intensive Care Medicine and Department of Anesthesiology, University Hospital Basel, 4031 Basel, Switzerland

**Aude de Watteville and Claudia Heidegger**
Division of Intensive Care, Department of Acute Medicine, Geneva University Hospitals, 1205 Geneva, Switzerland

**Alexa Hollinger**
Intensive Care Unit and Intermediate Care Unit, Intensive Care Medicine and Department of Anesthesiology, University Hospital Basel, 4031 Basel, Switzerland

**Nicole Goetz**
Endocrinology, Diabetes and Metabolism, University Hospital Basel, 4031 Basel & Department of Anesthesiology, University Hospital Basel, 4031 Basel, Switzerland

**Paula Ravasco**
University Hospital of Santa Maria, 1649-035 Lisbon, Portugal
University of Lisbon, 1649-028 Lisbon, Portugal
Centre for Interdisciplinary Research in Health (CIIS) of the Portuguese Catholic University, 1649-023 Lisbon, Portugal

**Cristina Cuerda and Loredana Arhip**
Nutrition Unit, Instituto de Investigación Sanitaria Gregorio Marañón, Hospital General Universitario Gregorio Marañón, Calle del Dr. Esquerdo, 46, 28007 Madrid, Spain

**Filomena Gomes**
The New York Academy of Sciences, 250 Greenwich Sweet, 40th floor, New York, NY 10007, USA

**Philipp Schuetz**
Medical University Department, Division of General Internal and Emergency Medicine, Kantonsspital Aarau, Tellstrasse 25, 5000 Aarau, Switzerland
Department for Clinical Research, Medical Faculty, University of Basel, 4001 Basel, Switzerland

**Julie Mareschal**
Clinical Nutrition, Geneva University Hospitals, 1205 Geneva, Switzerland

**Najate Achamrah**
Department of Clinical Nutrition, Rouen University Hospital, Normandie University, 76000 Rouen, France
Nutrition Department, Rouen University Hospital Center, 76000 Rouen, France

**Laurence Genton**
Clinical Nutrition, Geneva University Hospital, 1205 Geneva, Switzerland

**Dorothee Volkert, Franz Großhauser and Eva Kiesswetter**
Institute for Biomedicine of Aging, Friedrich-Alexander-Universität Erlangen-Nürnberg, 90408 Nuremberg, Germany

**Anne Marie Beck**
Department Nutrition and Health, University College Copenhagen, 2200 Copenhagen, Denmark
Herlev and Gentofte University Hospital, 2703 Herlev, Denmark

**Tommy Cederholm**
Clinical Nutrition and Metabolism, Department of Public Health and Caring Sciences, Uppsala University, 701 05 Uppsala, Sweden
Theme Ageing, Karolinska University Hospital, 171 76 Stockholm, Sweden

**Emanuele Cereda**
Clinical Nutrition and Dietetics Unit, Fondazione IRCCS Policlinico San Matteo, 27100 Pavia, Italy

**Alfonso Cruz-Jentoft**
Servicio de Geriatría, Hospital Universitario Ramón y Cajal (IRYCIS), 28034 Madrid, Spain

**Sabine Goisser**
Heidelberg University Centre for Geriatric Medicine and Network Aging Research (NAR), University of Heidelberg, 69126 Heidelberg, Germany

**Lisette de Groot**
Division of Human Nutrition, Wageningen University, 6708 WE Wageningen, The Netherlands

**Kristina Norman**
German Institute for Human Nutrition Potsdam-Rehbrücke, Department of Nutrition and Gerontology, 14558 Nuthetal, Germany
Research Group on Geriatrics, Charité Universitätsmedizin Berlin, corporate member of Freie Universität Berlin, Humboldt-Universität zu Berlin, and Berlin Institute of Health, 10117 Berlin, Germany
Institute of Nutritional Science, University of Potsdam, 14558 Nuthetal, Germany

**Maryam Pourhassan and Rainer Wirth**
Department for Geriatric Medicine, Marien Hospital Herne – University Hospital, Ruhr-Universität Bochum, 44625 Herne, Germany

**Ilse Reinders, Marjolein Visser and Hanneke A.H. Wijnhoven**
Department of Health Sciences, Faculty of Science, and Amsterdam Public Health Research Institute, Vrije Universiteit Amsterdam, 1081 HV Amsterdam, The Netherlands

**Helen C. Roberts**
Southampton NIHR Biomedical Research Centre, University of Southampton, Southampton General Hospital, Southampton SO16 6YD, UK

**Yves Rolland**
Gérontopôle, Centre Hospitalo-Universitaire de Toulouse, 31059 Toulouse, France

**Stéphane M. Schneider**
Nutritional Support Unit, Centre Hospitalier Universitaire de Nice, Université Côte d'Azur, 06200 Nice, France

**Cornel C. Sieber**
Institute for Biomedicine of Aging, Friedrich-Alexander-Universität Erlangen-Nürnberg, 90408 Nuremberg, Germany
Department of Medicine, Kantonsspital Winterthur, 8401 Winterthur, Switzerland

**Ulrich Thiem**
Centre of Geriatrics and Gerontology, Albertinen-Haus, Hamburg, and Chair of Geriatrics and Gerontology, University Medical Centre Eppendorf, 20246 Hamburg, Germany

**Stephan R. Vavricka**
Center of Gastroenterology and Hepatology, CH-8048 Zurich, Switzerland
Department of Gastroenterology and Hepatology, University Hospital Zurich, CH-8091 Zurich, Switzerland

**Thomas Greuter**
Department of Gastroenterology and Hepatology, University Hospital Zurich, CH-8091 Zurich, Switzerland

**Ilka A. Dähn**
Cereneo Schweiz AG, Center for Neurology and Rehabilitation, Seestrasse 18, 6354 Vitznau, Switzerland

**Marta Delsoglio and Claude Pichard**
Clinical Nutrition, Geneva University Hospital (HUG), 1205 Geneva, Switzerland

**Mette M. Berger**
Service of Intensive Care Medicine & Burns, University of Lausanne Hospitals (CHUV), 1005 Lausanne, Switzerland

**Emilie Reber, Zeno Stanga, Lia Bally and Rachel Strahm**
Department of Diabetes, Endocrinology, Nutritional Medicine and Metabolism, Bern University Hospital, and University of Bern, Freiburgstrasse 15, 3010 Bern, Switzerland

# Index

www.ingramcontent.com/pod-product-compliance
Lightning Source LLC
LaVergne TN
LVHW081018210926
848485LV00004B/896